My Tango with Cancer

A Dancer's Journey of Breast Cancer Survival and Growth

CYNTHIA SWAN

GOBEYOND PUBLISHING
SIOUX FALLS, SOUTH DAKOTA

Published in 2011 by GoBeyond Publishing.

Inquiries regarding orders or bulk order discounts should be directed to GoBeyond Publishing:

GOBEYOND PUBLISHING
401 E. 8TH ST., STE. 214-547
SIOUX FALLS, SOUTH DAKOTA 57103
WWW.GOBEYONDPUBLISHING.COM
INFO@GOBEYONDPUBLISHING.COM

BOOK DESIGN BY C.L. MILLER

Library of Congress Cataloging-in-Publication Data

Swan, Cynthia.
My tango with cancer: a dancer's journey of breast cancer survival and growth / Cynthia Swan.
p. cm.
ISBN 978-1-61425-005-0
Library of Congress Control Number: 2011928593

Printed in the United States of America

My Tango with Cancer

To my parents, for whom I was determined
to survive breast cancer,
and
to Artie, whose untimely death became
the source of my determination to survive.

This book is for all women diagnosed with breast cancer.
You are not alone.

The love of my family is
why I survived cancer.

Tango is *how* I survived.

My Tango with Cancer

A Dancer's Journey of Breast Cancer Survival and Growth

Contents

~ Act I ~
Diagnosis

~ Act II ~
Treatment

~ Act III ~
Survival

Prelude. The Show Must Go On

It's all an act. I do not speak for every woman that has ever had breast cancer, but I can tell you that for me, it was all an act. Since the day I was diagnosed with breast cancer, I have been playing the role of **The Good Cancer Patient** as convincingly as possible.

Performers are raised to be this way. No matter what happens, the show must go on. Sick, sprained, exhausted, broken . . . the show must go on. Which basically means—to the performer—put on your game face, get out there, and give that audience the best show they ever experienced. No one in that audience should have the slightest inkling that you have so much as a sniffle, and don't you drop that beaming smile for an instant, because that audience did not come here to see you plod through the motions. The audience is here to see you perform, so you get out there and *perform*.

Maybe I wouldn't have had the success I did in putting on The Act if I weren't a lifetime musician, public speaker, and professional Ballroom, Latin, and Argentine Tango dancer and instructor when I was diagnosed with breast cancer at 32.

While all of those things involve an element of performance, they are all based on something deeper. A love of music, enjoyment in learning and teaching, a fascination with dance . . . taking any of those things to the next level to challenge yourself involves being in front of people in some way, performing. Argentine Tango is different, though. Actually, though I danced Argentine Tango in shows, unlike most other ballroom dances I performed, Argentine "Show Tango" isn't really Argentine Tango at all. Especially if you're in Buenos Aires.

Argentine Tango is very different from other dances for a lot of reasons. It's a very old dance steeped in Argentine tradition. The actual origin and evolution of the dance in Buenos Aires is not particularly suitable storytelling for all ages, so we'll skip the 1800s and just take Argentine Tango for what it became, and has been, for the past hundred years or so. The old-fashioned social etiquette established in Buenos Aires shows great respect for the dance, the music, the musicians, and the dancers. If you want to dance with someone, you don't walk up to them and verbally ask them to dance, and you certainly don't just grab their hand and drag them to the dance floor. Instead, you silently make eye contact with the person, from anywhere in the room, and with a slight nod or eye movement you give or receive a "cabaceo," which is a non-verbal invitation to tango. When this happens from across the room, the pair meets on the dance floor. In the same manner, if someone sits far away from the dance floor and is decidedly NOT looking you in the eye, then you know without asking that the person does not want to dance with you at that time, so you keep looking around until you do make eye contact with someone, give them a cabaceo, and off you go.

Another special thing about Argentine Tango is the way the two dancers begin together. There is no designated "first step" in tango like other dances, at least not beyond the novice stage (teaching dance has to start somewhere, after all). In tango, the couple shifts weight together, the girl sensing when the guy is changing weight and following by shifting her weight to the same side, and the guy feeling when she changes weight so he knows which foot she is on and when she is ready to respond to his lead. Then, if he's a tanguero and not just a dancer, he will feel the music, take a long slow breath that the tanguera breathes in with him, and then they start to move together in the exhale and in rhythm with the music, completely connected in energy, breath, and movement. There is nothing more true than the statement "It takes two to tango." If either partner is just going through the motions, the dance is a plane wreck and you will probably not see those two people dance together ever again. As one of my favorite maestros likes to say, tango is "Four legs, one heart." Argentine Tango is a beautifully connected dance and has become a rock of foundation in my life. I am a tanguera.

Cancer did not change that. As chemo and radiation treatment gradually constricted away so many things, tango remained. Like everything else about my life during treatment, it changed, but that's kind of how life is. Life knocks us around with challenges and adversity, and we adapt. Life is never quite the same again.

Anyone who has ever faced adversity and run into complications along the way will understand *My Tango with Cancer*, because even when I thought I understood what was coming up in terms of treatment, I never really knew what was going to happen next. Not only is that statement excessively true for cancer patients, caregivers, and their families and friends, it also reflects a basic element of life that everyone has dealt with over and over again. Even when you have a plan, even when you know what is supposed to happen next, life rarely goes exactly where you expect it to or in quite the way you thought it would. Life is a journey, after all, an experience, and we all live it through good times and bad. I hope that anyone that has or is facing cancer, helping a loved one with cancer, or facing any extreme life challenge can feel encouraged and inspired by

My Tango with Cancer to keep going, to take it as it comes, and to know that we can survive and even grow through this unbelievable journey called life.

As my cancer journey became more and more challenging, I began living two lives, one documented on my website for family and friends, and one locked away behind layers of security, journaled only to unburden my heart into welcoming blank pages. During cancer treatment, I pulled excerpts from my private journal each day to post to a Web log called *The Cielem'el Cancer Journal*. Cielem'el, by the way, means "the sky's the limit," and it's one of many, many mottos I use to encourage myself when life is discouraging. Though I made daily posts to the public Web log, many of the more difficult challenges I was actually going through never escaped the pages of my private journal. In reality, no one—absolutely no one—ever knew the whole truth of my cancer treatment experience, and if this book is going to be of use to other people dealing with cancer or severe adversity, it must be honest—without the wig and makeup, so to speak.

The honest but rather ominous "Cancer Day 123" notation I used while journaling during cancer treatment is still very fitting. One way I got through treatment was by counting down the days until the current difficulty should be over and I could move on to start on the next thing, or, eventually, start a new life when cancer treatment ended. Maybe I think that way because, as a dance teacher, I am so accustomed to giving beginning students the count to taking their first step: "five, six, seven, eight!" Seriously though, as you see the counting of the days in the journal and become aware of the inconsistent nature of time—condensed and expanded as it can feel to a cancer patient—you are much closer to understanding and experiencing this emotional journey. Reading each day as it happened relative to every other day gives you a more honest perspective of what it would feel like if you were living the experience yourself.

To allow such honesty, the names of locations and individuals have been changed throughout the story with two exceptions: Artie, my boyfriend that died in a motorcycle wreck several years ago, and Brian, a lifetime friend and probably the best quality person I know. I just cannot pull the curtain on either of them by changing their names. But, you know, the names of people and locations and buildings and hospitals are irrelevant. The story is my own personal Truth, and is not meant as a reflection upon anyone else. You don't even need to know *my* name to read this and experience my journey, right? Of course not. (That's kind of funny, actually, since I was called Baby Cherrie until my parents adopted me and named me Cynthia.) What's in a name?

Which brings us back to The Act. *My Tango with Cancer* is the fusion of an emotional journey through cancer treatment that had two distinct and separate faces, one for the public and one kept hidden, offstage behind the curtain. I didn't plan it that way, I didn't expect it to happen that way, but that became the truth of it. There was the public visage of the professional tango dancer getting through cancer treatment as best she could, and there was the private secret little me stifling and hiding as much of the badness as possible so that my family and friends would not worry about me.

Why did I even need to engage in this masquerade? What was I protecting anyone from? Who was I to judge what my family and friends should or should not know about how I really felt and what I was really going through? I can't answer those questions, except to say that I have been on stages and performing most of my life. I'm not an actress, but a stage is a stage, a show is a show, and I simply grew up this way. No excuses, no defensive explanations. When you walk on stage, "you" disappear and all the audience should see is a performer.

So, I always have a game face at the ready. It is what it is.

It's not good for you, keeping so much locked up inside yourself. I know. Journaling it out definitely helped me get through some difficult moments. But when you're a performer, no matter what happens, the show must go on.

~ Act I ~
Diagnosis

Chapter 1.
Begin the Beguine

CANCER—DAY 0 MINUS 7 FRIDAY, APRIL 17, 2009

Shock. And not shock. This was the phone call I was expecting.

It ***looks*** like cancer.

CANCER—DAY 0 MINUS 6 SATURDAY, APRIL 18, 2009

I'm too young for cancer. I'm too healthy for cancer. I'm a professional dancer and instructor. I'm a full time supply chain management consultant with a very busy day job, rushing off to dance at night and all weekend. I'm an adjunct professor teaching graduate courses twice a year. I live in a national forest two hours from any major city. I don't have *time* for cancer.

I'm too young for regularly scheduled mammograms, so last Wednesday was just the "as usual, no big deal" annual physical exam. At 32, I am nearly a decade from the age of regular annual mammograms and concerns of developing breast cancer. My doctor and I talked about all the same usual stuff in my physical exam . . . that I'd been losing weight while practicing so much with my pro tango partner after working all day at my consulting job, having some stomach issues. I assumed all that was because I haven't been eating well recently because I don't find time to eat enough given how physically active I am. Physically, I am in amazing shape—think Latin dancer body, platinum blonde hair and a bright smile and you've got it. I went from being a lifetime runner doing 10K races to being a professional Ballroom and Latin competitor and instructor, then an Argentine Tango instructor and performer. Lately, I've been working with a professional partner four to six nights per week in preparing for a 4-night series of shows we have coming up in two weeks. So my doctor and I were chatting about all this activity during my annual physical on Wednesday.

But then she found this lump during my breast exam. I couldn't feel it while standing up, but lying down, when she told me where to feel for it, there was definitely this hard little ball, like a marble but in pretty deep so you couldn't really guess how large it was. She ordered a mammogram and an ultrasound for the very next morning.

Internet digger that I am, I was online late into the night learning about what mammograms are and how ultrasound is used for breast cancer diagnosis. I know absolutely nothing about this stuff. Zero. But I needed to get up to speed before morning so I could comprehend what was happening in the tests. The mammogram stuff on the Internet wasn't very helpful; the pictures were just these gray areas without any particular discernable shape as far as I could see. But on the ultrasound pictures, certain cancers were totally obvious because of the spiky star shape of the tumor.

Sheesh, do mammograms hurt! The ultrasound at least wasn't painful. I knew the techs wouldn't be allowed to say anything about a potential diagnosis, even though they might recognize the tumor as cancerous right away. But I had a pretty darn good idea what they were looking for, so I simply asked easy little questions like: "Where do you look on the screen?" I asked questions that would help me see what they were seeing without pressuring them in any way for a diagnosis I knew they couldn't give.

I saw a darkened area in the mammogram that was pretty meaningless, but the unusual spiked star shape in the ultrasound was unmistakable. I knew what that meant, so when my gynecologist called the next day to say it looked cancerous and we were going to do more extensive biopsies, I was not surprised. Freaked out, absolutely, but not quite as freaked out as the day the lump was found. Wow, did I lose it on my pro partner, Marco, when I told him why I had to cancel rehearsal that night. That was one of the biggest freak-outs in my entire life, I think. It was too much to comprehend.

I mean, come on. Cancer? At 32? Are you *kidding* me?

CANCER—DAY 0 MINUS 4 MONDAY, APRIL 20, 2009

But what can you do? It is what it is. Life moves on. I had four hours of dance lessons to teach on Sunday with one of my favorite students who was getting ready to perform in the showcase next weekend; we were working on this great pro-am tango I choreographed for us, with lots of attitude and sass, classic show tango.

Marco, my Argentine Tango pro partner, was to DJ (disc jockey) for a milonga (Argentine Tango dance party) on Sunday, so after I taught my lessons we went to that instead of having our regular practice session.

We went, and danced, and I had a really good time, actually. Dance is great for that—getting your mind off of harsh realities and giving you something to lose yourself in, if only for a moment in time.

CANCER—DAY 0 MINUS 3 TUESDAY, APRIL 21, 2009

Monday was back to work and a "normal" day. Well, normal on the outside, anyway. My brain, however, has apparently evolved overnight. I often get lost in what I'm working on in my consulting job because it's interesting stuff, and at night I shift into full-on dance teacher mode, rarely giving my body much rest or thought. A "normal" day for me means thinking about work and thinking about dance. But my mind was decidedly distracted today. Go figure.

The time I normally would have spent in rehearsal with Marco yesterday, I spent with a surgeon instead. I had an appointment with the surgeon for a consult on what was going on and what the process would be if the lump turns out to be cancerous. He seemed so cold at first, sterile, and I really wasn't sure I liked this guy Dr. Thatcher at all, but I wasn't convinced that I didn't like him, either. The better he is in surgery, the less I care about his patient rapport, and he had a great reputation for his surgical work. So we go with the flow, and Dr. Thatcher will be my surgeon.

CANCER—DAY 0 MINUS 1 THURSDAY, APRIL 23, 2009

Somehow life is still clicking along like a freight train—my usual mode. Tons of e-mail to catch up on, a Board meeting to run Tuesday evening in prep for the GSCMA (Global Supply Chain Management Association) event next Thursday (now how am I going to get through *that*?), dance lessons and classes to teach . . . Work, work, work . . . busy, busy week.

Now the big biopsy day is here. I guess I should have been terrified going in to this appointment because of what the results may be, but I was less afraid than I thought I would be. The thoughts were a bit chaotic in my head, but I did manage to keep myself fairly calm given the situation. I told myself it was just a medical procedure and the sooner it was done the sooner they would know what we're dealing with. I wasn't looking forward to it, but I told myself that just because you don't want to be diagnosed with cancer doesn't mean you should avoid the tests and surgical procedures to find out if you have cancer. I know they have to figure out what this lump is, and a biopsy is the way they do it. OK, so, I'm having a biopsy. People have biopsies every day, this doctor has been doing this for a long time, and I have nothing to fear except fear itself, right?

I'm not fearless—it's a generally scary situation—but today was the day that would give them the information needed to move forward. Moving forward knowing what has to be dealt with is a lot less scary to me than sitting frozen in a staring contest with a life-threatening disease.

So, more concerned about the results than the procedure, I had only a general understanding of the surgical procedure for a biopsy in advance. I didn't really know much going in. That was probably a good thing since I'm pretty sure it did not go according to plan for the doctor.

It started with an MRI of both breasts, which went fine. They wouldn't let me see the screens, so I couldn't do any self-diagnostic guessing like I did with the ultrasound, trying to prepare my mind in advance to handle the news when it comes. The MRI process, lying on a table while this huge machine clunked and clattered around me, was not a big deal, just noisy.

The biopsy was a mess, though. They cut me up pretty badly and snipped out tissue too close to my chest wall so they had to put some stitches deep inside to stop the bleeding afterward. The biopsy was this ridiculously painful thing, mostly because they didn't use enough local anesthetic, as I understand it. He took out a lot of tissue, so they should certainly have enough to test for cancer. Bottom line though: this seems a stupid amount of pain to go through just to gather the little sample they need for proof that it is a cancerous tumor, or if it's a malignant lump, or just a benign lump. I have my suspicions regarding the cancerous nature of the lump, given the clear star shape I'd see in the ultrasound, but I'm still holding out a little hope that the lump is benign.

Marco drove me to the biopsy. We had been strictly professional dance partners for several months before this health stuff came up last week. He had made more than a few attempts to get into more of a romantic relationship than a friendship and partnership, but I had always kept the partnership professional, trying to treat his advances as unfounded playful gestures while maintaining a professional partnership. It's a fine line. One of the reasons I had avoided a personal relationship with Marco had to do with a conversation we had one afternoon when he was having a particularly hard time getting into the proper mental state for tango because he was stressed about the ending of a relationship he had been in for a couple of months. We sat there on the dance floor and he told me all about what he wanted in a relationship in terms of commitment and expectations of co-dependence. He just needed to talk about it, so I listened without offering up any contrary opinions, just being a supportive friend. In the back of my mind I kept thinking "this is soooo not me." Knowing that pretty much everything about my independent lifestyle and self-sufficient personality made me a very poor romantic partner for Marco made it pretty easy for me to keep the dance partnership professional (that, and I generally avoid relationships, my most frequent excuse being that I have zero spare time).

On the day my doctor first found "the lump," I was scheduled for several hours of rehearsal with Marco that evening. I had to drive directly from the doctor's office to our rehearsal studio if I was going to be on time, but I was shaking so badly I pulled over. I tried to call my parents . . . voicemail. I certainly wasn't going to leave this news in a voicemail message! I would have to call them later. Then I texted Marco, and instead of meeting him for practice I went to his apartment for comfort, and, well, after that we were closer than just dance partners or friends and we literally shifted into a romantic relationship overnight.

Everything happened so quickly after my doctor found the lump, it all runs together in my mind, like spilled paint. My stance of avoiding romantic relationships pretty much flip-flopped as I realized I may be in a situation that will be incredibly difficult to manage alone, and here's Marco right by my side, my dance partner and thus the person I spend the most time with on a weekly basis. Marco has probably become my closest "local" friend over the course of the last several months. "Local" meaning, in Sacramento where I teach and dance, the closest major city to where I live. I do my consulting work primarily from my home in Volcanoville in El Dorado National Forest and I drive two hours each way to go to Sacramento for dance. I love the peace and quiet of my little place in the mountains (as I like to refer to it), and when I moved out to the forest a couple of years ago, I thought I wouldn't be teaching dance anymore but it turned out I can't live peacefully without dance in my life. Still, I love where I live and how I live, and I don't mind driving two hours to Sacramento for dance, because I love to dance. I've never felt like having a secluded place in the mountains was a disadvantage or a bad decision. I don't even feel secluded in the sense of not being around people, because I interact with people all the time. I know a lot of people down in Sac (Sacramento) and I've made a lot of friends in the tango community (SacTango), but my "closest" friends are, ironically, geographically far away. My best friend Brian has a place in Sacramento but he flies all over the world for work so he's not what you would call a "local." Like most of my closest friends who actually live all over the country, Brian is absolutely there for me, but he can't be physically around on a daily basis to help me if I need someone to be with me at a doctor's appointment and such. Meanwhile, I practice with Marco almost every day, I like him and he wants to get more involved, and I knew I needed someone really, really close to me for this. Malignant or benign, I needed a hand to hold and Marco was there, holding out his hand.

Knowing that I needed relationship-type of support in order to get through whatever the heck this cancer thing may be, I finally let the professional dance partnership become a relationship, and suddenly Marco and I were a couple. We'd been friends and dance partners for many months, so the transition seemed logical enough . . . if you didn't know me and my history of concerted effort avoiding romantic entanglement.

CANCER—DAY 0 FRIDAY, APRIL 24, 2009

So here we are again. Shock. And not shock. I'm not surprised by the news, but it's shocking news regardless of whether or not you think you're prepared for it.

I spent my entire day chasing down the biopsy results. I didn't think it would be quite so difficult to get an answer out of the medical community. They'd done this core biopsy the morning before, cut me up and had me in all this pain so that we wouldn't have to reschedule and delay diagnosis which they promised they would have for me today because they felt so bad about the way the procedure went. And yet, because the surgeon who had ordered the biopsy was out of the office (on his way to a long weekend ski trip in Tahoe) and apparently "he only gives this kind of news in person," they were going to make me wait all weekend for the formal *in-person* answer from the surgeon about the tumor, on *Monday*.

Well, that was not going to cut it for me, and I started making phone calls, and then I started making threatening phone calls, because I was not going to wait three days after test results were available to get an answer just because the surgeon wanted to tell me "in person." I am not such a baby that getting bad news in person is any different than getting bad news over the phone. After multiple phone calls with the office of every doctor the slightest bit associated with this thing, finally I got a call back from my gynecologist who found the lump in the first place. She is also my primary care physician and thus received a copy of the lab results first thing this morning.

The answer: Cancer. Not really a surprise at this point.

A little extra bit of bad news as well . . . the MRI identified two more potentially cancerous tumors, so they want to do several more biopsies and also get me into surgery as soon as possible.

I have an infiltrating ductal carcinoma, which is an invasive malignant cancer, as well as an area of what they hope right now is ductal carcinoma in situ, and another area that they hope isn't even malignant yet. This is all in my right breast. The two additional biopsies I'm having on Tuesday will tell us about the latter issues. We won't know until surgery whether they consider the cancer stage 2 or stage 3. They don't think I'm stage 4, which was the good news, but they don't know for sure yet. The staging actually depends on what they find in surgery. Stage 0 mean there is no cancer, stage 1 is the lowest stage, and stage 4 is the highest, most life-threatening stage for cancer diagnosis.

Here's the last bit of bad news for the day . . . breast cancer is both rare and more aggressive in young women (younger than 40), so they are definitely going to put me through aggressive treatment with chemotherapy and radiation because the first time a cancer appears they want to do everything possible to prevent a recurrence.

I'm not a baseball person, but Dr. Thatcher used a great baseball analogy to stress the importance of taking an aggressive stance to treatment. He said "We basically get one time up to bat with this thing, so we want to knock the ball out of the park on the first swing."

CANCER—DAY 1 **SATURDAY, APRIL 25, 2009**

It looks like I have a new tango partner, so to speak. I've been so stressed out and have so much coming up with doctors, oncologists, surgeons, tests, medical research and on and on . . . dancing is surely coming off my schedule. I definitely can't put my consulting work on hold since that's the job that pays the bills. My surgery will very likely be on what would have been the first night of the four tango shows Marco and I were doing (and the showcase I was supposed to dance in with my students). I made other arrangements for all that to happen without me, and I would have had a much lighter teaching and rehearsal schedule for a while after that anyway, so aside from missing the show the timing isn't so bad for me to take a little break from dancing. I always go light on dance in June anyway because that's the busiest consulting month of my year. So, I'm probably taking a little break from dancing tango.

But now I'm starting a new dance, balancing my full time consulting job with an equivalent or greater full time job of managing cancer treatment. My tango with cancer has begun.

Chapter 2.
Learning a New Routine

CANCER—DAY 9 SUNDAY, MAY 3, 2009

I've mostly been OK emotionally in the week or so since diagnosis, or at least I think I have. I had one good breakdown this morning because it's just getting harder every day to pretend life is normal, that's all. My life of course is not normal, but I act that way to make it easier for the people around me. And it helps me too, in a way, acting normal. It's not like I don't admit to, or avoid thinking about, having cancer, but at the same time, the medical process is thorough and therefore requires some time. It doesn't seem like a lot of time—we're still talking about a matter of only a few weeks from the lump being found to getting me in surgery—but still . . . While I do have a doctor's appointment or test or procedure of some kind pretty much every day of the week, I still have lots of time every day that I could wallow in self pity . . . or I can try to do my job, try to tango, and try to keep living my "normal" life as long as I can.

The breakdown this morning was overdue, because I've been pulling off the "life is normal" thing pretty well, apparently, and it finally burned me out a little too much. It didn't help that I was awake all last night thinking about Artie and his family.

I dated Artie for about five years when I lived in San Francisco, then he was suddenly killed in a horrific motorcycle wreck on the freeway. The pain of that kind of grief is utterly indescribable, except to say that I believe the only emotional pain greater than losing your spouse or significant other is losing your child. The pain I've seen Artie's parents go through in the last five years has been just heart-breaking.

So besides the general strain of pretending "life is normal" while I tried to work around all the medical appointments and so on, the other thing that came to a boiling point in me emotionally was that I've been trying to call Artie's mom (my mother-in-law, basically) to tell her what's going on, but I haven't been able to reach her or his dad or his brothers. I needed to tell them in person about my cancer diagnosis, I couldn't just leave a voicemail about this. Then, all of that got me thinking about how awful every year since Artie's death has been for Artie's parents and all of us who grieved when he died in the motorcycle wreck, and I just can't stand the thought of putting my family through that.

When I talked about it with Marco this morning, he unknowingly said something innately profound yet obvious: "That's why you're going to survive." I doubt he realizes how very deeply *true* that statement is. I will survive because I will not make my parents suffer the loss and grieving that comes with having to bury your child, not when there's a shred of a possibility that I can prevent that from happening. There was a time when I promised myself I would never let someone suffer over me the way I have over Artie these last five and a half years, and that kept me out of a lot of relationships. Well, that, and plenty of other issues. Isn't it ridiculous how hard we can make it for ourselves to have a good lasting relationship? Or maybe that's just me—I don't really know. It's been well over 18 months since there was a guy in my life that could be called a boyfriend. I've become pretty good at avoiding involved romantic relationships. Life's so much simpler that way.

CANCER—DAY 10 **MONDAY, MAY 4, 2009**

This is going to sound strange to some people, but for those of you who know me well, professionally as well as personally, you're going to totally get a bang out of *this* little story.

I met with the radiological oncologist today. I thought it would be a typical 15–30 minute medical consultation, but it was two and a half hours! You wouldn't believe how much I know about cancer radiation treatment now. And it's pretty fascinating stuff, how they model and analyze and simulate prior to radiation treatment. They do the same thing for chemotherapy treatments I guess, though we didn't talk about that too much because I will meet the medical oncologist separately for the chemo talk.

But here's the funny part—two and a half hours of talking cancer treatment, and I came out of there and called my parents to tell them that it was FUN! I haven't totally geeked out in a while, and we really got into all the details, seriously. We were talking mathematical modeling and simulation and quantum physics and negatively charged electrons jumping and how that affects the relation to the cell nucleus . . . all kinds of geeky details. I think the radiation oncologist was really getting into it—maybe these guys don't get to talk much about the quantum level of how this stuff works, and they must get a little jazzed when they get to talk about it to someone new who finds it interesting. Maybe that's why the appointment took so long. On the other hand, my gosh! How do people get through all of this and comprehend it all and understand what's happening to them and figure out how to deal with what's going to happen to them in treatment and recovery and all this mess that is cancer treatment? Let's be real. The cancer patient doesn't get eight years of medical school and three or five years of residency to learn all about their type of cancer, and most cancer patients are in surgery within a matter of weeks after diagnosis. It's unbelievable how complex it all is and how many extremely educated specialists are involved for just one patient. Maybe the doctors always have to spend lots of time discussing all this with every single patient. I kind of think it was the geek in me that made this *particular* appointment exceptionally long, though.

One nice tidbit to share . . . the radiation oncologist made a comment at the end—he said that it's good for my treatment and recovery that I'm taking such a proactive position in understanding and addressing the cancer and the possible scenarios we may face and the likely treatments and everything. He said it's really good because the more active a patient is in their own treatment and recovery, oftentimes the better their recovery. I thought it was nice of him to say that. And Yes! There *are* advantages to having a Type A personality!

Of course, afterward, my parents and I joked on the phone for a good twenty minutes about how these poor doctors just don't know what they're getting themselves into, taking me on. I'm not exactly someone who accepts a vague answer, nor am I particularly tolerant of someone intentionally withholding information, nor do I sit around waiting for assistants to call me to schedule appointments. I think that my being such a get-it-done person in business is making me quite the handful for my doctors and surgeons. But at the same time they seem to love it, once they get used to my asking so many questions and always following up and being informed. Altogether, I think that's really saved us quite a bit of time in the "process" while still being able to be pretty thorough.

I heard that these doctors basically have weekly or even more frequent meetings to discuss their shared patients and the surgeries and treatments and stuff, to coordinate everything. My mom joked that they must really get a kick out of talking about me, and I told her that they probably always talk about me first to get it out of the way because there's always something going on with me. It was a fun conversation.

Actually, aside from the fact that I was up working at 6 a.m. on just four hours of sleep, pounding through my work in order to get out of my office and drive to the radiation oncologist's office this afternoon, and then spending waaayyyyy more time there than I'd expected—aside from feeling like I'm working two full time jobs to do my work and also "manage" my cancer—I actually had a really good day, and it was even fun for me. And tonight Marco and I went and practiced at Firehouse 9 like we used to on Mondays, even though we're not doing the shows now because of my surgery and all of this. Getting to practice again was a treat, spending some focused time in tango with just Marco and the music and no distracting lessons going on in the sidelines. We were the only ones there, and though I wasn't dancing as well tonight as I was just before all of this came up, tonight was still actually the best dancing I've done since the day my gynecologist found the lump. So all around . . . a pretty awesome day.

Tomorrow morning I have two more biopsies that will determine if I am to have a single lumpectomy, bilateral (dual) lumpectomies, or a radical mastectomy with or without a lumpectomy or (possibly) even a radical mastectomy of both breasts. Yep, this case is keeping a lot of doctors on their toes and putting them through their paces. But Humanity Medical is supposedly one of the top medical centers in the country, and they've been pretty great with all of this mess so far.

Of course, the road ahead is long and winding, and it could easily be next February or so before I'm back to a pseudo-normal, non-chemo, non-radiation, cancer-remissive state, so I'll take my amusement where I can . . . like in the geeky quantum level radiological discussions. Man, that was fun!

CANCER—DAY 11 TUESDAY, MAY 5, 2009

You know, if it weren't complicated, the name on the chart couldn't be Cynthia Swan.

I stayed up too late last night, given that I knew I would have to be up early to go to the biopsies. But Marco had to work after dinner, he had a conference call around 9:30 p.m., and so I spent some time responding to e-mails from people who had sent me notes after hearing about the cancer (more on that later, I promise), and next thing you know, it's 11:30 p.m. and too late for me to take an Ambien to make sure I get a full night's sleep before a long medical morning. I took a half a pill, though, to help me fall asleep.

My alarm went off at 6:15 a.m., as I had to be at the RAS building at 7 a.m. for the first biopsy. This is a different radiology place than the one that did the biopsy last week. That place was a lot closer to my home, but no one was sending me back there, and they seem glad I can easily stay in Sacramento as needed. Thank goodness RAS (radiologic something-something) is only about a mile from Marco's house; that was the whole reason for staying at Marco's last night. (I hate getting up at four in the morning at home because of an early appointment in Sacramento!) So, Marco drops me off at 7 a.m., and I'm supposed to call him around 10 a.m. when I'm done so that he can come pick me up. They said I could drive, but Marco said it was just as easy for him to drive me and he wanted to make sure I was OK this time, after the mess the first biopsy was.

The first tech this morning put in the catheter for the contrast dye that they were going to use in the MRI biopsy. For some reason I didn't remember that little detail from the last MRI. Yuck, I'm already so sick of needles, and here we are, stabbing my right arm again just a few days after an IV for the colonoscopy (Did I mention that I had to have a colonoscopy too? Completely unrelated to the cancer but it had to be done, yuck). Granted, today's needle poke was in a slightly different spot on my vein, but the tech still had a hard time getting the needle through . . . she said I was building up scar tissue there. So of course I offer up my left arm, because I have "good" veins on both arms (good, meaning, the veins are large and easy to see so a medic is less likely to need multiple strikes to get a needle in the vein). But then she said that since the primary cancer is on my right and that's where we have the possibility of lymphedema (a swelling of the arm that makes blood draws very difficult, among other things), I should keep using my right arm for all the needles as much as possible now because they'll have to use my left arm for everything for the rest of my life after this. If they remove even a few lymph nodes, it affects the circulation of blood for that arm, so it won't have "good" veins anymore. Dr. Thatcher, my surgeon, is definitely planning on taking out lymph nodes on my right side. Better to use my right arm for IVs and blood draws as much as possible now, that's the MRI tech's advice.

Careful of the catheter sticking out of my arm, they take me in for the MRI biopsy. (The catheter was securely taped to my arm, but I didn't want to jostle it, nonetheless.) I have to lay face down again on the MRI table, but this time they have to pinch my right breast to keep it completely still for the scans and biopsy. But the least pressure on my right is painful because of the complications they had in the first biopsy and how tender it still is as a result. So I'm in tears because this little bit of pinching is so painful. They asked if I could tolerate it for a little while and when I asked how long a "little while" was and they told me 30 minutes, I was like, "yeah, ummmm, NO," so Dr. Martin came back in and loosened the pinchy thing. He actually took it off completely, I think. So then they told me that I had to be completely still, and take shallow breaths because if I moved it would throw off the MRI scans and mislead where they were putting the needle for the biopsy. OK, that I can do if it keeps me out of the breast vise.

Dr. Martin was much more adept with the Novocain shots than the last guy, and though the Novocain injections hurt, it wasn't nearly as bad as it was for the biopsy last week. Dr. Martin was also very careful to make sure that the area was *really* numb for the MRI biopsy so I wouldn't feel that part at all. So aside from the weird metallic taste and smell of the contrast dye they inject during the procedure, the MRI biopsy wasn't horrible in terms of pain. But it did cause additional trauma to my right breast, it required a larger surface incision, and after the biopsy it took a long time to get the bleeding to stop—about 30 minutes. But eventually the bleeding did subside, and they took me upstairs for the ultrasound biopsy on my left breast.

Unfortunately, Dr. Martin had to do another MRI biopsy before he could come up to do my ultrasound biopsy, and he wasn't letting anyone else do mine, so I ended up having about an hour to wait. I asked the ultrasound tech a bunch of questions while she found the spots for the biopsy again, and we talked about what makes the tumor look different from normal ducts and stuff. Meanwhile, the anesthetic was wearing off and my right breast was getting more and more painful. She brought me some Tylenol, but the pain kept notching up, and here I was with tears streaming, in pain, really struggling with it, when Dr. Martin finally came in. He offered to delay the left side biopsy a day or two to let my right side recover so I'm not in so much pain, but I didn't want to do that—I wanted to get it over with so we don't delay the surgery we already know is necessary for the two tumors in my right breast.

So they told me to "hold very still" again, and they got to work. But man, my pain threshold was already really pressed, and while he was doing just the Novocain prep on my left breast I again had tears flowing like a river and I actually choked out a word or two ". . . please . . . stop . . . " He said, "just a little bit more" and kept going just a second or two longer with that injection then moved the needle to another spot to do more, and this painful process continued.

Well, the amount of pressure it took to punch the needle through my skin didn't surprise me, after having to give my cat Kingsford sub-coetaneous IVs every day last year while he was dying of kidney failure. But even after punching the biopsy needle through the skin, it was incredibly difficult for Dr. Martin to get the biopsy needle through my apparently *very* dense breast tissue and that did *not* feel good. I swear, this guy was getting a major workout trying to wrestle that needle through to the tumor. Seriously! It was like trying to shove open a heavy steel door when you're a puny little kid, except Dr. Martin also had to be exceedingly careful not to press too hard either, because the slightest excess could drive the needle a fraction too far in and puncture my chest wall again or worse yet my lung, and then we'd have all kinds of trouble.

Well, that didn't happen, thankfully. But a biopsy is painful, and he actually had to do four of them on my left side. You wouldn't believe how hard he had to pull to get the needle out each time, too. Man, that tissue must be *ridiculously* dense. Ack! Each biopsy was more painful than the last, and by the fourth one I was practically writhing in pain, except I had to stay completely still. Tears streaming, gritting my teeth, my body entirely tensed to keep my chest from moving, I was so tight that I realized at one point that my backside was barely on the table because I was squeezing every bodily muscle so taut against the pain. My limbs shuddered with the effort of keeping my chest entirely stationary to minimize the pain and let them work. I held still and let the silent tears flow and scrunched up my face to bite down on the pain when I couldn't stand it, but I didn't move because if I moved it would screw things up, and this is a very delicate situation. I didn't make much noise—some little swallowed whimpers when I couldn't bear it was all. I was starting to think that it was never going to end—they were going to keep pushing these huge needles in and out of my body until I passed out and then some.

When he finally set the clips in place at the end (they put tiny little metal clips in to mark where the biopsy was, to make it easier to find the exact same spot later), my whole body was trembling from the strain against my muscles, and I was nauseous with pain. And all along the ultrasound tech, Mia, kept telling me how brave I was, how good I'd done, and I was like, "Oh please, I'm such a baby, I seem to have no tolerance for pain." But she told me lots of biopsy patients are much worse, screaming and jerking so that it's much harder to actually get the sample they need. And most people are only having a single biopsy, four like we were doing. Hmmm, OK, maybe I was doing better than I thought. I did hear a woman screaming earlier, and they apparently anesthetized her because her pain was so intense. She also sounded incredibly frightened to me, but the anesthetic probably helped with that too.

Wait a minute, why didn't they give me anesthesia? Not that it matters now. It didn't occur to me to ask for it at the time, I was just trying to contain myself until it was over.

Finally they tugged the biopsy needle out of my left breast for the last time. Finally.

So, we're icing my left breast now, and Dr. Martin wants to check the right breast with the ultrasound. But OMG did it hurt, and just having the slight pressure of the ultrasound sensor there made the earlier incisions start bleeding again. He injected some other stuff in the right breast to help stop the bleeding, and maybe a little Novocain or something to dull the pain somewhat.

Another 30 minutes of pressure and ice, and the bleeding has finally stopped. They re-pack my ice, bind me up in my sports bra and their bandage wrap, which again brought tears to my eyes as they wrapped it tight to keep pressure on that damn tender bleeding right breast. It hurt to take a breath, because the slightest expansion of my chest sent searing pains through my right breast. But they tell me I'm done, and I text Marco that he can come get me. It's a beautiful day outside, and Marco pulls up to the loading area and comes to take my bag and walk me to the car, then we head toward his house, just a mile away. So close and yet so far.

About six blocks from the building I say to Marco, "Darn, my ice pack is leaking and they only gave me enough ice packs to swap, not any extras in case one leaked," and I felt inside my shirt below the bandage to see how badly the ice pack was leaking. My hand came out all bloody, like when someone gets shot in a movie. I guess I learned how to react to this sort of thing from the movies too, because I was confused in a dumbstruck way even though I knew what had happened to me. I speak: "Marco, go back." He glances at me quizzically and I tell him, still keeping my voice calm, "It's bleeding again, a LOT. Take me back." He starts to flip out and immediately pulls over to make a tire-squealing U-turn as I'm slumping down in the seat so I'm more lying down than sitting up in order to bleed on myself instead of the car, and I blurt out "No, no, it's not an emergency, but we have to go back." His driving calmed down reasonably for the remaining three blocks, and just as I was telling him that he could just drop me in front and I'd go in right at the door, we pulled up to a parking spot right in front of the building (funny how that spot at the door was available right when we needed it). Marco said "No, I'm coming in with you." He helped me out of the car and grabbed my phone for me (I don't know why I remember that detail so clearly), and we hustled in the front door.

We get inside to find a short line of three or four people at the registration desk right in front of the entrance. I took one look at that and said to Marco, "I'm going in the back door; I'm just going to walk in and find Mia or someone to help." And off I went. Typical tenacious Cynthia Swan, not willing to bloody well stand politely fifth in line waiting to tell the registration person I'm back because I'm still bleeding, rather profusely now, from the MRI incisions made five hours ago.

I'll try to shorten the rest of the story . . . it's getting late and wow, am I tired! I waltzed right in the back door and kept going until I found a nurse, who in turn grabbed two more attendants (including Mia). They bustled me into a room and gown immediately, to get to work pulling off the gauze and getting new ice and putting lots of pressure on my chest again to stop the bleeding. Then they tell me that Dr. Martin is going to see me, and ultrasound me *again* to make sure what's going on. He finds a hematoma building up in my right breast from the MRI biopsy and decides that he needs to inject those bleeding vessels with a coagulant to help the blood clot. More needling, more pain. Just when you thought it was over and I was going home to rest, right?

Twenty minutes later, I'm still bleeding. As soon as they unwrapped the bandage, I knew this wasn't going to be a quick in-and-out, so I had texted Marco to go on home and I'd text him later when I could leave. And so I text him again now to tell him that it'll be at least another 30 minutes, but then the nurse tells me that they've brought Marco in and they're going to have him sit with me while I keep pressure on this to make sure the coagulant worked before they wrap me back up. Good thing we're dating now, eh? We were there another hour or more, and eventually Dr. Martin decided he'd have to sew up the third incision with real stitches instead of just using steri-strips, and then it seemed to finally stop oozing blood. Finally.

We got back to Marco's at 3 p.m. They had originally told me that I could drive myself there and back for these biopsies, that I wouldn't need heavy-duty pain pills like the last biopsy, and that I could work all day that day because I'd be done in just a couple of hours. Of course by the time we left they had called in a Darvocet prescription to the pharmacy and told me to do nothing for the rest of the day—lift nothing, don't raise my arms, don't do any vigorous moving, and don't sit upright at my computer, just rest. What was supposed to be a simple set of routine early morning procedures for them had turned into an entire day of work on me involving about ten different techs and nurses with Dr. Martin.

What a day. And holy cow, it's just the beginning. But hey, I learned way back when, with my blood pressure and heart condition, that if something was a simple medical case, then it probably wasn't the name Cynthia Swan on the chart. Some things never change.

CANCER—DAY 12 WEDNESDAY, MAY 6, 2009

We got our first truly good news today. The four left side biopsies all showed normal (but very dense—duh!) fibrous tissue. None of those biopsies showed additional malignant tumors, at all. Great news!

The extra biopsy on the right side tested as benign but they think it's cancerous (I don't know how they know when the test result is wrong, but they're the experts and I trust that they know what they're talking about even when I don't understand it). They're going to take a big chunk of this suspiciously malignant-looking area during surgery (besides the primary lumpectomy for the cancerous tumor they're sure about). They'll do a more extensive pathology on this suspicious tissue afterward, but they'll probably just cut it all out in the lumpectomy, rather than put me through two such surgeries. That sounds like a positive spin on a bad bit of news.

Surgery will be Monday or Tuesday next week, and this Friday I'll have the surgery prep where they'll do all the blood work (*again!*) and a nurse will go through everything that's going to happen in the surgery. There are actually several surgical procedures for my "surgery." First they have a surgeon who puts in the lead wire that will guide the surgical staff to the clips marking my tumor, then they take me into radiology to get radiation markers to identify the seminal lymph node so they can do the next procedure—which is to remove and biopsy that lymph node and a couple other lymph nodes to run pathology to find out if the cancer has already spread to other parts of my body—*then* we finally get to the surgery where they will remove the tumor and other iffy tissue, and then they will finish up with reconstructive surgery with an implant.

A month or so later, I'll go to Nebraska to stay with my parents for three to six months of chemotherapy treatments, then a month or so after chemo is done, I'll be back in Sacramento for daily radiation treatments for 6-1/2 weeks. So all in all, we're looking at somewhere between six and nine months of all this cancer stuff.

Besides all the cancer and medical things to manage, there's still all this life stuff going on, you know? I don't know how people handle it all at once. I'm sort of getting through by taking things one at a time. If I think about everything at once, it's just mind-boggling.

CANCER—DAY 13 THURSDAY, MAY 7, 2009

Oh boy. My cardiologist, Dr. Wolver, is NOT happy, at all. Because of the Adriamyacin, which is a cardio-toxin drug typically used in chemotherapy, a person's heart can be weakened by chemotherapy treatment. Dr. Wolver says I have to be taken off of my heart medicine during chemo because the chemo drugs could cause a negative reaction with my heart medication, so there are some worries concerning my heart anyway, besides the dangers of Adriamyacin. We have to do an echocardiogram before the chemo starts, and again when the chemo is done, and if the post-chemo echo is good, then they will put me back on my heart medicine. If not, I guess it's time for a pace-maker.

Most people don't know I have a heart condition. It's not exactly something that comes up frequently in common conversation. My heart condition is called neurocardiogenic disorder. I have medicine that I take every twelve hours (I have an alarm set on my phone for it). The medicine basically regulates things so that I don't have an "episode," a.k.a., heart failure.

My first heart failure happened while I was playing the flute for a Catholic Mass. Right in the middle of the Lord's Prayer, I blacked out. I don't remember anything between the blackness and coming to as paramedics lifted me onto a gurney and wheeled me out of church, and then the priest finished up the Mass. The paramedics had actually been having lunch with the guys at the firehouse about 100 yards from the church (both were out in the country a little bit), so when they received the 911 message they were there within two minutes, I swear. They had hooked up some tubes and an IV drip, and we were at the hospital within ten minutes. During all this, I feel faint and woozy, but I'm awake.

In the emergency room, they immediately hooked me up to all kinds of monitors for my breathing, heart rate, brain waves, you name it, I was plugged in to it, or so it seemed to me. I was lying down the first 30 minutes or so while they made sure my vitals (heart rate, blood pressure, breathing, etc.) were stable. When I had been in there thirty minutes without a hint of anything being wrong, they sat me up to take my vitals. But when they sat me up, I blacked out again. This one was more woozy, with everything turning a fuzzy gray and then somehow colorful, instead of going all black like the first episode back a the church. I must have sat up too quickly.

They said my heart rate elevated so quickly as I sat up that they were trying to lie me back down before I blacked out again, but even lying down, my heart rate was still increasing. Until it blew a fuse, in a way, and stopped beating, setting off all kinds of alarms on the machines they had me hooked up to. The ER doc was on it, though. They injected something or another and got my heart going at a reasonable rate again without too much trouble. They also sent for the on-call cardiologist. So I laid still another half hour, and my vitals were fine and stable. We decided to do the sitting up thing, very, very slowly. Two male techs raised me to a sitting position while the on-call cardiologist and the ER staff kept strict watch on the monitors. It seemed OK. I was sitting upright, and I didn't black out. My heart rate had increased more than it should have needed to for me just to sit up especially given that I hadn't actually even raised myself, the techs had gradually lifted me to a sitting position. They kept me there a while, sitting up, watching my vitals on all the machines. They had brought in a wheelchair with a toilet in it because I had been begging to go to the bathroom and I couldn't seem to use a bedpan because it was just too foreign to my body. After I had been sitting up with constant attention and my vitals remained unchanged for more than 30 minutes after the cardiologist arrived, the cardiologist said he would let me use the wheelchair thing but only with the techs and everyone in there, and staying attached to all the machines. I was OK with that, so the cardiologist held my right arm while a tech held my left arm, and a nurse helped lift my legs slowly to hang over the side of the bed. They all watched the machines. So far so good. The cardiologist said, "OK, good. Slowly now, just let your legs reach down to the floor. Slowly now." And I slid forward to the edge of the bed.

No alarms went off. So I tried to reach my legs down to the floor and hold my own weight so I would be standing. The monitors started beeping faster just as I was trying to let myself onto my feet, but I collapsed. As I blacked out again, I could hear the heart rate monitor accelerate like a rocket and then become a constant wail. And then I was . . . somewhere else. It was a very interesting experience, actually, with all kinds flashes of life and colors and the big bang and—after seeming to experience the entirety of the history of our universe in a flash—I found myself in this completely peaceful state of oneness, sitting Buddha-like on a mountaintop feeling fully connected to all energy. It didn't seem strange at the time, but it was weird to remember after they got me back. I had never explored spirituality before, but I became curious about it after this particular heart failure.

This time it took much longer for them to get my heart beating again, and they had to shock my heart with those electrical paddle things several times, but they did get it going again. As my head cleared, the on-call cardiologist told me that I was not allowed to sit up, I was not allowed off that bed, and if I so much as moved an arm too quickly he was going to have me bound to the bed. He winked as he said that last one, so I don't think they really would have tied me down. Besides, I never disobey doctors orders, and if he says don't sit up, I'm not going to sit up. Easy enough. Then he told me, "If you have another heart episode like what just happened, you're going straight into surgery and I'm putting in a pacemaker with or without your permission." I promised I would stay still and asked him to please try to hold off on any kind of surgery until at least my parents could get there the next morning.

They moved me to the ICU where I no longer had a curtain, because the ICU nurses keep such vigilant watch over ICU patients. It was very quiet there, though. The nurses told me it's unusual for them to have a patient like my in the ICU, someone awake and able to make conversation. That was when I noticed how very quiet it was, even though it was essentially one enormous circular room with the nursing station in the middle.

It was getting late, about 11 p.m., when the on-call cardiologist came in to introduce me to another, specialized doctor, an electro-cardiologist. Even though it was Sunday, the on-call cardiologist had stayed at the hospital with me all day, and felt this was serious enough to ask for the electro-cardiologist to come see me that night rather than wait until morning. The specialist seemed like a nice enough guy, and told me to lie still and rest while they went to go over my charts and readings from my "episodes." He came back around 7 a.m. to tell me that he didn't think surgery was the right action to take at this time. Lucky for me, this guy happens to be one of the top electro-cardiologists in the country, and he knew exactly what was going on with my heart and also that we didn't have to go straight to a pacemaker. He said I was too young and if I was going to keep dancing in competitions and shows, I wasn't going to want a pacemaker making my chest all lumpy. Besides, pacemakers don't last forever, they have to be replaced at some point (every ten years?), so he didn't want to give someone in their twenties a pacemaker if it could be avoided. He had just led the successful testing, evaluation, and FDA approval on a new medication for this particular heart condition, the neurocardiogenic disorder, and he was going to put me on that and watch me carefully for three months (during which I wasn't allowed to drive a car because I might have an episode and cause a car wreck!). If things looked good to him after three months, he'd keep me on the medicine but we wouldn't have to talk pacemakers or anything else for a very long time, if at all.

Keeping it fairly simple, the problem is in the electrical connection between my heart and another muscle/nerve called the vagus. As I understand it, the vagus is located just behind the heart, and it is supposed to tell the heart when it is going fast enough for the current activity. In my case, that electrical connection wasn't happening, and my heart would accelerate itself until it simply locked itself up in a constriction and couldn't beat any more.

He actually marveled a bit at my recovery from the third episode in the ER. He said they shocked me twice more than he would have expected (is there some kind of standard number of shocks before they pronounce you dead?). That was a little freaky, having a doctor marveling at the simple fact that I was alive and making conversation with him. I couldn't remember who the state senator was, but that wasn't because my brain was damaged. I knew the important ones, like the President's name and my own name and where I lived. They did a bunch of brain tests too, after the day I died three times. What a weird thing to be able to say, eh?

After three months on the medication without any complications, side effects, or heart episodes, he was content that I could stay on this medication for the rest of my life and I quite probably would never need to do anything else as long as I stayed on this every twelve hours. I was a little surprised. I asked him, "Do I really have to take this for the rest of my life?" He leaned forward and pulled his glasses off and shook them at me as he said "You don't understand. Your heart stopped for *long* periods of time. They could have pronounced you but they kept trying and luckily they brought you back that last time. Yes. You will be on this medication for the rest of your life. End of discussion." Well, that settled that!

Until now. My heart medication cannot be mixed with the chemotherapy meds. Now cancer is a bigger threat to my continued existence than the possibility of my heart stopping. I hadn't even thought about my heart stuff, because it's been fine with the medication. And I didn't know until today that Adriamyacin makes doctors very, very nervous when you already have a heart condition.

The other thing that upset Dr. Wolver today is the plan for me to go back to Nebraska to do chemo. He softened on the idea when I told him who my medical oncologist is here (they know each other), and that the medical oncologist here in Sacramento will be in charge with the medical oncologist out in Nebraska just executing the chemo under his direction. But Dr. Wolver is unhappy about my being away for chemo, in case anything comes up with my heart while I'm not on my medication. He doesn't want me so far away from where he knows I can get the best care, since he doesn't know of any electro-cardiologists with his specialty out in Nebraska. And Sidney is not exactly a grand metropolis of a city.

This just keeps getting better and better, doesn't it?

CANCER—DAY 14 FRIDAY, MAY 8, 2009

Tomorrow and Sunday, there are Argentine workshops in the City, which Marco and I are going to, although I don't know if I'll be able to dance by then. My right side, especially, is still hurting quite a bit from the last biopsy. Either way, it's not much of a weekend for Marco and I to spend any time "together." My parents are due to arrive on Sunday. Surgery is Tuesday. So, I guess no real Marco time again until after Mom & Dad leave. I wonder when that will be—maybe a couple or a few weeks. Then, maybe a little time alone with Marco before going out to Nebraska for chemo. Then . . . no more Marco. I'm kind of sad about that—I don't expect him to still be thinking of me after I've been gone three or six months. He'll probably have both a new girlfriend AND a new dance partner by then.

Sheesh, I have GOT to get a new attitude before I ruin this weekend for myself!

CANCER—DAY 15 SATURDAY, MAY 9, 2009

Wow, what a painful day. My stitches both hurt and itch, my entire right breast is yellow with bruising, and my left side is getting strained from overuse while compensating for my right. I tried to only take Tylenol so that my mind would be clear for the Argentine workshops today, but it just hurt too much. Then, in the workshops, well, trying to focus and learn and dance was not easy this afternoon.

We went back to Marco's for a while afterward. I rested a little, we had dinner, and then we went back for the milonga. I only danced the first two tandas with Marco (a tanda is a set of three tango songs), then later a tanda with Szak (my previous tango show partner), and at the end of the night one more tanda with Marco. My body was just done in from the workshops, and I knew there were more workshops the next day, plus my parents were coming in, so I knew I shouldn't push it at the milonga.

My dancing with Marco just keeps getting more and more connected though, and it's ever easier to slip into that state of shared consciousness with him. Oy vey, I can't tell you how close and personal it is to feel that kind of connection with someone. That's where the real sensuality of tango exists for me. Not in steps and moves, but in moving with my partner in the heart connection. Four legs, one heart.

CANCER—DAY 16 SUNDAY, MAY 10, 2009

I'm sad that this was my last morning waking up with Marco. After the tango workshops, I rushed home to Mom & Dad, who arrived in the early afternoon.

And wow, I haven't slept in my master bedroom in more than a year I think, not since before my cat Kingsford died a year ago last March. I had switched to my guest room bed when Kingsford couldn't get up on the big bed anymore, and I just hadn't had the heart to switch back after he died. Besides, the view from the guest room has more trees, which is nice to wake up to.

Mom & Dad were at the ready when I got home. They were out on the front porch before I even got out of the car. We started chatting and next thing you know it's late. So the cats and I are all snuggling in together on half of my bed now because I'm too tired to finish folding my laundry. Mom restrained herself admirably to not start cleaning immediately upon arrival today.

Seoul's a little confused because this bed is significantly higher than the other one, and she doesn't yet understand about using the steps to graciously step up onto the bed instead of leaping and scrambling from the floor like a wildcat. It's also pretty hilarious to watch her climb down, not trusting the steps. Kittens, gotta love ‘em.

Both of the cats are being pretty skittish tonight, though, with visitors staying overnight. I can't remember the last time anyone other than me has stayed here at my house in the forest. My parents came out to visit was when I first moved in two years ago, but that was before Seoul was born. Mizzou is totally comfortable with my parents. Seoul, not so much.

I imagine Marco is probably feeling a bit relieved, having his room in the new house to himself for a while. (Did I mention that, on the day after I got the phone call confirming that the tumor was malignant carcinoma, we moved Marco out of his apartment and into a house with a friend of his? Probably no, it’s just another example of how busy life already was *before* cancer). I wonder if it might feel lonely to him now. But heck, it's not like we've been together a long time; it's just that we've been together a lot *lately*. Well, together *constantly* a lot lately.

I'm usually the one bugging out from those situations, but in hindsight, I think it's been pretty important that I haven't been home alone for any great length of time since diagnosis. The times I was especially low or stressed, Marco generally brought me back to a calm that I really needed to be in. I hope doing that wasn't too hard on him. Sometimes I get really drained when people need a lot of bolstering up from me, especially these days—it seems people can drain me really quickly now. Like the day after I was diagnosed when Marco and I had lunch with a friend who’s just starting to think divorce instead of separation—she needed to talk about everything, and we were there to listen, but wow, was my energy ever wiped out after that hour.

Chapter 3.
Surgery

CANCER—DAY 18 TUESDAY, MAY 12, 2009

Surgery is tomorrow . . . I'm a bit nervous but also relieved to get it over and done with. Today I preoccupied myself with drafting and sending an e-mail to my family and friends who don't yet know I was diagnosed with breast cancer. I filtered through my contacts in Outlook taking off people I have just zero contact with any more and never expect to have contact with again, but the send-to list was still more people than I can count. But there are so many people I *do* need to tell, and I can't go person by person through every e-mail address before tomorrow, and for a lot of people I feel like a message was long overdue even though diagnosis was only, what, a couple weeks ago? Anyway, it's a good summary of where I'm at in treatment at the moment.

> *I am sorry to send you this news in an e-mail blast, but I wanted to let you know that I was diagnosed with an invasive malignant breast cancer (infiltrating ductal carcinoma) on April 25. Since then I've had a multitude of additional tests, procedures, and more biopsies on both sides which thankfully have so far shown the cancer to be contained enough for a single lumpectomy surgery. We will also do a sentinel node biopsy then, which will tell us whether the cancer has spread to other parts of the body so they can stage the cancer. So far what they've seen of the lymph nodes in my MRIs and such look clean, but they're doing another biopsy to be as certain as possible.*
>
> *My surgery is tomorrow afternoon, Tuesday, May 13 at the Humanity Medical Center in Placerville (about 45 minutes from Volcanoville where I live). I actually have a bunch of medical stuff before the surgery tomorrow too. It starts with an echocardiogram at 8:15 a.m., then I'm having a stint (guiding wire) put in at 10 a.m., a radiation treatment and the sentinel lymph node biopsy at noon, and then the actual lumpectomy and reconstructive surgery at 2 p.m.. It's a busy schedule, and it's all outpatient. I should be sleeping in my own bed next to Mizzou and Seoul (my two cats) again tomorrow night, how wild is that? My parents are here and will be staying at my house and taking care of me during the surgery recovery.*
>
> *Because it's rare for someone my age to get breast cancer, and because it is both more aggressive and more likely to recur in younger women (under 40), my surgeons and doctors are all telling me that I will undergo aggressive*

chemotherapy treatments regardless of the results of the sentinel node biopsy. Chemo will start about a month after surgery, and the current plan is that I will go stay at Mom & Dad's place in Nebraska during the chemotherapy, which will be three to six months in duration. About a month after that I'll start radiation treatments in Sacramento: fifteen minutes a day five days a week for 6-1/2 weeks. I guess all that means I may get back to a normal life around January or February, give or take a month.

It's a serious diagnosis, to be sure, but we're doing everything that can be done, and the technological advances in the past ten years or so have been truly amazing, so much so that I have every confidence that this is essentially just another medical process I have to go through, and I will be fine when it's over. Heck, I'll generally be fine while I'm going through it too, especially with the friends who have been my support so far and of course my family who is taking such an active role in my treatment and recovery and all of their friends who are wishing me a complete and speedy recovery as well.

I have started an online journal, so if you want to keep track of my progress and get a dose of my personal opinions on the process, what I'm experiencing, and what's going on in my life during this time, feel free to check out my blog now and again at www.cielemel.com.

Best regards,
Cynthia

I summed it all up in the e-mail, but the whole time I was writing it, my mind wanted to go back into shock mode, to hide from the reality behind a curtain of disbelief. But cancer isn't exactly something you can hide from.

There's this saying that I use a lot, but I didn't come up with it. Close to ten years ago, I worked for a software company in Toronto. They had just sent me to do a workshop for a prospective client in Melbourne, Australia, and from there I had to skip California and fly straight to Toronto, landing there just two hours before the week of training I was scheduled for. Needless to say, I was more than wiped out. I was physically present, but the huge time zone change and lack of sleep was having a serious impact on my ability to think. There was a new guy from Chicago sitting next to me in the training, and we chatted during the breaks, talking about why we joined the company and stuff like that. He was going to be doing essentially the same job as me but based in Chicago, so he asked a lot of questions about what it had been like for me so far (I had only been there a few weeks myself, at that point). I told him about the Australia trip and that I didn't think every week was going to be as crazy as that with travel, usually we can schedule travel with a little more cushion but when something comes up that is urgent for a client or prospect, you pretty much just have to go do it and keep going. He said, "Yeah, I can relate to that. You know, it is what it is, so you just do what has to be done."

"It is what it is." This has been one of my sayings for almost ten years now. I've always found it a good perspective on life when you can't change what it is and you just have to deal with it. In life, it's an acceptance of your current situation and knowing that, because you can't change the facts, you simply have to move forward from where you are.

That training in Toronto actually contained several people I work with today at my current consulting company. Back then, we all reported to John, who was the Director of Marketing back then, and who is our CEO today. There was a product manager in training with me who is now the VP of the division I work with in my current company. And there are at least three other people from then that I work with now.

Back in the day, starting from that week of training in Toronto, we all kind of took up that saying, "it is what it is." What's kind of funny now is that my VP uses it *all* the time, and quite a few of our newer consultants fresh out of college hear the saying from him and take it up as their own. So now it's both a saying and kind of a joke for everyone in my consulting company. "It is what it is." In other words, you can't change the facts. That saying has always resonated with me ever since I first heard it from the guy from Chicago, almost ten years ago, and I keep thinking about it now.

Raw data can't lie, facts are facts, and you can either go with it or knowingly ignore it. Well, I cannot knowingly ignore cancer, it isn't going to go away if I ignore it. The cancer simply is.

"It is what it is." All right, then. Having breast cancer is simply a fact now, a new starting point, and all I can do is move forward from there. So, off to the hospital I go.

CANCER—DAY 19 WEDNESDAY, MAY 13, 2009

Just got home from the hospital. Because they couldn't get the pain under control, I was admitted to the hospital overnight. They kept giving me morphine every hour throughout the night. No real sleep, but I did doze in and out of consciousness, which was very strange. I'd be in the middle of texting Marco, then get too drowsy to finish the message . . . and then I would reawaken and turn the blackberry toward me again (I didn't get drowsy enough to actually let go of the blackberry) to finish the text message.

Ahhhhh . . . so nice to be lying in my own bed now. I didn't sleep worth a darn in the hospital, but at least they kept the morphine coming in little doses all night. So, you must be wondering, just what *did* happen to Cynthia yesterday?

Well, the first task during the morning of the surgery was to get an echocardiogram done for my cardiologist. After the echocardiogram, we went to have the stints put in, and that's where the fun started. I should mention now that if you have a weak stomach or can't stand the thought of me in severe pain, you should probably skip the rest of this journal entry.

You have to keep in mind that I have had four biopsies on my left breast and two biopsies on my right breast in the last two weeks, with the second one on the right requiring a larger incision and more cutting that unfortunately led to uncontrollable bleeding and created a fairly severe hematoma in my right breast. To paint a picture of this, think of a softball sized bruise at the just-turned-yellow stage, and that's what it looked like yesterday morning. Since it's just one big bruise, it has been ridiculously sensitive to even the slightest bit of pressure. Now, try to imagine compressing that breast for a mammogram and then compressing it further to insert large needles that allow wires to be set into my tumor clips (I had two tumor sites to be excised from the right breast, so, two wires), then set those wires with lead weights, and do it all without pain medication. That was my morning. Then we had to go up the hill to the hospital.

By the time we got me in a wheelchair and in the hospital, I was in agony, tears everywhere, teeth clenched, every muscle tense to the point that I could barely gnash out the words "I can't tolerate this much longer." I thought I was going to pass out. And it was tearing my mom apart, having to see me in pain like this. The look of agony on her face was unbearable, and I tried to signal my dad to take her outside. Then a surgery nurse came rushing up with morphine, which helped ease the pain to a barely sufferable level, and we got me out of the wheelchair and onto the x-ray table.

Then it gets worse. The next thing they need to do is inject this radioactive material in my breast so that it travels from the breast to light up my lymph nodes and identify the sentinel node (first node from the breast) via x-ray. So they have to give me more shots, which was a lot like getting Novocain only there's this radioactive stuff burning in me. Mind you, the morphine shot merely eased the previous pain somewhat, but not significantly. As if all this radioactive stuff wasn't bad enough—they then had to use tape to pull my breast toward my sternum so they could take an x-ray straight down to the lymph nodes. Then, to block the blazing light of the radioactive material that they just inserted in my breast tissue, they put a *lead weight* on my breast, and took a whole bunch of x-rays. They made marks on my body to direct the surgeon to the sentinel lymph node, then x-rayed again to check the marks. So there I was, with this lead weight on my just-turned-yellow tennis ball bruise of a breast for 20 minutes. It was awful.

They took me to a surgical staging room and said that my parents could come in if I wanted them. The pain is generally unbearable at this point, and the thought of Mom seeing me like that made me tell them to keep my parents out until after the surgery. They didn't want to give me any more painkiller because it was only 45 minutes or so before the surgery. Forty-five minutes? Of feeling like this? They left me alone to wait.

I can't stand it and I text Marco. "Oh baby this sucks!" He reminds me to breathe and focus (a little trick he used on me during a tango rehearsal once, right before my conference in Atlanta when I was so stressed out about work that I couldn't dance). So now I'm in the surgery prep room, trying to breathe and focus on the breath. But it's just too much. I text him again: "Suddenly wish I had your hand to squeeze, all alone in here." He's on his way, and my surgery is in 30 minutes. I tell the nurse who he is and she goes to tell the desk clerks to let him in right away when he arrives. *But not my parents.* I can't bear the look on my mom's face after she sees the look on *my* face.

Meanwhile, my mom is apparently fussing at the clerks, saying that she wants to come back to be with me. They try to tell her that I asked them to give me privacy, but Mom wasn't taking "No" for an answer. (No more wondering where I get *that* little stubbornness characteristic from, eh?) Marco arrived, the nurses gave up trying to dissuade Mom, and all three of them came to my room.

I was relieved to see Marco, but asked Dad to take Mom out almost immediately. A quick hug and "I love you's" for them both, and then "Please, go." I ended up with just a few minutes to clench Marco's hand, not talking, before they finally took me in for the surgery.

I, of course, don't remember the surgery—I just woke up in the recovery room where they were monitoring me closely before releasing me back to the surgical prep room. Then they took me back to my room, Room G, which was apparently the kids' room—it was painted in bright colors, with fish and such on the walls and ceiling. My parents and Marco came back in, and the pain was getting bad again as the anesthetic wore off. Bad, as in, if I moved I shrieked out in pain before clamping my mouth shut to swallow down the pain and not agonize my parents beyond the worry they already felt from my surgery running more than an hour longer than expected.

I never thought about it in this much detail, but the hospital had a pain chart on the wall next to my bed:

0 no pain
1 some pain but ok
2 mild pain worse
3 annoying pain
4 distracting pain
5 pain too bad to ignore for long
6 pain can't be ignored at all
7 pain makes it hard to think and sleep
8 pain limits activity
9 I cry out in pain
10 passed out

The nurse comes in and I ask her how much pain I'm supposed to be able to tolerate as I study this pain chart. The nurse asks me to tell her what level my pain is. I scan through the levels and descriptions, and choke out "Nine." That was clearly not the number she wanted to hear.

But they couldn't get the pain under control. Morphine helped—that brought it down to a seven, but it was getting late and they needed to have me on oral painkillers before they could send me home. We tried some Tylenol No. 3, which I guess has codeine in it, but it didn't do a darn thing to lessen the pain. They were trying to decide whether to send me home or not, and all I could say was, "I can't even get to the front door of the hospital from the bed; there's no way I'll be able to handle the 45-minute ride and bumpy dirt road to my house."

The nurse told me that she wants my pain down to a three before she sends me home, and I tell her I'd consider a five tolerable enough. But clearly even *that* wasn't going to happen any time soon, so they called my surgeon, Dr. Thatcher, and he had me admitted to the hospital overnight. Then they gave me some more morphine, and after another 30 minutes or so, it finally started becoming bearable (a six). Marco had been with me this whole time, letting me squeeze his hand when the pain surged, brushing the hair off my face, doing his soothing calm thing, and really comforting me. It was one of those times I think I'll never forget how much his being there meant to me right then. My muscles finally relaxed somewhat, I wasn't trembling anymore, and I could breathe without scrunching up my face in pain. They had a room for me, my parents came back in, and Marco left to go teach. My parents took me upstairs to my hospital room, and then left to go back to my house for the night before returning for me in the morning.

I have another whole story to tell about the rest of my hospital stay, but I've been writing too long already tonight, so I'll have to leave this for now as . . . to be continued . . .

CANCER—DAY 20 THURSDAY, MAY 14, 2009

Technically, this entry is more about day 19 for the cancer journal, but the surgery day got me a bit off in my scribing. Still, this is one story my parents will never forget, and I can't very well leave it out of the journal, so I'm going to tell you about the night and the morning in the hospital after surgery.

During my overnight at the hospital I had a wonderful aide, Amy, and a fantastic nurse, Tracy. My nurse was actually the charge nurse who usually runs the floor, but that night she was working the floor because she needed more nurses. They were great. Amy made sure that I ate, and she came in to check my vitals on a schedule. I would ask her questions and she would chat with me a little bit about what she does and what kinds of patients they get—you know, small talk—but she and I have the same opinion on stuck-up doctors and people who think they're better than anyone else (apparently many people treat hospital aides, like young dance instructors, with about the same level of respect that some executives treat the mailroom clerk). And since I couldn't sleep, Amy would check in on me and try to get me to eat some crackers or soup whenever I got a shot, and we'd chat now and again. She even came in to say goodbye to me in her street clothes in the morning as she was going home.

My overnight nurse, Tracy, was amazing—somehow very caring and amazingly efficient at the same time. I suspect this is what my mom was like as an RN before she retired. Tracy talked with me early on about how much pain medication Dr. Thatcher had approved per hour (up to 10 milligrams of morphine per hour—woweee, would that have been a druggie trip or what?), and how she is perfectly fine with giving me the full amount per hour even though she prefers to dole it out in smaller doses more frequently so we can adjust the medication to how the pain shifted during the night. This made perfect sense to me, and so whenever the pain started to be too great, I would push my little call button and Amy would come on the speaker to see what I needed, then Tracy would come in a moment later to talk about the pain and we'd decide the dosage (usually two to four milligrams).

She'd be back a moment later with the shot and administer it with some saline to help prevent nausea from the morphine. Tracy is from New Zealand, and her accent was amusing to me. Same sort of thing as with Amy—since I was up most of the night—Tracy would check in on me sometimes between patients, and we would chat a little. With Tracy in charge and Amy aiding, I felt safe and protected, and completely trusted their care. I also really empathized with their rationale for working nights . . . the workload is more calm and controllable, and very little of the daytime hospital politics or attitudes seep into the night shift.

Their shift change was at 7 a.m., so I had my last shot from Tracy at about 6:50 a.m. She told me that they needed to get me switched over to oral meds in order to let me go home, so we decided to up my last dose to six milligrams. She was encouraging it, which I didn't completely understand at the time, but an hour later it was obvious that the day staff is very different from the night staff at Humanity Medical.

My new aides came in at 7 a.m. to take my vitals. There were two of them, because one, Cheryl, was in training. Cheryl had been an aide in convalescent care for many years, but had only been at the hospital for two days, so she was new to how the hospital does things. The aide training Cheryl, Arynne (pronounced Erin), was very busy telling Cheryl what and how to do things, and when she asked me what my pain level was, she apparently didn't hear me say "5" because she wrote zero on the chart. Zero, HA! What I wouldn't give to remember what it feels like for pain to be at a zero, when pain doesn't exist. Anyway, the aides seemed too busy to actually take care of me, and, uncharastically, I didn't ask them any questions.

A few minutes later my day nurse, Susan (Sue) came in. She and I butted heads almost immediately. The first thing she said was "I understand you're in a hurry to get out of here." Which shocked me, because, aside from asking someone the night before if there's a typical time they release patients (so I could tell my parents when to come back), I had never suggested to anyone that I thought I didn't need the pain shots or that I was anxious to go home on oral meds. So I told her "No, not at all, I just asked if there's a time I should tell my parents to be here because my house is far away. I definitely prefer being where I can be cared for and have my pain controlled." She asked about my pain and I said it wasn't too bad at the time because I'd had six milligrams of morphine just 30 minutes ago but that we'd been dosing it in smaller more frequent doses all night. She pooh-poohed that, like it's just a hassle to do small frequent doses.

But morphine wears off after about an hour, and so just 30 minutes or so later, I was ringing the call button for Sue to come in and give me my shot. It took her about ten minutes to show up, but she went straight to it and gave me four milligrams without asking how bad the pain was or how much morphine I thought I needed. This woman was clearly not the caregiver that Tracy is. But, hey, she did bring my shot, and an hour later I buzzed for her again, and so on through the morning.

At ten o'clock she brought me pills instead of morphine and said we needed to get me onto orals so I could go home later. It was Darvocet. I took it, but I told her that I had been given Darvocet after the last biopsy and that it had started causing me stomach problems and not working very well after I'd had it a couple of days, and that the nurses yesterday in post-op had said I was going to have Tylenol No. 3 with Codeine instead of Darvocet or Vicodan (which also has made me sick in the past). She was annoyed by this, and flipped back in the chart saying that Darvocet is what Dr. Thatcher ordered so that was what I was going to get. I tried to ask her when that order was written because the Tylenol decision hadn't been made until late in the day yesterday, but she fussed about having to call in a different prescription and left the room. Not long after that, my parents showed up. I told them about the Darvocet thing and that I was worried about getting sick from the medication when we got home, and they told me to make sure that Sue changed the prescription so we wouldn't have to worry about that. When Sue came back in (while Mom & Dad were with me), I mentioned again the conversation the nurses and Dr. Thatcher had while I was in post-op and that I was supposed to have Tylenol No. 3 because Darvocet hadn't worked well for me before and caused me stomach trouble. She snapped, "Well, how do you feel now?" I told her I felt about the same as when she gave me the pills an hour earlier, a six on the pain scale. And she said the pills were obviously working because the pain hadn't increased since I took them. I pressed her on the prescription thing anyway, and she said she would have to call Dr. Thatcher to get the Tylenol No. 3 prescription approved. I told her "Well, yes, I think you need to do that then." And she kind of stomped off, obviously annoyed that I had increased her workload by requiring her to make an extra phone call to my surgeon and also call the pharmacy to change the prescription that she'd just called in. Mom & Dad agreed, though—I had to push her to do it—we couldn't go home with Darvocet knowing that it doesn't work for me. It would take Dad 90 minutes to go get another prescription if the Darvocet didn't work, and we would have had to call Dr. Thatcher from home to change the medication. So it's 12:15 p.m. now, and we're waiting for the aides to bring my lunch and then wait to make sure the pain pills work before I can go home with Mom & Dad. They were hungry too, and Dad was getting antsy. I suggested that they go downstairs to get lunch, so they went. I was trying to rest and snooze a little, but not long after that, the pain started going up, because the Darvocet wasn't working.

So once again, I pushed the call button, got the aide station, and asked them if I could get some pain medicine please. They replied with the usual "OK, I'll let your nurse know," and I waited. The pain went from a bearable six to a muscle-tensing seven. No nurse. Ten minutes go by. I page again. In a slightly more agitated voice this time, "Can I please get some pain medicine?" They said they already told my nurse, but would tell her again. I wait.

The pain goes up to a nauseating eight, and ten minutes go by. My phone chi-gongs (it makes the sound of a chi gong when I receive text messages, such a soothing sound) with a text from Marco "still drifting?" I text back "almosrrt aa 9 waaiitng 4 nurrrse" my hands trembling so much I can't type into the blackberry properly. Pain rises to a face-wrenching shrieking crying nine, and still no nurse. I'm alone in my room. I press the call button again. I can't control my voice, I'm crying and my voice is hoarse and I beg them, "Please, I need some pain medication. PLEASE!" They start to tell me they're looking for my nurse and I croak out, "I don't need SUE, just send in a nurse, just send in *anyone's* nurse. Please!" They start babbling about how Sue is my nurse or something, as she finally enters my room. "Never mind, she's here," I gasp, and collapse back on the bed. I can't even look at Sue, I can't even see through the tears, and my whole body is shaking uncontrollably. It's been 35 minutes since I first pressed the call button, which I didn't even do until the pain was more than I could take. Sue says something about having been on the phone calling in my new Tylenol No. 3 prescription and I just scrunch my eyes closed and try to stop trembling. She administers her decided standard dosage of 4 mg of morphine and disappears without a word.

I can't imagine how awful it would feel being a caregiver and finding your charge in that state from your neglect. Apparently it didn't seem that awful for Sue, though, now that I think about it. She seemed fine with me being in agony.

Mom & Dad came up about fifteen minutes later when the morphine was working and I was back to a 7-1/2, tears still drying on my red cheeks. I didn't tell them everything right away, just that it took Sue over 30 minutes to bring my pain meds and I was hurting, badly. As you can imagine, my Director of Nurses mother and Hospital Administrator father have an opinion about the minimum quality of care one should expect of nurses in a hospital. I didn't want to upset them by telling them how bad it had gotten.

The next time Sue came in the room it was to confirm the Tylenol No. 3 prescription and make sure the morphine was working. Her tone had changed completely, and she was almost meek in her efforts to be helpful now, in front of my parents. At home, later, I told Mom & Dad how bad it had gotten, and I told Dad that I couldn't tell them at first because he would have gotten her fired then and there if he'd known. After all, he'd just been downstairs chatting it up with the Humanity Medical hospital administrator, who was cooking for the hospital barbecue where my parents ended up having lunch. Dad and the administrator hit it off. Go figure. And apparently one of my nurses from the day before had remembered my parents, and came over at lunch to tell them that she hoped I was doing well, which made Mom feel good. Meanwhile, I'm upstairs begging for pain medication from a nursing desk that is unresponsive even after three buzzes. Ridiculous.

Anyway, we got me out of there around 2:30 p.m. or so, and now I'm thankful to be home even if the pain isn't down to a three like the first nurse told me it should be for going home. I can live with a seven for now. Just please, please, *please*—no more nines.

CANCER—DAY 21 FRIDAY, MAY 15, 2009

I am deformed.

Why I thought they would be able to do this lumpectomy surgery and not leave me deformed, I don't know, but I honestly had not thought I would turn out like this. I should have done more research. I should have asked more questions. Why didn't I know this kind of deformity was a possible outcome of the lumpectomy?

I had the follow up appointment with Dr. Allondry today. He's the plastic surgeon who inserted the implant after Dr. Thatcher did the lumpectomy. This was my first time out of the house since we got home from surgery, except for a couple of little walks that Mom made me take around the house and to the end of my driveway. But today, we went out and had lunch with Marco in Folsom before going to the doctor's appointment. My parents were fairly excited to see that I wore my contacts and a little makeup. Mom kept saying how pretty I looked. I must have looked pretty awful the past several days, eh? I'll probably hear that from her a lot during chemo when I'm bald and trying not to look like a freak. Anyway, we had lunch with Marco, which was really nice because I'd missed him and we had a good time. Dad says his laugh is infectious. Good grief, what in the world will I do with a guy that my dad actually likes? Dance, I guess!

So then Marco went back to work, and Mom & Dad took me to Dr. Allondry's. He took off the bandages, and I got to see for the first time what I'm going to look like from now on. It wasn't pretty. OK, yes, fully clothed with a stiff padded bra with a sock or something in the cut away area, no one would know what has happened, but bikinis are certainly going to take a lot more bravado than in the past. Or maybe swimsuits will just be eliminated from my wardrobe altogether. Uff da, and Latin dance costumes.

Without getting too personal on the details, Dr. Thatcher basically removed the right half of my breast, and the way implants work is that they're placed underneath the current breast. So even though the implant basically fills out the bra cup size, there's still this weird missing space for the right half of my breast, which makes everything sort of . . . point right, for lack of a more detailed description. Of course, it's especially gruesome right now with stitches in three places and all the bruising in addition to the misshapen form.

I let my mom see (she is an RN, after all), and the look on her face was clear confirmation that this is not a pretty sight nor one that will probably get much better. She had that kind of skeptical look on her face before she asked to see—it was that look you get from your mom when she thinks you're faking being sick to get out of going to your brother's basketball game or something. But when she saw the damage, hers was definitely a look of "Oh, dear" and sympathy.

What bugs me now is a part of the conversation with Dr. Allondry today, after I asked him if this is what it's always going to look like. He said something about how some people opt to have more breast tissue removed from across the entire breast so that when the implant is put in it can have a more natural shape, and he asked me if Dr. Thatcher had mentioned that as an option to me. Dr. Thatcher is my cancer surgeon, and his focus of course has been on diagnosing and defining the extent of the cancer and getting it removed. But it bugs me. Surely Dr. Thatcher has done many lumpectomies before, and surely he knows that it turns out misshapen like this. And surely he knows that by removing a little more of the breast tissue across the entire thing they can allow a more natural looking final result. Why didn't he talk about any of that with me? And how the heck did I miss THIS little detail in all my Internet research?

I know that Dr. Thatcher's singular concern was removing the cancer, making sure that there isn't any more cancer, and making sure we treat it aggressively and completely. And I agree with everyone out there who's wondering why the hell I'm whining about this when I should just be thankful that the cancer was successfully removed with a clean margin, that they got the second tumor out completely (even if it turns out to be benign), and that they were able to remove the sentinel lymph node and only one or two additional rather than removing *all* my lymph nodes and possibly causing irreparable damage to my right arm and circulation. It's true, all of that is vitally important, and this thing about being deformed after the fact is a small price to pay for saving my life.

But still, if the doctors know that this happens, and they know how to prevent it or make it less of an issue, why wouldn't they have talked about it with me as part of the whole process? I thought I had done some good research and asked a lot of good questions of all the doctors, but I obviously completely missed this one. Dr. Allondry said today that the long-term answer is that if the cancer is really gone, and after months of chemo and radiation I still really hate this misshapen thing next year, I can elect for more plastic surgery to possibly make it more normal looking.

Ach, well, I was pretty upset about it this afternoon, but I seem to be calming down on the whole thing now. After all, it could be worse. It could always be worse, and I can remind myself of that often when I get too down on any one part of my situation or treatment/recovery.

In general, I've been feeling somewhat better each day since surgery—less foggy in the head too. The pain stays around a five almost all the time now, so I actually think my parents are going to let me go to (or take me to) the milonga in Sacramento tomorrow night. I will probably only dance with Marco, but it would be so neat to go even just for that tiny bit of dancing with my old partner. Also, I had promised my students *months* ago that I would take them out to this particular milonga as a congrats for all of their hard work in class as well as their work and practice for the show last weekend. I made this promise to them before we even knew that I had cancer, but at my last night of classes before surgery, I told them that I was still planning to attend this milonga, even if my parents had to come along to babysit me. I hope that some of my students still show up—it would be so nice to see them social dancing after having taken my classes all year.

On the other hand, selfishly, I really want to go to this milonga because I know I'll be leaving for Nebraska soon, and there won't be any Argentine Tango in my life for a long time out there, so I really want to absorb as much of it as I can before I leave for chemo.

Chapter 4.
Mixed Emotions

CANCER—DAY 21 FRIDAY, MAY 15, 2009

It's nice to be home in the forest a few nights, away from the craziness, in my secluded little house surrounded by hundreds of pine trees, peace, and serenity. But even here my mind ponders the challenges ahead.

A more personal concern I've been having is that, happy as I am to see Marco when I do, I'm getting more and more sad about the poor likelihood of us actually having a relationship because of me going to Nebraska for chemo. Sure, he cares about me a lot right now, but it also seems I am not much of a consideration in his thought process to do what he wants, with whom he wants, when he wants. I always feel like I go overboard the other way, putting a guy's feelings ahead of my own interests too much of the time and giving up my personality for them. Maybe that's something I'm supposed to learn from Marco, to try to keep my own life, my own personality, even when I have a boyfriend. Of course, with my current situation, I don't expect to have a lot of energy to invest in personal growth goals. Enter boyfriend, exit Cynthia's life at home in the forest.

This thing with Marco is a little weird—I go from one extreme to the other, from thinking that he loves me to thinking that he doesn't care about me at all. Is this just me being cancer-emotional, or is it that I am letting my imagination getting the best of me when it seems he cares deeply about me? And why even think about it? I'm leaving in a matter of weeks, my parents are here now, and I'll be gone who knows how many months while his life continues as usual. Surely he'll find a new girlfriend, probably a new dance partner, too, and forget all about me. Because really, there's nothing so great about me that anyone should entirely give up dating to wait for me to return months later when it's only been a short time together to begin with. Heck, there's no reason for him to be faithful to me now, even though I haven't left yet.

He said something like "we'll see" when I made some comment about our relationship not long ago. I paused, uncertain. I wasn't sure he really said what I thought I heard. He repeats himself: "I *said*, we'll see how it goes." Wow, *that* didn't feel good. But what can you expect of a brief new relationship? Eternal commitment? I wonder if this is what a military person goes through emotionally after getting orders to go overseas. Will our relationship still be alive when I return? That is, of course, assuming I survive to return. That's what I would think about, if I were leaving a relationship by going off to war.

Not that long ago, before diagnosis, I thought that I was all independent and happy with my single life and that I was all wrong for

Marco because he seemed to so desperately want to fall in love with someone he could be with forever (which I just didn't ever worry about), and now it's like our roles have reversed.

Marco has a rule to *not* say "I love you" before he's spent six months with someone. I think I see it in his eyes all the time, but that does me zero good when I'm away from him like this at my own home in the forest. And in Nebraska? Forget it, Cynthia. Let it go now, get your life in order to leave for unknown months of time, and forget about trying to work this guy into your life. You have no life now, you're going home to live like a teenager again with no freedoms and no place for a boyfriend. Let him go. Let him have a life. Don't drag him into the mess your life has become and may be for the next year.

Think about something else, Cynthia.

CANCER—DAY 22 SATURDAY, MAY 16, 2009

WOW! I can't believe how many people responded to the e-mail I sent to let them know about my surgery. Nearly 90 people wrote to me at my home e-mail account, and that's not even counting any of the SacTango community or work people who have been wishing me well throughout all of this as well. Amazing! I don't actually know how many people I sent that surgery e-mail to—I think it was maybe 20% of my Outlook Contacts. I just looked on my blackberry, and there are 1,546 contacts in my address book. Holy cow. I didn't know I knew that many people! I have a lot of voicemails, too. Gosh, a lot of people have really been sending me a lot of good thoughts and intentions this week.

I don't know when I'll catch up on all this e-mail. Today has been my most alert day since surgery so far (least nap time), but still, I've been in bed five of the six hours I've been awake. I was up chatting with Mom & Dad a little. We made plans for dinner and for them to take me to the milonga for a little while tonight, and after making dinner reservations and getting the addresses into my GPS, I was pretty tired! So now I'm ready for another nap.

I'm planning on working Monday; we'll see how that goes. My head has been less foggy each day, so maybe by Monday I'll be able to stay awake and think. Wouldn't that be nice!

On Monday we also have the post-surgery follow-up appointment with my surgeon, Dr. Thatcher. He's planning to take out the stitches from my last not-so-smooth, couldn't-stop-the-bleeding, leave-her-with-a-nasty-hematoma bruising biopsy, but I don't know if he'll remove any of the surgery stitches just yet. Mom and I were a little concerned about the stitches over one of the lymph node incisions . . . it doesn't look very secure (the skin puckers out funny compared to any of the other stitches) and it's really, really red. But it's not bleeding and doesn't look any worse today than last night, so we'll probably leave it for Dr. Thatcher to check out on Monday.

I don't see the medical oncologist, Dr. Sloe, until May 27, which seems *foreverably* (like my new word?) far away at this point, since finding out my chemo schedule will basically determine what my life will be like for the next six months. That's the current frustration. It bothers me, not being able to determine how much I'm going to be able to work when I *do* know for a fact that I'll start chemo two or three weeks from now. I hate to suddenly disappear and leave my company in an unanticipated lurch. On the other hand, I want to take as much time as possible to focus on the treatments and healing, rather than stressing about the typical work issues of rerunning reports because so-and-so gave us bad data, or chasing down signatures, or writing agreements for new companies I don't have time to manage.

Now that the surgery is over, I should be focused first on healing and recovery. But just because I'm sick doesn't mean the company won't still have deadlines. We just don't know what I'll be able to do and what I need to train other people to do until I meet with the medical oncologist and find out about the chemotherapy plan.

Ah, look, I've come full circle, back to the original frustration—that it's going to be ten days before I even *meet* the medical oncologist. Full circle on the thought process . . . that means it's time to stop complaining, right?

CANCER—DAY 23 SUNDAY, MAY 17, 2009

That was a strange dance experience. I guess in hindsight I should have just stayed home and kept resting, but sheesh, I've been cooped up for days—and getting better every day—and even my parents thought it was OK for me to go (but they wouldn't't let me drive). The best I can figure about what felt so strange is that maybe Marco didn't think I should be up and trying to dance yet, and that really affected his dancing with me. I was nervous to lift my right hand to his to dance, that's true, and I didn't trust my feet or balance (heck, that bit of time at the milonga last night was the longest stretch of time I've been upright on my feet since a week ago). Maybe all of that was why I felt so disconnected from him. After the first song that we danced, Marco asked why I was shaking. I *was* shaky, unsure of my feet, and during the second song of the tanda—when I did finally start feeling it a little and dancing a bit to the music—I threw him off and then I felt bad for getting in the way of his lead by feeling the music. I was disappointed in myself. By the third song, all he did was walk, waiting for the tanda to end. After all the hours practicing with Marco for the show and having it become easier and easier to slide into that tango shared-energy nirvana with him almost every dance, then to have that suddenly so far from comprehension last night made me feel bad, like I'd really let both of us down. Maybe I can blame it on the painkillers. Listen to your parents, kids, Tango and drugs don't mix!

I didn't sleep much last night. I was lost in thought, which is usually why I don't sleep . . . sometimes I just can't stop the mental wheels from churning. I think I have my mind all wound down and then more thoughts get in the way. Now that surgery is over, I keep getting stuck in this frustration of not knowing how intense or how long chemo will be—whether I'll be able to work no-problem, or with difficulty, or not at all—and how to shut down my life here for an as-yet-indeterminate length of time . . . a time which we don't even have the start date for, though it's supposedly in the next 2–3 weeks. I've already found someone to substitute teach my dance classes, so that's taken care of, but there's still all the GSCMA (Global Supply Chain Management Association) stuff: being on the advisory committee, running my programs team, being president of the board for this new roundtable in Sacramento that still has a lot to learn. I'm supposed to be in meetings and speaking at a GSCMA seminar in Chicago on June 6–7, and I don't even know if I can go because I don't know when chemo will start.

When it does start, how incapacitated will I be? Will I be able to see Marco for his birthday on July 1? And dance? I haven't done West Coast Swing, Ballroom, or Latin in weeks anyway, and soon, no more tango either. And when I come back, will I still have my tango partner? Will I be physically strong enough to do shows again, or teach again? While I'm gone, what happens to my relationship with Marco, my friendships, all the people I've gotten to know and care about out here in California? If chemo were only three months long, well, I don't think that would be a big deal at all—three months go by before you know it. But six months? Nine? And radiation treatment after that, every day for 6-1/2 weeks. I could be back before the GSCMA conference in October, and this could all be over by Thanksgiving, or I might not be through with chemo and radiation treatments until Easter of next year. The range and number of unknowns really frustrates the analytical me.

What I've realized this morning is that I'm clinging. I'm clinging to my life out here in California. I'm clinging to Marco and all the things that make my life what it is here. The only thing I don't have to worry about leaving is teaching at the university, as the academic calendar recently changed and they're not offering my Business Intelligence graduate course again until January (I think). I should be able to do that. At the very least, it's not something worth worrying about now.

Everything else has to be decided, and soon, but I don't want to cancel the June Forum presentation, I don't want to step down from my board position with GSCMA or turn over my programs team to someone else, I don't want to quit the advisory committee, I don't want to pack up weeks and weeks worth of clothes to let Mom & Dad take to their house for me, I don't want to close up my house or take down my hammock or pack up the cats . . . I don't even want to make any decisions about whether I should drive or fly out to Mom & Dad's house when I have to go, and whether I should go alone or ask Marco or someone to travel with me, like Mom wants me to. My parents just moved to Sidney, Nebraska a few years ago, to live closer to my brother's family (they have three little kids) in the Black Hills (close but not too close, from a grandparent's perspective, I think). Not knowing anyone out there and the town not having a dance community means I'll be in chemo with nothing to do and no social life if I have good chemo recovery days when I should really get out and do something rather than sit around just being Chemo Girl.

What if the medical oncologist tells me on May 27 that I only have to have chemo once every three weeks and it's only going to slow me down for a day or so when I have a treatment? Shutting down my life here and going to Nebraska for that really seems like overkill, but it seems as though waiting until May 27 to make these decisions is silly, too. For someone who's always been the get-things-done person, I certainly don't seem like myself right now. It's unusual for me to be so indecisive.

But I also know that staying here in California for chemo would be hard on my family because they are worried about how difficult chemo will be, and it means so much to them to have me close and be with me when I'm in chemo. Who am I to deny them that with some selfish desire to maintain the façade of my normal and far-away independent life? So I have to go be with them for this thing, and it's about time I stop trying to postpone the inevitable and just go ahead and step away from all these other things. Hopefully the new life I can start after all of this will be greater than anything I could have achieved or contributed if I stayed here instead for treatment.

I had a long online chat with Marco tonight, and at the end of it I felt so much better—we had gone up a notch in understanding each other better, and he said he realized how tenacious I am (in general, sure, but specifically about not giving up easily on him is what he was so impressed with in me) and why I am tenacious about that (because I appreciate and respect him). Apparently, this made him realize that he's probably underestimated me, and he seems to have realized that he shouldn't think of his relationship with me as a superficial passing fancy. There's more to us than that. Who knows what will happen with chemo and all, but at least we'll keep learning more about each other and enjoying each other in the meantime. There's a possible future for the relationship, and it seems a positive one.

CANCER—DAY 24 MONDAY, MAY 18, 2009

Good news!!! The sentinel lymph node and adjacent lymph node biopsies were both negative for metastic tumors!!

I'm hoping this means a less tortuous chemo program, but I won't know what the chemo schedule will be like until at least May 27 when I see the medical oncologist, Dr. Sloe.

As for the surgery, they completely excised the invasive ductal carcinoma tumor, which was just barely a stage 3 cancer based on the size of the tumor. They also took out that area of questionable tissue and tested it after surgery. The second tumor did turn out to be another invasive ductal carcinoma, but smaller. So they completely removed two tumors—one classified as stage 3 and one classified as stage 2. No lymph nodes were involved, and *that* is fantastic news.

But Dr. Thatcher kept harping on the point that cancer is more aggressive in young women, stage for stage. He did say there was a slight possibility that the medical oncologist may not require chemo, but I got the impression from Dr. Thatcher that he would insist on a second opinion that *did* require chemo, if Dr. Sloe doesn't treat me with it. Dr. Thatcher is adamant that we do everything possible now to prevent a recurrence. He told me once that studies show that they basically have one really strong chance at bat when a cancer is first discovered, so with young women especially, they do everything possible to hit the ball out of the park on that first up at bat. Dr. Thatcher is definitely more of a baseball fan than I am, but at least I understood his analogy, right?

Altogether, it was the best possible news we could have received today. The cancer has been completely excised and was removed before it metastasized to other parts of my body. Technically, at this moment, I am cancer-free!

CANCER—DAY 25 TUESDAY, MAY 19, 2009

Aside from being ridiculously busy, today was kind of like a normal day. I started work at 5 a.m. (most of my clients are on the East Coast, so starting work really early works well for them, besides allowing me greater flexibility with the evening hours). I barely wrapped up by 3 p.m. in order to spend a brief hour with my parents before leaving for the two-hour drive to Sacramento for my GSCMA board meeting. Then I got out of that around 8 p.m., had another short meeting with one of the board members after that, and finally headed out of the city a little before 10 p.m. to get home a little before midnight. And that, ladies and gentlemen, is a fairly normal work day for me, with the exception of taking an hour break and visiting with my parents a little. I don't have meetings down in the capital every day, thankfully—our GSCMA board meeting is in-person only once a month or so. Usually if I'm driving in to Sac, it's for tango (for future reference, locals often abbreviate Sacramento to Sac or Sacto).

One frustrating thing since surgery, or maybe since diagnosis . . . I don't feel I'm nearly as efficient as I used to be, work-wise. I don't specifically think about cancer stuff all the time, but I suspect it's pretty close to the surface of my subconscious most of the time, generally raising my stress level higher than it needs to be for whatever I'm working on.

Then again, a week ago right now I was nearly incoherent with pain from the surgery. So to be back at my desk all day, driving in to Sacramento by myself, and running a board meeting pretty much like usual, well, dang, that's pretty amazing. What a strange illness. I wonder what chemo will be like, in terms of effect on my work, ability to think, and so on? I'm sure I'll be wiped out for at least some period of time after each chemo treatment. I'm also not sure about how this *not* taking my heart medication is going to fly. Ah, still so many unknowns with chemo. I'm apparently still wondering about that a lot even when I think I'm working or thinking about something else!

CANCER—DAY 26 WEDNESDAY, MAY 20, 2009

WhooHoo! Going to Cell Block in San Francisco with Marco to tango tonight! It's one of the neatest places for NeoTango or Tango Nuevo. Cell Block is something of a warehouse sort of space with cement floors and an artist's loft kind of vibe that's perfect for Tango Nuevo, which is kind of a clubby, showy sort of tango with unusual movements and balances in addition to the strict traditional tango. Apparently, no one except Marco and my parents can tell from looking at me that I'm ill or in pain (everyone at the board meeting Tuesday night, and also my surgeon on Monday, kept commenting that I look great . . . gotta love what a little makeup and a big fake smile can hide, eh?). I'll have to be careful who I dance with—I'll tell them to take it easy on my right arm and watch out for how tightly they embrace me, but I am still sooooo excited to be going to Cell Block again. I don't think I've been out there even once since the cancer diagnosis. Then again, we only found out about the cancer 26 days ago, so it hasn't really been that long since I went to Cell Block, but honestly, it seems like the last four weeks or so of my life have actually contained several months worth of experiences and emotions, you know?

CANCER—DAY 27 THURSDAY, MAY 21, 2009

Mother Nature must be having a bad hair day, or maybe she and Father Time had an argument, but whoa! My parents called from Laramie, Wyoming (on their drive home) to tell me that they just saw a semi blown over at the side of the road and that they've been driving through high winds and hailstorms, and now tornadoes! They were hiding out with a bunch of other folks in the ballroom of a Holiday Inn where the power was off. Apparently it's a mess out there tonight! Mom called again later to tell me that they now have a full blanket of snow covering the ground. Sheesh, doesn't Wyoming know it's the end of May and there shouldn't be any more snow? Do I sound like a Californian or what?

I'm definitely having some pain today, but I also managed to get through the entire day on normal Extra Strength Tylenol, instead of the prescription Tylenol No. 3 with codeine in it. So while the pain still feels at about 5–6 today, I know it's getting better because I didn't have to take as many pain killers. Last night I was getting sick to my stomach from all the pain medicine that I took without enough food. I have gotten pretty good about keeping little snacks in my messenger bag—trail mix or balance bars or something—but last night I had forgotten them, so I had to take pain pills on an empty stomach.

Wow, tomorrow's Friday. Where has the time gone?

CANCER—DAY 28 FRIDAY, MAY 22, 2009

I lost it on my MIT guy a little bit yesterday because, even though it's been four weeks, he's not responded with something that should have taken him an hour to do. Now I'm in this ridiculous, massively past-due time crunch on a report to all the clients. I told him that I may be out for 3–6 months starting on June 9, and that this has to go out next week even if I have to incorrectly tell the clients that he's going to do all the analyses I have spec'd out (which is of course impossible). I copied his boss on the message, our VP, and he flipped out about the 3–6 months thing, which of course I'd told him on the phone just yesterday but he apparently didn't hear clearly. My employer doesn't seem to understand how severely this may impact my ability to work, possibly to the point of complete disability in the short term.

I've been too optimistic with my co-workers about the prognosis and how well I could be during chemo, because I didn't want to let them down or worry them. And in the meantime I've been preparing the area I manage so that they will be able to execute the work in my complete absence, should that be the case. Now I'm concerned, and trying to figure out how to get my company in the mindset of not expecting very much of me over the next several months—they seem to think that me having said a month ago, "You'd think I'd be able to work part-time during chemo," means that I'm going to work just as hard and just as effectively during chemo as I did before I was diagnosed. It almost feels like, because they're also all old friends and colleagues of mine, that my co-workers are in a kind of denial that I'm going through this thing at all.

I was talking about it with Marco, and his response was that companies always want more than is realistic. Not completely untrue, I mused. I said, "Sure, and historically that has worked really well for any company I worked for, since I'll push myself beyond the limit to deliver on an excessive expectation, if I committed myself to doing it. But I can't do that anymore." Marco's next point was a big "duh" moment for me. He said, "True. Have you explained that?" Apparently not, eh?

CANCER—DAY 29 SATURDAY, MAY 23, 2009

Last night I went to a wine club party with Marco. He's been in this wine club for a year or so, I think. Once a month, they get together and everyone brings a bottle of wine. They have this tasting party, like the one last night. It was often uncomfortable for me because Marco would leave me alone to go talk to his friends, or to take pictures, and I didn't want to follow him everywhere to be introduced and impede his conversations. Interestingly, most of the people I met and talked to were also on the fringe of the group, a past roommate of the hostess, a woman from Germany here for two weeks visiting her friend who's in the wine club, that sort of thing. Apparently all the people who knew each other in the wine club were talking to each other so that the people who didn't know anyone met the other people who didn't know anyone—funny how that works. Making small talk with so many strangers feels like I'm at work or a GSCMA function doing business networking. I never know what to talk to people about. It seems like the only thing I can think to ask them about is their work, and yet I don't like talking about *my* work in a social setting. Catch 22, eh?

Eventually, there was music and some freestyle dancing though, and then I had a really good time. Later I commented to Marco that I could see why he was concerned about me going to Nebraska and not dancing. It was so great just to randomly freestyle with a bunch of people last night. I can't really imagine not dancing for months. Then again, if chemo is bad, I won't feel like dancing anyway, right?

CANCER—DAY 30 SUNDAY, MAY 24, 2009

Judging from my recent activities, you could almost look at me from the outside and not believe there's anything wrong with me. Not so by 3 a.m. this morning, though. I had gone to a barbeque in Sacramento, and then last night Marco, Rachelle, and I went to an all-night milonga in Berkeley. Don't ask me why I went to an all-night milonga so soon after surgery. By 3 a.m., the pain in my breast and underarm had risen to an 8, and I was nauseated from the pain. Unbelievable. The pain was not just from dancing, though. I didn't take enough pain medication with me and just taking more when I got home around 7 a.m. didn't seem to help. It took forever to get it under control again and my whole day has been a mess of trying to catch up the pain medication with the pain . . . the pain was finally reduced to something tolerable sometime this evening, 16-18 hours later. Insane.

CANCER—DAY 31 MONDAY, MAY 25, 2009

Now this is annoying—I definitely have a cold. Since Wednesday, I've been feeling dehydrated and tired, and yesterday I started to cough, and now today Marco and I are both in full-fledged, want-to-stay-in-bed-all-day sick mode. Thankfully, it's Memorial Day, and my company has a holiday today. So I did sleep in, and, after a couple of errands with Marco, I laid down again and tried to rest a little before going to a tango barbeque party that Marco committed us to. Man, Sacto is a busy place!

After 30 minutes of trying to get my energy up to go to the barbeque, I decided it wouldn't be good for my health to go, so I stayed in bed. Marco refused to go to the barbecue without me, saying that he's sick too. He does have a nasty cough. He and Randy played some computer games—very low key evening.

My stress level has been rising a little today, and now tonight I'm really noticing it. The medical oncologist appointment is tomorrow. This is the guy (Dr. Sloe) who is going to determine what my chemotherapy will be. But I have no idea what the appointment tomorrow will be like. I tried to ask Dr. Thatcher if this guy Dr. Sloe would already have my chemo plan prepared when I came in, but he said, "Probably not." Turns out the guy didn't even have my chart from Dr. Thatcher at that point, but I imagine he'll have that by tomorrow.

Ach. If I'm this wiped out by a little cold now, what is chemo going to do to me?

Chapter 5.
Chemo Options

CANCER—DAY 32 TUESDAY, MAY 26, 2009

Well, that was an interesting appointment. I didn't really think I was going to have chemo options, but there are actually several different regimen options. The medical oncologist was not as personable as the radiologic oncologist, but certainly knowledgeable about the standard chemotherapy regimen. He had my chart, and he was scanning it as he walked in and during the beginning of the appointment. He was a little pressed for time, I think, which made it a bit difficult to interact with him because he didn't explain anything in any kind of detail unless I asked elaborating questions, and it's hard to do that while you're taking notes and trying to absorb what someone just said when it's such foreign material as this. But, here's what we know now . . .

The fact that my cancer may be hormone-receptor positive is both a good thing and a bad thing. It means that hormone therapy can help, but also that the cancer can be dormant a very long time and yet still recur, even 20–30 years later. This oncologist said that my probability of recurrence is about 20 percent right now, after having had surgery. I believe he meant that as a 20 percent probability within the next five years, rather than over the course of my entire lifetime, because he also made a point of telling me that "recurrence will happen," even if it's not for twenty years, and that I will have to be on the lookout for this constantly, for as long as I live. OK, I can deal with that. I'd already figured that out on my own actually. After a cancer diagnosis, regardless of your age, surely the vigilance to catch any recurrence earlier rather than later becomes a lifetime commitment.

So anyway, the reason for chemotherapy is to reduce the probability of an acute recurrence, meaning "a cancer recurrence within five years of the original cancer." An unfortunate side effect of chemotherapy on a hormone-receptive cancer is that it damages the ovaries so they won't produce enough estrogen, which unfortunately is important for bone density, blood pressure, and cholesterol. Oh, and the damage would probably also lead to early menopause, so we had to have an entire conversation about whether I'm married, have kids, plan to have kids, and all that. I already had all those conversations with my cardiologist several years ago because he doesn't think bearing children would be wise given my heart condition. I don't really care, though. I was adopted, and I've never had a problem with the idea of adopting kids if some day I wanted them but couldn't bear children. The part about the ovaries doesn't bother me too much, though I do not like what I've heard about what menopause does to your body. I guess that's just another "oh well" in the process. It is what it is. Another thing about this cancer is that it's likely to recur in the ovaries, and we talked about possibly having my ovaries removed in the future. Who knows—that's so far down the road at this point. But still, better to know it's out there than get blindsided a year from now.

Going through chemotherapy reduces the five–year recurrence risk by about five or six percent, he said. After that, there's another drug therapy called Tamoxifen, which reduces the risk further, as does radiation treatment. So, my ultimate recurrence risk five years out after doing everything possible, is about 10 percent lower than if we did no further treatment at all after the surgery. Longer term, they're not so sure about recurrence probability, or else he's just not telling me all the details about that yet. (I wonder, are doctors required by some kind of oath *not* to tell a patient certain bad information unless the patient knows what questions to ask?)

You know, 10 percent doesn't sound like a high probability of recurrence until you think about lining up ten women you know and saying, OK, we're going to lose one of them. All of a sudden, 10 percent sounds like a lot. And 20 percent, well, let's just not bother focusing on the 20-percent possibility; we're definitely going to go the chemo route and do everything the doctors recommend to reduce the risk of recurrence as much as possible.

My heart condition is a serious concern. Dr. Sloe ordered another special heart test, which they're doing before chemo, in the middle of chemo, and again after chemo. I have to read up on this one more; it's called a MUGA, and I have to go to a nuclear medicine facility to have it done. That appointment is scheduled for Friday.

Before chemo starts, I'll go back to my surgeon (Dr. Thatcher) to have a receptor port put in before I start chemo treatments. They usually refer to it as a port-a-cath, which I was confused by at first since what I heard was "portacath" and I couldn't find any information about what that was. The port is a little receptacle thing they put just under my collarbone and then use to inject the chemotherapy drugs into, instead of sticking me with IV needles every time I go for chemo. Inside my body, the port is connected to a catheter that goes through a vein and into my heart. This way, you don't have the risk of someone missing a vein or having to have a new catheter put in your arm for every chemo session. Have I mentioned that I hate needles? I usually become faint whenever they draw blood.

During the appointment today, Dr. Sloe explained my chemotherapy options to me. Basically, there are three "generations" of chemotherapy, each greater in intensity.

First-generation chemo is 12 weeks of two drugs administered in three-week cycles. This is the most mild chemo treatment, and he doesn't recommend this for me because cancer is more aggressive in young women. That's all that he said about that, he didn't say anything specific about breast cancer. It seems that, at this point, what kind of cancer we're dealing with doesn't matter much.

Second-generation chemo starts with the same 12 weeks of two drugs administered in three-week cycles, like the first generation chemo. Then second-generation also includes an additional 12 weeks of one more drug, also administered in three-week cycles.

Third-generation chemo includes all three drugs at one time, administered every two weeks. It's much higher risk in terms of infection and how debilitating it is, but it's over with in 16 weeks as opposed to 24 weeks.

Dr. Sloe recommended either second or third generation chemo for me. He wants me to have all three chemo drugs. He told me that during chemo, I will basically go through a cycle of being sick from the drugs in the first week, and exhausted with fatigue the second week. If I do the second-generation chemo, I'll have a third week of recovery during each cycle and I may be somewhere from 50 to 75 percent of my usual strength but generally able to have a normal-ish life during that third week. With third generation chemo, the most aggressive regimen, there is no third week for recovery time between chemo rounds, and they say people get weaker and weaker throughout the treatment because there's no real recovery time.

Still, the idea of spending six months at Mom & Dad's with no semblance of my own life is rather depressing. Four months, even if it's four months of feeling like death, actually sounds better to me than six months of being away and feeling tolerably well. Six months just seems too long to abandon my life. I wouldn't be back until my birthday in December! This information is a lot to get your head around, especially when you have a cold.

The creepiest part of being at the oncologist's office was when they had me wait in the treatment room until they could draw my blood for the CBC. There were eight or so patients getting chemotherapy. A couple were chatting at the far end, while the others read magazines and such, with their little IV bags hanging up above, and all looking scary pale and worn. I was the youngest person in the room by at least 30 years, if not more, and for some reason, this scene really creeped me out. I couldn't wait to get out of there.

I've been doing more research on medical oncology and breast cancer treatment, and I'm going to see another medical oncologist in addition to Dr. Sloe. This other oncologist is down in Sacramento, and he's a breast cancer specialist at the Marshall Cancer Center. (Dr. Sloe is in Cameron Park, halfway between Sac and Placerville, which is considered close to my home in the forest, but not inside the 45-minute winding mountain road part of my drive.) The appointment with the second medical oncologist will be basically a second-opinion sort of consult, and I don't really expect to hear anything significantly different, but I think it will be good to meet with a breast cancer specialist about my treatment and/or any other different or additional treatment options and medical trials specific to breast cancer. Dr. Sloe didn't know of any medical trials going on for breast cancer, but I keep reading that there are always some going on, so I want to know if I am eligible for any. I like the idea of contributing to medical science that way, especially if it helps them find a way to stop breast cancer.

I'm not so sure about this medical oncologist, Dr. Sloe. Sure, he's an oncologist and knows about the various standard chemo options and he's geographically as close to my home as possible, even though it's still an hour and a half to get there. But I don't get a good vibe from him. He doesn't know anything about clinical trials for breast cancer, and he seemed vague in response to questions I asked that were specific to breast cancer as opposed to cancer in general. I told him I was expecting to live in Nebraska for my chemo treatment so we would need to coordinate his instructions with a chemo facility there and any appointments I would have had with Dr. Sloe would have to be with someone in Nebraska that will have to act as a go-between. He's didn't have any reservations about that—he thinks it's just fine—which actually makes me a little more nervous about him since none of my other doctors think leaving for chemo is a particularly good idea, though of course where I go for treatment is ultimately up to me to decide.

CANCER—DAY 33 WEDNESDAY, MAY 27, 2009

All the medical people keep asking if I have a family history of breast cancer when they find out how young I am. When I tell them I'm adopted and don't have a family medical history, they invariably say "That's not good. Can you get your family medical history?" I've never cared about finding my birth parents for multiple reasons, but that story will have to wait for another day. Today's story is about the administrative ordeal, trying to get the biological family history to know if I have a genetic history of cancer.

I asked my parents if they could do a little digging to find out if we can get my biological medical history. I have to agree with the medical people that knowing whether or not there is a biological history of cancer (especially breast cancer of course) would be useful. I don't need to know who my biological parents are or meet them or anything, but I thought maybe we could get some kind of medical history from the adoption agency. Unfortunately, the adoption agency that handled all my foster home placements and my eventual adoption by my parents is closed, gone.

With a few phone calls (being a retired hospital CEO does have its advantages), Dad located adoption services for the county in Wisconsin where I was born, and he called them to see if it's possible to get my medical history from an adoption agency that has closed. They called him back and told him that, unless I was incapacitated, they would need me to be the one seeking the information, so I left them a voicemail the next day.

Yesterday a woman called me back from the department of health and family services in Wisconsin, and apparently I have to fill out an adoption search application in order for them to search for my medical info. She told me that they have to send it in the mail. I explained to her the urgency of this, with the cancer treatment implications and all, and she agreed to fax the eight pages of paperwork to me. So, last night I filled it all out, thinking I'd get it sent off today on the drive between home and Sac. No problem, no big deal, right?

Well, getting it sent off proved to be much more hassle than I'd allowed time for. My signature on the application has to be notarized, so of course I went to the bank (where the adoption search people said there are notary services), but they would only notarize documents for use within their own bank.

So now I need to search for a notary, which I can do on my GPS, but I've also now remembered that in order to get an updated (meaning, everything from when I was adopted until now) family medical history, I have to "Attach physician's letter with application." That's all it says on the form. It doesn't say what has to be in the letter, just that there has to be one. I imagined this would take some time, so instead of looking for a notary, I drove to my doctor's office, Dr. Carmina, who is my general practitioner and the gynecologist who found my breast lump. She doesn't have the best staff in the world, but eventually I got them to listen long enough to understand what I needed. Of course there was no telling when Dr. Carmina would have time to do it, and her staff certainly wasn't making it a priority. She's out tomorrow, so they think I should just come back to pick up the letter on Friday. I explained the urgency of the adoption search for my medical history, and I told the staff that I would stop by later in the hope that they were able to get it taken care of. Sometimes knowing when a person is returning for something will get people to get that something done sooner rather than later, so I told them what time I would be back.

I went back out to the Jeep to use the GPS and find a notary. Turns out, there's *one* notary in all of Placerville, at a lawyer's office, and it's right where I just was: at my bank. So I drove back across town to find this notary office, which was tucked away out of sight around the back corner of a building so I walked all the way around the building before happening upon the right door. I went in, and there was a young guy with full-arm tattoos on both arms, in a T-shirt and shorts, talking with a guy who was trying to get his girlfriend out of jail. (Doesn't that sound like a fun way to spend a Wednesday afternoon?)

It took maybe half an hour to fill out all the forms and stuff, while making small talk with the notary guy. He especially scrutinized my driver's license and the long blonde hair in the photo . . . "When did you get your hair cut short?" he asks. I had decided to go short in anticipation of chemo, since I'll have short hair for a long time after chemo. I answered him, "Oh, gosh, just about three weeks ago, I think." Then he said "You wear it well." I look at him a bit quizzically, so he explains. "Most people going from long hair to a short cut are always fussing with it and looking uncomfortable." OK, well, like I said, we were making small talk. Then he noticed the motorcycle classification on my license, and we got into a long conversation about race bikes. Oh, did I mention that there's a big, dirty, friendly, bored yellow Labrador retriever looking for attention in there? Quite the law office, eh? Small towns—gotta love 'em.

OK, so now I'm in the law office's parking lot thinking about this doctor's note thing, knowing that Carmina's staff is *not* going to get that taken care of in any kind of timely manner. Then *duh*—it occurs to me to try Dr. Thatcher (my surgeon), whose office is three doors down from Carmina in the same building. Surely, the adoption search people will accept a letter from my surgeon instead of my primary care physician. It's not like they said what *kind* of doctor they want this letter from. So I pulled out my cell phone and called Dr. Thatcher's office and talked to Remé, his assistant and office manager. Remé and I are good buddies now; she's seen a lot of me with all of these appointments, and we have a good relationship. Remé tells me that Dr. Thatcher is in surgery this afternoon, but available in Folsom tomorrow. Did I need to schedule an appointment? I explain the whole thing to her, and she tells me, "Oh I can do that! Do you think they'll accept a letter with his stamped signature?" In the interest of avoiding further delay, I decided we should just send it with a stamped signature and see what happens. Surely it won't be *that* big of a deal. So I drive back across town again, to Dr. Thatcher's office.

Remé had already typed up this great letter and put Dr. Thatcher's signature on it:

"To Whom It May Concern: This letter is to inform you that CYNTHIA SWAN has been under my care. She has a recent diagnosis of breast cancer. In order to provide the best treatment for her, a family medical history is being requested. If you have any questions please contact our office."

Wow, it even sounded like how he would say it. That girl is really something. Oh, and this is neat, because Dr. Thatcher was out for surgery Remé had her daughter in the office with her. I got to hear all about the purple fairies in the garden and in her room. Too cute!

So, with multiple copies of my letter from Dr. Thatcher in hand, I walked back over to Carmina's office and of course her staff hadn't even told her that I need this letter written yet. I gave them a copy of the letter to put in my patient file, and walked out.

Amazing what can be done in a more expedited fashion when the patient is seriously engaged in her care, eh? The radiation oncologist would be proud.

Chapter 6.
The Decision: Choosing My Caregiver(s)

CANCER—DAY 34 THURSDAY, MAY 28, 2009

I have a decision to make.

Actually, I have several decisions to make, but the most complicated one is where to do my chemotherapy: down in Sacramento, or out in Sidney, Nebraska. I want to let my parents take care of me, but I don't want to abandon my life in California for six months. And of course, no matter what, I can't stay at my own house out in the national forest, 45 minutes from the nearest hospital and more than an hour from any of my local friends. I like the privacy and seclusion of the property where I live, but it's not exactly convenient in this situation. I don't expect to be able to drive myself an hour or two each way to and from each chemo session.

Another big decision, if I stay out here, is what oncologist to use. I'm meeting a new one next week, so I'll have a choice of where and with whom I do my chemo if I stay in CA.

And yet another big decision is whether to do six months of second-generation chemo, where the process and side effects are more drawn out, or four months of third-generation (that being the more debilitating, immune-system damaging one). Which ties—in part—to the decision regarding *where* to do chemo. If I go to Nebraska, the 4-month option is a lot more tempting. Get it over with in four months and get back to California for some sun before the truly nasty weather kicks in out there. Who wants to be in chemo in Nebraska in November? Surely that wouldn't be good for my immune system.

Being analytical and geeky, I've been developing a mental model to categorize my options and give me a framework for logically considering the various options. Still, this is complex, and I'm stressed, worried, and uncertain.

I was a little overwhelmed after meeting with the medical oncologist on Tuesday, and so I texted Marco to see if he had time to have lunch with me. We went for soup at Panera (mindful of my cold, which of course Marco caught from me, though I kind of think I caught it from him first, but anyway, we both had soup for our colds). I told him all about everything that the medical oncologist had said, and we talked about the different treatment options, and what it would be like being in Nebraska for treatment vs. Sacramento . . . what my life there is like, versus here. Basically, I have no life there. My parents moved to Sidney long after I had moved to California, so I literally know no one out there, just my parents.

Marco offered that I could stay with him for chemo, which I wasn't really expecting and I kind of brushed past conversationally with a thank you sort of statement, but no real response. I don't think he realized at the time just what he might have been volunteering himself for, in making that offer. And I needed to mull that over in my mind, before getting him into something as complicated as caring for a cancer patient. This wouldn't be as simple as, you know, just having me "stay over" for an extended period of time. He would have to actively participate in, well, *everything*.

After lunch, we stopped at the pet store to get some crickets for Marco to feed to his tarantulas (he has three of them), and then brought them back to his house. After feeding the tarantulas (well, the smallest one anyway, the crickets were too small to interest the big spiders), I was wiped out and fell asleep on his bed while he went back to his office in the back of the house to work. I went back there later, after a short nap.

I sat down on the floor next to Marco's chair and mulled over my choices. Go home to Nebraska for four nasty months of treatment or six months of not-so-nasty treatment, or stay with him in Sacramento and do the not-so-nasty six month treatment, staying closer to my life and even getting to participate in a little bit of "normal life" when I'm feeling well enough, as opposed to being in a quiet little town where I know no one and have none of my usual activities to draw me out of the house—namely, dance—but especially Argentine Tango.

So many things to consider, such an overwhelming decision, such an overwhelming situation to begin with . . . I finally dropped my head down and cried sitting there on the floor. I have a weird way of crying, a sort of keeping-it-all-in-while-letting-tears-fall crying with tears practically gushing from my eyes, but I make no sound, I barely breathe, and my body just trembles with the intensity of the emotion. I was leaning my head against Marco's knee, pretty much like a loving dog would. Marco let one hand down to pet my head and shoulder while he worked and it was comforting. He grew silent, then motionless, and eventually I glanced up at him to find that he was watching me. I asked him, "What?" He said, "I'm worried about you." Well, yeah, me too.

I told him I was struggling with what to do because I didn't want to disappear from my own life for six months. He considered that for a moment, and gently asked why it's so hard to decide. I tried to explain, but didn't have any substantial answers until I finally took a slow deep breath, looked up at him, and said, "I don't want to leave you." Pause. "Then don't," he replied. My response made him laugh when I said, after my own pause, "That's a very high-risk proposition." But he was serious, and so was I, and now there's another real option to consider, of how I really *could* stay in California instead of leaving for chemo.

Then, randomly, as he always seems to do at just the right time, my best friend Brian texted me, and I suddenly thought it would be really good to have dinner with him and talk about this stuff even though I have this awful cold. Marco had to be at the dance studio, and lo and behold Brian wasn't out of the country so we were able to take my sick bum out for miso soup and sushi. Brian and I talked about all the chemo/cancer stuff, and he ended up telling me many, many times that he thinks I should stay with Marco for chemo, with himself as my backup, and my parents as my final backup if things don't work out here with my care. Both he and my cousin Dane have opined that my parents will come around to letting me stay out here if that's what I decide to do. And I agree with both of them that no matter what happens, Mom & Dad wouldn't turn me away if doing my chemo out here just doesn't work and I end up needing them to take care of me later. They would never turn me away if I asked for help, even if it was the help that I had previously declined.

Still, it's an enormous decision, and I'm going to have to let myself have some time to think it through over the weekend.

I also wonder, is it really right to even try to be with Marco? Think about the very worst-case scenario. What if he really falls in love with me, loves me with his whole heart, and then I go and die of cancer in a few years, leaving him in agony like I was when Artie died? I can't put someone through that. No matter what it means for me, I cannot do that to someone.

I've been weighing it out in my mind. There are several facets to my where-to-do-chemo decision, including the location of all my medical specialists and my own (rather complicated) medical history, financial concerns, my cats, my independence, maintaining my life/relationships/friends, and trusting that my caregiver(s) will place my health as the utmost priority during treatment. After all, I'm entrusting my life to someone at this point (not that I'm going to die during chemo, but still, that's how important this decision feels to me). This is no small decision. There are several reasons I'm leaning toward staying with Marco in Sacramento for my chemo. One very large reason is that I would still have access to my life, and I think this will make me work harder to recover because I'll want to go out and do at least some of the things I would normally do, at least during that third week of chemo when I'm not so ill. I'll still see my tango friends fairly regularly, and be able to go to milongas, and dance. I think giving up dance would be the hardest thing about going to Nebraska. After all, dancing is both my physical and my social outlet. My doctors don't like the idea of me giving up both of those, even if it is so my parents can care for me while I'm feeling ill from the chemo.

On the other hand, no one in the world would care for me with the complete commitment and unconditional love of my parents. Feeling loved goes a long way in carrying me through emotional stress. Actually, it was my parents' love that brought me out of a suicidal depression after Artie died. With chemo, no matter how sick I get, no matter how crabby or whiney or discouraged or even demanding I may become when sick with chemo, they will always give me 100 percent unconditional love. Knowing that has always been a kind of emotional safety net for me to get through really difficult times.

My doctors, well, all of them except Dr. Sloe whom I am not sure I trust, have reservations about me going somewhere else for chemo—somewhere they do not know the doctors or what kind of care I'll be receiving. There may be fantastic oncological care in Nebraska, but still, my doctors are here, they know me, and they know each other. Staying with Marco, it will always be easy to go to any of them at any time. Plus he lives within walking distance of Marshall Memorial Hospital—not a bad thing. I worry about what will happen if I have a neurocardiogenic syncope episode in Nebraska and they can't find the right kind of heart specialist, and instead of doing what my cardiologist would do if I were here under his care, they suddenly dump in a pacemaker or something completely unnecessary and now I'm stuck with that thing for life, too.

On the other hand, staying with my parents has the financial advantage of costing me absolutely nothing, not even for food. I would have my own nice room downstairs with my own desk and walk-in closet and lots of familiar things and my cats there with me every night. At Marco's, I don't think I would have any space entirely to myself and I imagine he'd expect me to share household expenses, maybe even rent. My cats would have to stay at my house in Volcanoville or something else because Marco is allergic, so I would only see them once a week at best, when I am well enough to drive myself home to see them. Or I would have to let someone else drive me home to visit my house and my cats and my forest. At least I would have access to all of my stuff whenever I go to see my cats. I could swap out whatever I'm in the mood for instead of being stuck with what I thought to pack in terms of clothes. I could still go for walks in my woods and enjoy some of the things I love so much about where my home is, like lying in my hammock watching my trees move and whisper with the wind, and feeling the serenity that is so special to me in my special place. In the last two years of living out there, I've learned better how to keep that serenity with me when I have to be somewhere else. Still, it's so complete when I'm there, just an all-encompassing sense of peace beyond anything I can seem to capture anywhere else.

With my parents, though, I know with absolute certainty that they will put my health and safety above all other concerns, absolutely and unequivocally. I can't say that I know this about any other living being on the planet, at least not with such complete trust. And that makes it risky to trust my life to Marco like this. Granted, he won't be completely on his own in caring for me—Brian is close by (when he's not halfway around the world for work), I have lots of other friends here who keep asking how they can help, and my parents can always fly out and take over if it doesn't work out in Sac. But the possibility that Marco may, in some instances, let teaching or other concerns slip ahead of thinking first about my health and care does worry me. Even though I'm his girlfriend, Marco never puts consideration for me ahead of his own wants. It's a weird relationship, I have to admit, and scary in terms of support.

If I'm in pain or throwing up from chemo, taking care of me has to come ahead of the fact that it might make Marco late to teach a dance class with Debra. Doesn't it? That could mean he'll have to suddenly cancel out of a class or something else seemingly important, at the last minute. Will he do that for me? Surely not, in our normal relationship, but what about when he's supposedly my caregiver during treatment? And how will I handle the fact that he won't be there for me every minute of every day, and that he needs time to recover, too? Just because he's caring for a cancer patient shouldn't mean he has to abandon his own life—at least, I would hope that I wouldn't do that to him. What about when he wants to go to a milonga and I'm well enough to be home alone but not well enough to go with him, or my white blood cell count is too low for me to be out dancing and risking infection? What about when I get on his nerves, being there all the time? What if it turns out I'm really sick all the time from chemo and really need him all the time, driving him crazy, making us both nuts with the neediness?

Here's a completely honest personality flaw: I *hate* asking for help. I'm too independent that way, and it bothers the people closest to me, like my parents or best friends, as they all want to help me because they care about me so much. But I just hate telling anyone I *need* him to do anything for me. Obviously, I have to get over that. I would have to trust Marco, and do so in a way I have never trusted anyone in my life other than my parents. They've earned it in adopting and raising me, especially my mom, holding me for months, me, this crying, shaking, deformed, six-week-old abused shuffled foster child afraid of the entire world with a complete and absolute mistrust of all human beings. Any trust I've ever had of anyone in my lifetime has only been possible because my mom gave up her own life for those first several months to constantly take care of me and love me and show me that she would never hurt me or abuse me or stop loving me. And I've had that from both of my parents my entire life. I know that, in that regard, my life is truly blessed.

The more I think about it in those terms, the more stupid I feel for even considering staying with Marco. Why the hell would I do that to him, put him to what could be such an incredible life challenge? Why would I challenge myself like that? No matter how horrible it gets, no matter how hard it is, no matter how terribly it temporarily destroys their own lives, my parents will not fail me in this. Just like I would not fail either of them in the same situation. I would quit my job and sell my house if I had to, to be100 percent unfailingly there if someone I care about deeply were facing such an illness. Can Marco say that? Even if he believes he can, will he? Really? And can I get over my own trust issues that have plagued me all of my life, both isolating and protecting me from the world?

Aren't the next six months going to be hard enough as it is, without testing my own strength of character as well? Surely, surviving cancer is a challenging spiritual growth experience in and of itself, without me further challenging myself to make some specific intention to grow as a person in the experience. Ah, but therein lies the rub: it's in my nature to challenge myself, and to want to continually improve the positive energy I bring to this world. And, really, I can't imagine a greater life challenge or learning opportunity for me than this. To be humane and kind to others through a health crisis practically designed to bring out the very worst in our selfish human nature . . .

I've only been at this a month, and I already can't believe how hard it's been to be kind and patient to everyone around me (which has been a specific intentional goal of mine for several years now), and I know the exact moments when I've failed most miserably at that, though it's hard to disbelieve the people who have commented the very opposite to me with the utmost sincerity . . . so far those moments of patience and attempted kindness are outweighing the failings, I hope. But I know it's only going to get harder. I am completely naive to this experience.

Ugh, I feel sick to my stomach.

CANCER—DAY 35 FRIDAY, MAY 29, 2009

The MUGA test was today. They want to document the condition of my heart before chemo, and then they're going to check this again halfway through and again at the end of chemo, before putting me back on my heart medication. First, they drew two vials of blood (why the hell can't they make vials in different sizes to do just one draw, instead of wiggling the needle in my arm to swap in additional vials?). Then, they left me sitting there for half an hour with a catheter in my vein while they mixed some radioactive stuff into my blood. Then they reinjected this radioactive blood back in my vein through the catheter, and as I understand it, the radioactive isotopes attach to red blood cells and pass through the heart while in circulation, so the isotopes can be traced as they move through the heart. They took two ten-minute sessions of recordings from that. Toward the end of the second one, I had a coughing fit because of my crummy lingering cold, and they came in and said we'd have to do it over again. My response was, "OK, but can I please have a sip of water first?" I mean, come on. Where they seriously annoyed with me because I couldn't NOT cough for twenty minutes straight while I was sick? Actually, they were obviously busy with scans all afternoon, so they didn't have extra time to waste on me. And the old guy before me didn't want to go in because he was scared, so they were running late to begin with.

Basically, this MUGA test is supposed to show how well blood is pumping through my heart. I don't expect the test today to show anything abnormal at all. If it were necessary in terms of my heart, or if my cardiologist thought I had a weak heart, he would have already ordered this test. But if it makes the medical oncologist happy, so be it. What's one more radioactive injection in the big scheme of things anyway? I wonder how many times they can inject you with radioactive materials without giving you some kind of radiation poisoning?

The real reason they need the MUGA is because my cancer was HER2/NEU positive, which means that it is an aggressive cancer. Dr. Sloe would like to include another drug in my chemo called Herceptin, assuming my heart is strong enough and stays strong enough. Herceptin, as I understand it, is hard on the heart. (Gee, where I have heard that before? Would it be Adriamyacin, another drug Dr. Sloe intends to use on m?) They can't administer Herceptin it if your MUGA falls below a certain percentage or score. So while I expect today's MUGA to be fine, I suspect that if they give me Herceptin, the score is going to fall. Of course, everything else I read about Herceptin and what it does to the female body is pretty hellish, so let's just not go there yet. I'll cross that bridge when I come to it.

Surely, at some point the potential damage to my heart must not be worth the incremental improvement in the cancer recurrence prognosis, right? When do they take quality of life into consideration over the necessity of severe treatments? Or don't they? Am I the only one in this medical process concerned about my quality of life regardless of the overall *duration* of my life? I guess it's hard for doctors to think like that.

CANCER—DAY 37 **SUNDAY, MAY 31, 2009**

Same stuff, different day. Well, yes and no, really. With another day to think about it and one very long and very open conversation between Marco and I this afternoon, he says he understands the scope of the caregiver role, and he really, *really* wants to do this chemo-care thing. He got it worked out with his housemate that it's OK for me to stay with them, and he made a Google calendar so that Brian and everyone will know what dates are my chemo and which week I'm working (and supposed to feel pretty normal). He's looking at yoga classes for me, and even scheduling time each day to make me walk or exercise. He's going to go with me to my next medical oncologist appointment so that he can ask questions about how to take care of me. We hadn't talked about it all weekend because we've both been sick, so finally today I brought it up. I didn't expect the conversation to turn out this way; I thought he had decided against it because he hadn't said anything. But the reason he hadn't said anything was that he was still trying to figure out how he felt about it. Which is exactly why *I* didn't say anything about it until this afternoon. Now that I'm down to the wire, I really need to make a decision on this and take action very, very soon to move on whatever my decision turns out to be.

Now that I know Marco is committed to taking care of me—and is learning about what he will have to do and has thought about the details of how it will affect his life—well, what worries me most *now* is the relationship side of things. The primary reason I want to stay in Sac is to be with him. There are lots of other reasons to stay, but let's be honest, that's the first reason on the list. It's not a slam dunk decision though. This relationship is still very young; we've been dating for a couple of months, give or take a week. We *were* dance partners before that, so we were getting close even before we started dating and had known each other for a fairly long time in the tango community, but this cancer thing really pushed our relationship to a more advanced level more quickly than would ever have happened naturally. Circumstances (first, the cancer stuff, and now us both being really sick this week) have forced us to see each other at, and support each other through some of our much-less-than-great moments already, and we're still together. Man, he can be a beast when he's sick or stressed (which he totally admits to, btw).

But here's the problem: he's not committed to *me* yet; he told me his heart is still open to meeting someone else. That's exactly what he said during our conversation this afternoon, "I'm still open to meeting someone else." He doesn't know why—he's not sure if it's him or if he just hasn't met the right person. Personally, I think it's because he holds back all the time, worried about getting hurt because of his past experiences. How can you ever feel committed to someone if you're restraining your heart all the time? Relationship avoidance became an area of expertise for me in the years after Artie died. I certainly haven't let anyone deeply into my heart since then.

Even so, it did not feel good to be bluntly told that Marco is not actually committed to our relationship. After that blow in the conversation, we talked some more, and he told me he's inspired by me, and he said something about how I believe in him like no one else ever has. And he's inspired by me because of my tenacity and the fact that my tenacity also applies to him, that I really believe in him and appreciate him, and that's inspiring to him. As we talked about inspiration, I told him that he doesn't need me for inspiration—he has himself. But he says he doesn't inspire himself because he's never done anything significant or inspirational in his life, and that doing this would be really important. I agreed that doing this would be huge, and then I joked something about how it could also be a huge failure if he let me down.

He smiled at first, but then his eyes got watery and I hugged him and he started crying, then *really* crying, and I pet his head like we do and held him and told him it would be OK, and he choked out "I'm afraid." "I know, Baby, I know, it's OK," I told him. I held him in my arms a while and soothingly pet his hair. Eventually his breathing calmed down. After that he seemed to decide that he absolutely wants to do this caring for Chemo Girl thing.

After it was all calm, though, I still felt it was important to tell him that he should see the inspiration in himself that I do, that he brings joy to people every week and enriches their lives by teaching them tango, and his co-workers really appreciate him, and that every single time he laughs he makes someone else happy. (My dad really loved Marco's laugh when we had lunch; Marco's laugh is completely heartfelt and happy and infectious.) Hearing all that from me with such sincerity brightened up Marco. Why hasn't anyone ever told him these things before? It's not rocket science—everyone I've met who knows Marco has good things to say about him. And he has more tango friends in Sacramento than can even be counted, I think. And they all want to help him and help me with the cancer and chemo and everything. It's amazing.

I'm still torn though. Mom & Dad's house is so comfortable, and they love me so much. I have my own room there, and my cats can stay with me. I miss my cats. I've been down in Sacramento with Marco every weekend since this thing started, and I miss my quiet home in the forest, the beauty that surrounds it, and my cats.

I'm glad I'm going back to my own house tomorrow, right after the doctor's appointment with Dr. Thatcher to get the rest of the stitches removed. At home in the forest, I'll have some space to think this through.

CANCER—DAY 38 MONDAY, JUNE 1, 2009

Round and round and round I go. I'm almost there, but nobody knows.

I talked for more than an hour today with this woman, Catherine, who's basically a cancer caseworker. I think she told me she's an "Oncology Patient Navigator" when she called. How's that for a job title? She didn't really have any information that I haven't already read in my own research in terms of what to expect (sometimes on the common questions it sounded like she was reading to me from the National Cancer Institute Website, which she's probably recited a thousand times), but it was good to be able to speak with someone who's worked with hundreds of breast cancer patients and to ask her opinion on the things I'm thinking about right now, which go well beyond common questions like side effects or treatment duration. Specifically, of course, I'm still thinking about where to do my chemo: California or Nebraska.

Like all the medical professionals I've discussed my situation with, Catherine did not provide a direct answer to the fundamental question, but rather gave comments on the two possibilities I'm considering: staying in Sacramento at Marco's, or staying in Sidney at my parents' place. She really clarified some of the medical care points that I was unclear on, in terms of implications of leaving Sac for six months for chemo and then coming back.

All of my doctors have expressed concern about me not being where I can go to them for the necessary checkups and care throughout chemo, particularly my cardiologist. The point Catherine made that many of my doctors have alluded to but not said outright is about working with multiple medical oncologists. I was only so-so on the medical oncologist, Dr. Sloe, in Cameron Park last week. I have much higher hopes for the new one I found in Sacramento—Lombard—because of what I've read about him (he's actually specifically a breast cancer specialist, whereas the other guy is a general medical oncologist) and what I've read about the Marshall Cancer Center where Dr. Lombard practices and how they're active in some very current clinical trials and treatment options and oncology conferences. In general, I've felt better and more secure medically about the procedures that have been done down in Sac where they treat a ridiculously large number of breast cancer patients daily. They really know what they're doing. And they know what to do with a *young* woman with breast cancer. I know my parents have heard rave reviews about the medical oncologist in Sidney, Nebraska, and she's supposed to be young and up to date and have great bedside manner, but still, how many young women in Sidney, Nebraska, get breast cancer in a year? More than in Volcanoville where my house is of course, but still. Any? I'm sure there are plenty of cancer patients in Sidney, and chances are that 80% of them are over 60 years old with a lot of different cancers other than breast cancer. Let's face it: Sidney is a small town in the Great Plains, not a large city in a state with the world's seventh largest economy and the population that goes with it. How progressive and specialized to my situation can the oncologist in Sidney be, compared to Sacramento?

Catherine's real point though, came up twice in different parts of our conversation. When it really drove home for me was when she was preparing me to understand that while it's important to focus on one thing at a time, I should just focus on the next thing and not worry too much about what's far ahead on the treatment path (I had started asking her questions about side effects of the drugs after chemo and how those drugs and chemo drugs damage the ovaries and cause menopause). She also wanted to make sure I understood that this is not going to be over when chemo's over. It won't even be over when radiation is over, or after my hair's grown back. She said I need to get used to the fact that my medical providers are going to be very active in my life for the next year, and that they will still be working closely with me for the next two years after that, and still checking me frequently through the five-year mark (which is a hugely important milestone to make without a cancer recurrence), and even after that. This is my medical team.

As I understand from Dr. Sloe, my pathology showed them that my cancer is one that will recur. He said it with clinical plainness. It's not a question of if I will have a recurrence; it's a question of when and where in my body. He says we can do a lot with chemo and all this treatment stuff to make it a long time before that recurrence occurs, but it will happen someday in Dr. Sloe's opinion, maybe even 20 years from now. So, I need to be very comfortable with my medical team, especially with my oncologist, because they will be with me for a very, very long time.

And when I think about all that, it doesn't seem wise to have another oncologist involved for the chemo and then someone else do the rest. What if the two have different opinions on what drugs should be in my chemo? What if they disagree about how many rounds of chemo I need? What if something happens partway through and we need to involve my cardiologist? What if it turns out that I need more chemo rounds after the first six months, or later, after a period of time passes? Would I go back to Nebraska every time I needed chemo, to see the oncologist there? Would I have to fly back there every three months for the follow up appointments? So now, besides the fact that I feel better about my medical care staying with my cancer doctors here and my cardiologist here, I also think it's important to do my chemo with the medical oncologist who is going to continue to care for me after the first six months' chemo sessions are over. And I think that oncologist should be Dr. Lombard. This is precisely his specialty, he has a great reputation, and he's working with more breast cancer patients than I really want to know about even though the "headcount" is reassuring to me in trusting that he is up to date on the latest advances in treating breast cancer.

So, to what will surely be my parents' dismay, I am becoming convinced now that, medically, the best option for my chemo treatment is to do it in Sacramento. But I still have some other issues to resolve to make that happen. Logistical things like what to do with Mizzou and Seoul, and what creature comforts I may need in Marco's house. And then there's this underlying concern, not necessarily of Marco's capabilities as a caretaker, but rather of the strength of our still-new relationship.

Just like the chemo-care situation can put huge stresses on the relationship, any problems in the relationship could create stress that I'm not sure I would be able to handle gracefully during chemo. I mean, come on! Breakups are usually messy to some degree, making it hard to end a relationship gracefully anyway, but can you imagine going through that emotional stuff while your body's being beaten up by chemotherapy and you're basically trapped in the guy's house by your poor health while he's going out socially hoping to meet the next Ms. Right?

That's the extreme, but hey, I have a tendency to consider all possibilities before making a decision, like potentially having some huge relationship issue that interferes with Marco taking care of Chemo Girl. When I was still fretting about that while instant messaging with Marco tonight, he bluntly told me to "stop worrying about that." Well, if he's so completely not concerned about that the stability of our relationship, then he must have some reasonable faith that, whatever happens, we'll work through it so my care isn't compromised.

And at the end of the day, upset as they could be to find out I've decided to stay in Sacramento for chemo, my parents would take me back home in a heartbeat, or probably even temporarily move here to take care of me if things really went so terribly wrong with this plan. It's much easier to take on some risk of falling off the high wire walk of life when your net is as strong as my parents.

CANCER—DAY 39 TUESDAY, JUNE 2, 2009

Ironic. I was accidentally one hour early for my dentist appointment this morning. Because I live 20 minutes away, it didn't make sense to drive home and back, so I sat down and did my Runes journal while thinking through the last of this decision. Where should I do my chemo? There are so many things to consider, it's hard to get a perspective on the overall situation. But that is exactly what the Runes are for.

It's a little difficult for me to explain the Runes, and I'm always hesitant to talk about them at all because I know that lots of people are skeptical about a variety of spiritual concepts. Many people who know about Runes believe them to be an oracle. That is a subject which, after years of using the Nordic Runes, I still do not feel qualified to comment upon, but I do like how one author, Ralph Blum, says you shouldn't get caught up in the idea of an oracle as some kind of forecasting tool or predictor. Rather, an oracle points your attention toward those hidden fears and motivations that will shape your future by their unfelt presence within each present moment; Blum also believes you are the one responsible for selecting your future, but the oracle can direct your attention toward those inner choices that may be the most important elements in determining that future. At any rate, you don't have to believe the Runes are an oracle in order to benefit from using them, or to understand my story, but I'll explain them a little just in case.

Some people use the Runes when they are facing a particular difficulty or a difficult decision, like: Should I go for that promotion? Will I be OK if I quit my job to start my own business? Is it time to discuss separation/divorce with my spouse? I have to admit that, like many people seeking direction in life and worried about taking the wrong path, I wonder about relationships because they can seriously disrupt or wonderfully enhance your life. Getting into a relationship can be sort of like driving on an access road with a slower speed limit that runs next to the freeway, rather than taking the freeway and getting where you intended to go in less time without much distraction.

For example—when Marco started giving me the impression that he wanted to be more than dance partners and I was unsure of whether or not that was wise, I used the Runes to look for a perspective on the situation.

My Runes are small amethyst stones with the Nordic symbols carved into the stones and filled in with gold paint. I still use the little gray Ralph Blum *Book of Runes* that came with my first set of Rune stones I bought at a Barnes & Noble bookstore. I keep my Runes in a little embroidered Korean silk pouch, and when I'm pondering a situation I'll hold a question in my mind for a moment and then reach into the pouch and take out a Rune stone, then look up the meaning of the symbol in the little gray *Book of Runes*. Sometimes I take out the Rune that feels heaviest, or I'll sift the stones through my hand and draw out whichever one stayed in my hand. Sometimes it feels like a certain stone has a little magnetic pull or is sticky so that's the stone I draw from the pouch. Sort of like a horoscope can be interpreted different ways, no matter what the Rune stone is, it always gives me a perspective on my situation.

I draw a Rune every day, usually in the morning, and generally use it as a kind of guide to some personal thought for the day. I can't tell you how many times the entry for the Rune that I drew on a particular day came back into my mind when something happened later in the day as the thought, "Ah, so that's what the Runes were talking about; I know to be careful how I react to this." Each day's Rune is often something of a guide in how to react in a particular situation (in my case, usually by being more patient or trusting, or getting out of my own way to let life take its own course instead of trying to force it to be some certain way).

The day my gynecologist found the lump and I flipped out and my parents didn't answer their phones and I ended up going to Marco's to talk about it instead of dancing . . . well, that day my Rune was *Gebo*, which means both Partnership and A Gift. It never would have occurred to me that morning what that Rune could have been indicating. It was going to be a completely normal work day, I happened to have a normal annual doctor's checkup that afternoon, and then I would go to my usual dance rehearsal with my pro partner. Nothing was going on in my life that would have made me think ahead to the points that *Gebo* focuses on. But looking back on it now, that evening was what solidified my relationship with Marco a clear step higher than it was prior to that, and every moment he's helped me through this cancer process since then has been a gift. There are so many times when I told him after the fact that I couldn't have gone through this or that thing without him. It only occurred to me today to go back and look up the Rune for the day my doctor found the lump. Everything was happening so quickly then that I didn't really register it at the time, but that the Rune on that day had been Gebo, which is about Partnership and A Gift, and then things went the way they did with Marco. I'd been getting *Gebo* a lot in regard to Marco all spring, and I couldn't make anything of it except as a dance partnership because I didn't really see it becoming a romantic relationship. You could say the Runes predicted it all, or you could say it just happened to work out that way. You don't have to believe in anything one way or the other to understand my story. What matters is that the Runes give me a point of consideration and perspective each day, and that generally helps me keep trying to develop and grow as a being.

My Rune today was *Isa*, Standstill, which surprised me. I journaled, "Funny, I was just thinking that I'm about ready to decide to stay with Marco for chemo, but Isa is about stillness." And I realized that I was still unsure, anxious about the decision. I pondered it a bit, then decided to Rune for general guidance on the decision to stay with Marco in Sacramento for my chemotherapy, and actually, probably for my radiation treatment too. I thought to myself: "What guidance can the Runes give me regarding staying with Marco for chemo?" Then I did a three-Rune spread, which means taking out three Runes that, in order, give guidance with: an overview of the situation, the challenge to be faced, and the action to be taken. Here's what I drew from my little silk Rune pouch, along with a bit of what each Rune means in *The Book of Runes* and what I think is the message for me in each one:

Rune #1. Overview: *Wunjo*. Joy, reversed [upside-down]. This Rune says things are slow in coming to fruition [my relationship and trust with Marco]. The process of birth is long and fears arise for the safety of the child within [exactly!]. A difficult passage even if brief, is at hand [I told Marco I would decide by tomorrow]. Consideration and deliberation are called for [I need to think it through completely and be sure I'm doing the right thing]. Seen in its true light, everything is a test. And so, focused in the present, sincere towards others and trusting in yourself, know that you cannot fail [yes, this is definitely a test, but I can do it. We can do it].

Rune #2. Challenge: *Nauthiz*. Constraint, Necessity, Pain. The necessity of learning to deal with severe constraint is the lesson of *Nauthiz*. This Rune represents the obstacles we create for ourselves [trust is my biggest one] as well as those we encounter in the world around us [my cancer]. Both can be equally difficult to handle. The role of *Nauthiz* is to identify our shadow, our dark or repressed side, places where growth has been stunted. [Trust. Again!] The need for restraint is unquestionable here [I have to believe in Marco and control my emotions stemming from lack of trust]. Clearly there is work to be done on yourself. Let the constraints of the time serve you in righting your relationship to your Self. Be mindful that rectification must come before progress. And, as always, consider the uses of adversity [trust has been a lifelong issue for me and going through chemo will be difficult, but if I remember to learn from it and use it to become a better person, recognizing this as a real test of being a good person to others while undergoing personal adversity, I can grow enormously from the experience].

Rune #3. Action: *Gebo.* Partnership, A Gift. Drawing this Rune is an indication that some form of partnership is at hand. You are put on notice not to collapse yourself into that union [which I have a tendency to do in relationships, give up too much of who I am to fit the other person, though I control this well now everywhere else in my life and have definitely improved on it over time]. True partnership is achieved only by separate and whole beings who retain their separateness even as they unite. Remember to let the winds of Heaven dance between you [this always brings Artie to mind, only a breath away from me in spirit]. The path of partnership can also lead you to the realization of a still greater union—union with the Higher Self. [This is what I have to do. It will be difficult, but also the greatest spiritual development opportunity of my life.]

OK. Wow. That does it—I know what I have to do. Time to call my parents.

CANCER—DAY 40 WEDNESDAY, JUNE 3, 2009

Interesting. The number 40 is big in historical texts, especially the Bible (as any good Catholic schoolgirl knows), as an important period of time of passage, so it's interesting that today was cancer day number 40 for me.

I called my parents today. I was nervous about the conversation we needed to have, and I actually left a voicemail for my brother right before I called them to warn him that I was going to tell Mom & Dad that I'm staying in Sacramento. I figured that Mom would probably call my brother as soon as we got off the phone. I thought she would be upset. They *were* upset when I first suggested staying in California several weeks ago; that's for sure. But they surprised me a little today; we actually had a very nice conversation about the whole thing.

I hadn't posted my blog for several days. I've been writing in my journal a lot, but I think it's been three days or more since I posted any excerpts from my journal out to the blog. I didn't know what I was going to decide, and I didn't want my family getting unnecessarily agitated by my thought process before I knew what I wanted to do. But on the phone this evening, my dad said that he already knew what I had decided, from reading my blog. I guess that makes sense. I mean, they have known me for more than 30 years, so I suppose that having the information through Saturday's or Sunday's blog post would have been enough for them to figure out what I was going to decide even before I did. Funny, it took me days longer than my dad to figure out what I was going to do.

Apparently, lots of people, specifically people who have actually had chemotherapy, I guess, have been talking with my mom about what it's like. They've been telling her that even though there are times in the cycle when I'll be really sick for a few days at a time, there will be these recovery periods, at least the third week of each cycle (which is when I'm planning to work my regular consulting job stuff throughout chemo). Mom and her friends agree that I would be really bored during those third weeks in Sidney, away from all my friends and dancing. And lots of people seem to have been telling my parents that it would be better for me to stay closer to my own life rather than leaving it for six months. And of course, if things don't work out or I need more care or whatever, I can always go home to them then.

You know, I just have to state the obvious: I think I have pretty much the best parents on the planet.

Chapter 7.
Pre-Chemo

CANCER—DAY 41 THURSDAY, JUNE 4, 2009

Ah, United Airlines. Nothing like paying hundreds of dollars to be treated like disobedient cattle. Our pilots are cranky. Bad weather will justify our soon-to-be-late arrival in Chicago. Fun, Fun, fun. You know, I read not long ago that United has a 40-percent on-time performance record—meaning, 60 percent of the time, you as a passenger on a flight with United should plan on arriving late. Granted, gate scheduling and parts placement planning are not the easiest algorithms in the book, but come on—that's just probabilities and math. Even the crummiest planning software solves at a much higher rate of executable accuracy than 40 percent! Still, there are plenty of excuses for delays with airlines: too many planes, too many places to go, too many people to keep track of, too many repair persons and replacement parts to have in too many places . . .and so on.

Anyway, off in anonymity to the airport I went this morning, one of the countless hordes being rounded up and prodded into the flying cattle cars. Oh yeah, and don't you just love the guy who stands up to get his cell phone out of the overhead compartment while the plane is landing, totally freaking out the flight attendants?

Speaking of United and flying—here's a funny story: Years and years ago, I don't even know how long ago (way before Artie died, though), I had a trip to . . . where was it . . . home to visit my parents I think. They were living in Missouri then, and I was flying out of San Jose. Yeah, that was it. I was flying on frequent flier miles to go home for a visit. So, as usual I take a cab to the airport, check a bag (I always seem to take too much stuff with me when I go to visit my parents), and stroll over to security.

I was traveling a lot then, and I *always* got stopped by San Jose security to re-run my shoes in the scanner and run one of those little cloth things around my laptop bag. On this particular day, I noticed that there were two other young professional women right there with me, waiting to get their shoes, and one really tall guy right next to me. I joked to him something about "Which one of these things is not like the other?" You know, like the *Sesame Street* song. I rarely have the urge to joke while waiting in a security line or at the airport in general—usually I keep my earphones on to avoid conversation in airports—but for some reason I wasn't on the phone or anything this day, and it was just too ironic to be random that three young women were being stopped by security, and only one guy.

I had to chuckle to myself. This tall guy (about 6'5") just *had* to be an engineer, because while waiting for security to scan his computer bag he was picking up his loose stuff out of the bin and putting it back on, you know, the phone on the belt clip, the Bluetooth in the ear, the Intel name badge on the shirt pocket . . . Ha! I got a real chuckle out of that. Leave it to an Intel engineer to go to the airport from the office, forget that he has his name badge on, and then absentmindedly put it *back* on after taking it off for airport security screening. Too funny. Anyway, they're giving the guy his computer back and I've gotten my shoes on, and now we're heading down the same terminal, from which there is basically only one airline, United. Furthermore, about the only place United flies to from San Jose is Denver, then you have to connect to get anywhere else (like Missouri, where my parents were living at the time).

So, being in a wise-ass mood and highly amused because this guy put his name badge back on after security, I say to the guy as we're walking, "So, what are you going to do in Denver?" He looks at me, speechless. "Lucky guess," I said, and then pointed out to him that "There's only one flight out of this terminal at this time of day, United to Denver." He laughed, and he told me that he's from Denver, but that he was on his way to Albuquerque via Denver. We made small talk going out to the gate, and sat down to wait for boarding.

Then, being in a *very* impish mood, I decided to really throw the guy for a loop. I asked "So, what did you think of the casino party in San Francisco last weekend?" He gazed at me in utter disbelief, decided he hadn't heard me correctly, and asked "What?" I had expected that, and I replied "You know, the casino party that Intel threw in San Francisco last weekend; didn't you go?" (I had gone to the party with a friend who works at Intel, a guy that's a very competitive tri-athlete, big guy, all muscles, outdoorsy tan, blond hair . . . I think he'd just broken up with his girlfriend and needed some last-minute eye candy on his arm for the party, or something like that so he took me and we had a fabulously good time).

The tall airport guy is practically going into shock now, wondering who the hell this stranger is and how in the world she knows so much about him. "How did you know about that?" he asked, completely confounded. I told him simply: "I was there." He retorts, "Nuh-uh, no way!" He obviously didn't believe me, so I reached in my bag and pulled out my leftover casino chips. (How's *that* for serendipity, that I forgot to cash in my chips at the end of the night, and they were still in my bag?)

He asked if I'd seen him at the party and I was like, "No, I've never met you before." Which made him ask: "So how did you know I was there?" Ahhhhh, *finally*, here comes the zinger! I point to his shirt pocket: "Name badge."

And that's how I met Brian Bradford.

CANCER—DAY 42 FRIDAY, JUNE 5, 2009

I had an interesting realization while talking with my old friend Paul at this officer's workshop I was speaking at in Chicago. He commented that I looked more serene now than I did at the winter advisory meeting that we both attended in January, and I thought about it for a moment. Then I realized that, because I can't travel again for eight or nine months and I'll be living at Marco's during that time, and my life is pretty much dictated from now through January or February already . . . now that it's all settled and the plan is in place, it's actually strangely calming to have the stability of knowing that. Weird. I rarely know where I will be or what I'll be doing for an entire nine months out. I've always been at the ready for things to change, which is a different kind of life than that of Chemo Girl, who will have a stationary life and not a crazy one like the regular Cynthia Swan does.

And you know, people continue to just amaze me. After skipping half of the afternoon sessions today to nap because I was too tired to keep up all the interactions, I was starting to think that I shouldn't have come to the GSCMA leadership forum this year (I could have easily gotten someone else to give the presentation I'm doing tomorrow). But now, tired as I am, I'm glad that I suffered through the travel pain to be here. Tonight I was starting to question why I even come to this event anymore, because I was meeting the typical I'm-really-only-here-to-advance-my-career types, which definitely turn me off. (There was one woman in particular who bothered me tonight. I was sitting down trying to eat, and she was walking around "networking." She introduced herself to me and proceeded to tell me why she's so important to GSCMA, and essentially pressed me to validate that for her—oh yes, of course, you are important and here's why your role is invaluable [not]. But later on, I talked to other people, some old friends, and then I felt like this evening alone was entirely worth the effort to travel to Chicago right after surgery for this event.

People can be so inspiring! I had an amazingly motivational conversation with Christine, one of the Chicago staff tonight. I didn't know this before, but she's a five–year breast cancer survivor. I had always thought that she's a wonderful person, so now we're talking not just wonderful, but generally amazing, given what she's survived with such a great attitude. And it was sooo great to hang out with Kristin and Paul—we're just such kindred spirits. Somehow, now it seems even more valuable for us to be here because there don't seem to be as many go-getters in "The AC" as there used to be, so we have to stick together! I also had a really nice conversation with Christopher about his son's three years of chemo, and an interesting conversation with the

CEO of GSCMA about how this is really a life test and happened at this point in my life for a reason. I had no idea that he possessed such spirituality, and now I feel like we're really friends instead of just professional colleagues. Last but not least, I have to give additional credit to Paul Mearlo for being a good and true old friend, without whom I couldn't have made it through this event (even though he doesn't have time to read this to know that he's being thanked). You know that you're listening to a dull speaker when you're texting all of your buddies in other parts of the ballroom to stay awake, which Kristen and Paul and I tend to do, to our own great amusement. I'm bummed that I will probably have to miss the Conference in October this year, even though it's in Denver and darn close to home. That's supposed to take place during the fifth cycle of my chemo, and I've been told not to expect to feel well at all by that point, but I still have to wonder now: could I maybe be well enough to just go to the roundtable officers' events on Sunday to see my friends, and not necessarily stay for the whole conference? Maybe. Or maybe that's just wishful thinking.

CANCER—DAY 43 SATURDAY, JUNE 6, 2009

OK, here's a story that you either have to find completely amusing or else just stop reading what I write.

I am seriously an idiot. I meet so many people at these conference things. I have a terrible memory to boot, which is not good when you're at the airport waiting to go home, and no one has their name badges on anymore. Maybe you can guess where this story is going?

So I'm at Chicago O'Hare with three hours to kill before my flight, though it's worth the wait because then it's a direct flight back to Smurf instead of hassling through multiple airports, which my recently-post-surgery body definitely cannot handle (direct flights and wheelie bags were bad enough without having to hop planes besides). "Smurf," by the way, is how we frequent Sacramento flyers refer to the Sacramento airport because its three-letter code is SMF. Anyway, since I'm not in a hurry, I wander down the opposite direction of the concourse, away from my gate. Lo and behold, there's a McDonald's, and you know, I can't remember the last time I had those completely unhealthy, yet strangely addictive fries. I order some, and then meander to an empty gate area to sit down with my embarrassingly unhealthy snack. There's a flight boarding, so there are some people in line over at the counter, but otherwise the gate area is empty. As I sat down, I glanced up at the line of people, and had a zing moment of eye contact with a guy standing in the line. I'm usually pretty careful to avoid eye contact while traveling; it's just easier to get through airports when you don't have strange men trying to chat you up.

Well, next thing I know, the guy from the line is standing right in front of me and says, "Can I have one fry?" I can honestly say no one's ever used that as a pickup line on me before! He's a good-looking guy, nice smile, possibly familiar but I have no clue who he is or if I know him from somewhere or if he's a total stranger just hitting on me with some originality. What could I say? I pulled out a single fry and handed it to him saying something like, "They're like Pringles—no one can eat just one." I set the package of fries back down on the bag and went about getting out my Sudoku puzzle and such, but the guy sits down in front of me. Now what? He says, "Sacramento, right?"

Damn, I *had* met this guy and not remembered. Worse yet, he wasn't just one of the roundtable officers I met at the event I just presented at, oh *no*, that would not be embarrassing enough . . . this guy works for my consulting company! I've even advised him about how to get involved with GSCMA and the roundtable boards, albeit via e-mail, so I didn't know what he looked like then. But I *did* meet him briefly yesterday. He specifically found me in order to introduce himself last night, and here I didn't have a clue seeing him today at the airport. Pathetic! Let's blame cancer stress and lack of rest for the ridiculously embarrassing mental lapse.

On the up side for the day, people really seemed to enjoy my presentation this afternoon, which is always nice to hear afterward. It's tough to be the last speaker of a conference—the only thing between people and their flights home is you! At least no one left while I was talking; that would have been mildly embarrassing even though it's to be expected. And they were pretty engaged, now that I think about it.

Now I just have to keep my fingers crossed that the tornados north of here and thunderstorms south of here don't create huge delays for the long west coast flights. Uh oh, here comes the rain. Pouring!

CANCER—DAY 44 SUNDAY, JUNE 7, 2009

Well, Marco finally read some of my blog while I was in Chicago. He brought it up at dinner after he had picked me up at the airport. He's not quite comfortable with the personal details I included in the blog (specifically the entry where he cried, of course) because it's so intimate. But unfortunately, that's exactly why it was so important to include that in the blog. He said it's compelling to read and the intimacy is part of why it's compelling, but it's also written in a way that the overall story in and of itself makes you want to keep reading it. He said it's compelling to read about the journey I'm on. I would have been more impressed with his compliments if the conversation hadn't started out as a criticism and the suggestion that I withhold even more personal information while pulling excerpts from my journal out to my blog.

I knew it was coming. Marco has never read my blog, much as it would tell him about who he's dealing with here. I knew that someone someday would say something to him about it, though, and then he would finally read some of it. I also knew that this is how he would react. I thought long and hard about whether to include any intimate details of the "crying" conversation, and I decided that it was simply too important to the emotional journey to leave it out. It was integral in his decision to keep me here, important in my decision to stay, and a pivotal point in our relationship.

It's interesting that he's obviously fine with me writing about myself crying and him comforting *me*, but apparently that doesn't go both ways. Is that because he's a guy? I told him that as a result of the blog, I won't be the only one who thinks he's amazing anymore. Actually, that's already happened—my co-worker Rachel thinks that Marco's the best thing since sliced bread. She reads the blog religiously and often sends me text messages about it. I told her privately about the six-months-to-say-I-love-you rule and she said, "It's going to happen sooner than that." I told her that the only way that would happen was if I was dying, which isn't going to happen. But then, tonight, it was all over his face when he came to pick me up—he was so happy to see me, he was just glowing with it and gazing at me with those lovey-dovey eyes. And he missed me. I know he loves me. But he has this six-month rule, which basically means that by the time the requisite pre-I-love-you six months have passed, we'll be so used to not saying what we feel that I'll never hear it from him anyway. Which doesn't matter, except that it does. I love saying "I love you" to someone. It makes them feel good, and it makes me feel good. Except when I'm the only person saying it.

It's a little scary to realize that I'm going to be living with him for eight, well, *nine* months. Both comforting and scary—comforting because of the stability of it, committed to staying in one place with one person so long, which is pretty unique for me these days. I'm just a person always ready for different paths to appear and have the wherewithal to go off in a new direction for a great opportunity or life experience when one presents itself. It's not that I'm always looking for the next thing, but I'm always ready, mentally, for change. And now I'm going to be settled in one place for nine months.

I still go back and forth a bit on this whole thing—staying with Marco and having to trust him with so many things in order for it to work. I have these moments of frustration when it appears that he is thinking only of himself or what he wants to go do . . .and then there are these completely opposite moments, when, even though it's not really necessary, he completely takes over in caring for me as if his own life didn't even exist. I have to wonder if having either one of those extremes is really a great thing. I hope he's still feeling his way around this whole subject—how much to consider my health while trying to stay sane somehow through everything he's doing for me. Either extreme will probably destroy him; he needs to find his own balance as a caregiver.

There's another interesting side to this in that it's presenting Marco an opportunity to take better care of himself. For example, we're going to start yoga as soon as my arm is strong enough and I can actually reach over my head. And he wants us to plan on going for a walk at lunchtime every day, except on my very worst days. He's talking with my oncologist about what kind of foods will be best, and thinking about not just looking after *my* health, but better looking after his own which will probably improve his emotional state. It's an odd exploitation, Marco using my illness to improve his health. But I like feeling like other people are benefitting in some way from my experience, especially if they benefit emotionally or spiritually.

CANCER—DAY 45 MONDAY, JUNE 8, 2009

Uff da, I had the worst nightmare about Marco this morning. We lived in this little village, where the main home was owned by a dentist and his life partner while Marco lived in a guest house on their property. I got really sick and had to be gone a long time. I couldn't remember very well the circumstances of my leaving, but Marco was avoiding me when I returned. I went to meet him at what used to be our favorite restaurant [only in the dream, we don't have a favorite restaurant in reality]. He was there with friends from his wine club, and he pretended not to see me. I didn't want to make a scene, so I went to see the old dentist because I needed a place to stay that night, and he let me stay in a guest room of the big house. He was telling me to go talk to Marco in the morning before work, that Marco loved me very much and that all I had to do was go talk to him and everything would be fine. Then I went to my room, and in the middle of the night I woke up because I could feel Marco there watching me. I wondered why he would come and be there in the room but not talk to me. The next morning [we're still in the dream here], I overslept, so I was running out the door in my pajamas as I heard the shuttle bus start down the road to pick up everyone from the little village to go to town where they all worked. Marco wasn't with the crowd. I started running toward where he lived, and at the next block I saw him coming up the side street, so I turned to run toward him, but he crossed to the other side of the street! He was walking really fast to catch the shuttle, and wearing this long black trench coat that was open and blowing back with the speed of his pace. And he had these roundish big plastic framed glasses, like my brother used to wear in school, only reddish brown colored. And then I was at his feet begging him, "You won't even speak to me?" In my nightmare he said something like, "Isn't it obvious?" and then pushed past me. I fell on the ground and watched his back as he hurried to escape me. Then I woke up.

Darn it, why do my dreams have to be so real to my brain that I don't know it's a dream? I woke up crying—it was an awful dream. I feel nauseated.

Good grief, I haven't had such a nightmare in a long time. What's wrong with me? Well, besides cancer, of course.

CANCER—DAY 46 TUESDAY, JUNE 9, 2009

Sadly, it's my last pre-chemo regular full workday at my home in Volcanoville, out in El Dorado National Forest. It's a beautiful day here though, 70 degrees and perfect. A huge jackrabbit was hanging out in the yard, and Mizzou was ready to leap through the office window screen to catch it when the thing finally hopped out of sight. They have such HUGE ears! I know my property probably doesn't look like much to other people; there's nothing fancy or impressive about my little place out here surrounded by trees, but I really love it here, and I'm really going to miss my house and my cats and the sound of the wind in the trees . . . without city and people noises filling in all the space and pressing uninvited into any semblance of tranquility.

I wonder how many people sink into depression while going through this? Through cancer treatment I mean. I think I'm holding on fine, and then—whammo! Everything seems miserable. One problem tonight is that I pushed myself too hard to get more work done instead of calling it a day when I should have in order to spare my body and mind. Granted, it was a bit of a sad day to start with because I have this fear that I won't get to be here much after this, though getting to come home at all is better than six months straight of being completely away from California. But with a ton of work to do and feeling bad for leaving my company during the busiest month of the modeling report cycle, I was in crunch mode all day. I started working before 6 a.m. today and didn't stop until I could hardly focus my eyes anymore, which was around 9 p.m. I have myself totally stressed out with what I've probably overcommitted to get analyzed and written for the company before chemo starts. I don't feel prepared for the oncologist appointment tomorrow, even though I've already had an oncologist appointment and Marco says it will be fine. (I get tired of hearing that said without any substance behind it. Sometime it would be nice to hear *why* it's going to be fine, but Marco just gets too busy with work or whatever to really do any sincere comforting if I'm not standing right there in his office waiting for more than a blank "It'll be fine.") I mean, I know he's right, it *will* be fine, but today I definitely don't know how. Well, no, wait, let the brain tick tock a little; I guess I do know how. I'll end up canceling things that I want or need to do, I'll give up time that I had hoped to have to rest or relax at home, time will pass, and next thing you know, the first week of chemo will be over. It will be fine. But getting there, that's not feeling so fine.

So, it was around 9:30 p.m. and I was finally having a salad (cleaning out leftovers from the 'fridge that were about to go untouched for who knows how long) and filling out doctor forms and disability forms in front of the television, letting a recording of *So You Think You Can Dance* play. Not that this is the world's greatest show or that I'm really into it, but as someone who loves dance, I can't resist the opportunity to see so many styles and ability levels, along with the personalities that show through. On the commercials (which I normally zip skip with the DVR clicker) I'm unloading the dishwasher and cleaning up after the cats and, you know, just doing house stuff, though my house still seems a mess to me. And, this is the weirdest thing (if you've never felt depressed a moment in your life then this will be completely nonsensical to you): well, I just felt like it was getting darker. It had already been dark outside a while, and of course I don't mean this literally. But I can feel a darkness pressing in, and I know where that goes and it scares me. The emotional roller coaster of this thing has definitely gone from a peewee to a 48-inch-height-requirement this week. It has to be the stress of worrying about chemo and what that's going to do to me, of course, but knowing that's why I'm worried doesn't make it much easier.

There are too many things going on, and I'm doing too many things at once for the level my brain is functioning at right now. Six months ago, the variety and complexity and volume of what I got done today would have been no big deal, but these days it feels like a ridiculously large effort to accomplish my typical workload, and I get frustrated with how long it takes me to do things that I *know* don't take me this long: doing analyses, writing things up, answering questions for clients, multi-tasking constantly while keeping the foreground of my mind focused to get each thing done. Yet today's frustration is during what will probably be my best physical state for the next eight or nine months! I can't even imagine right now how I'll get through a day two weeks from now when I have chemically-induced fatigue, as opposed to whatever they call what I'm in right now, which is just plain stressed, I guess.

There's still sooooo much to be done before Monday: getting Marco's house ready, packing and closing up my house (leaving my cats behind, man that sucks, it's been so nice to be back with them on my desk today after I've being gone nearly a week with travel and stuff), more doctors appointments, doing my tenacity thing to make sure they all have all the pathology reports and test results and whatever they need to make sure my chemo is right and as non-heart damaging as possible, hoping they can do something about the growing numbness in my right hand from the lymph node removals in my first surgery, and another surgery on Friday to put in the port (port-a-cath? whatever they call the thing that they're inserting below my collarbone in order for them to do my chemo and draw blood through and all that). This means that, even if I'm allowed to drive on the pain meds this weekend, I probably won't really be in any condition to be packing or loading things into the car to take to Marco's. Heck, now that I think about it, I couldn't do that tonight if I wanted to, with how my right side is still hurting. And as allergic as Marco is to cat dander, I am absolutely loathe to ask him to drive me out here again to help me (the one time he did come out here was a real mess for his allergies, although if I remember correctly, he also had forgotten to take allergy medicine that morning).

Writing about this stuff, though, getting it out of my head, has helped to put it in perspective and clear away some of the foggy darkness that I had felt coming. Interesting. I mean, I've always journaled, but it's not usually so immediately self-correcting. (You know *that* from how long it took me to journal and think through to decide about where to do chemo, staying at Marco's versus staying with my parents in Nebraska. Then again, that was a little more complex than a bit of potential oncoming depression.) At any rate, journaling through this is a pretty interesting experience both for myself and for all the people reading my story and experiencing it with me.

Chapter 8.
Gene Testing

CANCER—DAY 47 WEDNESDAY, JUNE 10, 2009

Holy cow. So my MUGA was good and the FISH wasn't positive, and today Dr. Lombard told us that I don't necessarily have to go through chemo! He's issuing another test on the surgery tissue, an oncotype test. This is apparently a very expensive test (I hope my insurance is really good and not just OK). The oncotype test checks a panel of 21 genes in the tumor to establish a Recurrence Score that is exactly that, a score of the probability of a recurrence within ten years.

Now, one thing to keep in mind is the thing that Dr. Sloe (the first medical oncologist I met with) brought up about the positive hormone receptors and how that pathology tells us that the cancer feeds on estrogen & progesterone, which tells them that my cancer will definitely recur. It could be in 20-30 years, but it will happen.

One specific new stat that Dr. Lombard mentioned, which I hadn't found in my research, was the specifics on how rare breast cancer is in someone my age. Instead of a one in eight chance (12.5%), which is how many women will get breast cancer during their lifetime, for a woman my age the probability of getting breast cancer is one in *six hundred* (0.16%), less than two-tenths of one percent of women.

Dr. Lombard also told Marco and I about a clinical trial that I can participate in to help advance breast cancer research. It's designed to further the oncotype research so that fewer women are unnecessarily treated with aggressive chemotherapy when it won't actually help prevent a recurrence at all. So this oncotype recurrence score tells us how likely my cancer is to recur within ten years, which (I think) is already five years past the time period in which chemo is known to be effective (I think it's five years for chemo, anyway). And here's the really wild part: if my recurrence score is 26 or higher, then they know with certainty that chemo will contribute to reducing my recurrence risk. And if my recurrence score is 10 or lower, they know with certainty that chemo has absolutely NO impact in improving my likelihood of survival and I won't have to do it! So, let's all put really positive energy towards my recurrence score being really, really low.

The clinical trial is for the in-between range, for those recurrence scores of 11 through 25, where they don't have any clinical evidence one way or the other regarding whether chemo is beneficial, or if women can just take Tamoxifen without doing chemotherapy. The way the trial works is that I have to agree, before knowing my recurrence score, that I will be in the trial. Then, if my recurrence score is 10 or lower, I go on Tamoxifen only, but if my recurrence score is 26 or higher I go on chemo and Tamoxifen. If my score is between 11 and 25, then a computer's random generator will determine whether I am to have chemo or not.

There are a couple of issues I have with this. I'm really glad that Marco was with me at this appointment, because he and I were looking at it from different perspectives. I was thinking about it all in terms of the possibility that I would have a score on the high end of the range, say 25, and then the computer would randomly select me to NOT have chemo. The problem with this option is that, if I were in control of the decision, I would probably have chosen, with a 25 recurrence score, to go ahead with chemo, rather than risk a recurrence that I could have prevented by getting chemotherapy. Marco looked at it from the opposite perspective, which was, what if I come back with a score in the low range, like 11, and the computer assigns me to chemo? He's really concerned about me not being on my heart medication and what to do if I have an episode where my heart stops without the medication that I normally take every 12 hours. And he doesn't want me to put myself at risk of that for a low score where I would choose, if it were my choice, not to have chemo.

But I completely understand the research and how important it is for them to get women to participate in these types of clinical trials, and I really want to contribute to the advancement of a cure for breast cancer. Ach—the agony of big decisions. I was sooooo ready for a break from big decisions when we thought I would be starting chemo on Monday. But now, here we are, another really big decision to make regarding my care and treatment. Do I want to risk participating in the trial and being randomly selected for an option I wouldn't choose for myself?

Sheesh, I'm such a hypocrite, eh? I finally got what I wanted, a doctor specialized in breast cancer and the leading edge in research and developments in the field, and now I'm mentally resisting getting involved in a clinical trial he's offered to me.

CANCER—DAY 48 THURSDAY, JUNE 11, 2009

I called Marshall Cancer Center this morning and told them that I'm not going to do the clinical trial. I just couldn't stomach the idea of being randomly selected for chemo when I wouldn't have done it, or randomly selected not to have chemo when I would have opted for it. I also called the place that does the oncotype test to make sure it's covered by my insurance, because I guess this test is really expensive (they said "thousands of dollars" yesterday), but they have a contract with my insurance company so that's all good. Now, in two weeks I'll see Dr. Lombard again and find out what my recurrence score is, and then we'll know with much greater certainty whether or not chemo is going to do me any good. And if I'm still in the gray area where they're not sure, well, then I'll have to take into consideration the fact that I will have to come off of my heart medication for chemo, find out what level the recurrence score is at, and make my decision. Oh, and we're still following up on the medical history of my birth mother and her family to find out if there is a history of breast cancer. I don't know if we'll be able to get that information in time, so I'm still thinking about getting the other genetic test done to see if I have the BRAC 1 or BRAC 2 gene that shows a hereditary inclination for breast cancer, which I think would possibly skew me toward being slightly more aggressive about choosing chemo if my recurrence score is in the mid-range where I will have to choose.

Then again, my recurrence score could be a 10 or less, and then we know for sure that chemo won't help prevent a recurrence.

We're in a holding pattern again, and unsettled again. It's a relief not to have to start chemo on Monday, and I'm honestly ridiculously relieved that I have two more weeks to work and get the market report done and out to clients, because I felt so bad dumping that on my company; it bothered me to know that the report would either be late or of lesser quality than in the past if I were suddenly away the last two weeks of the modeling and report cycle.

I didn't have any doctor's appointments scheduled today, but I ended up going out to El Dorado Hills to Dr. Allondry's (the plastic surgeon) this afternoon. Both of my surgery incisions had under-the-skin absorbing stitches, but the incision on my breast had a little bit of stitching poking out, which had started getting pulled by my clothes when I moved. Today it started to sting and look red, like it might be getting infected. Marco thought we should just pull it out, but a little bit of the knot was showing under my skin. I didn't want to take a chance that we may pull on a stitch that wasn't quite done dissolving (since I'm a bleeder). So Dr. Allondry took it out, and covered the area with an antiseptic goo that's also supposed to help the scar. Plus, he wants me to massage the scar tissue to help it heal. Ugh, the scar under my arm from the lymph node removal is sooo sensitive; I am loathe to press on it to work the scar tissue. But it's sooooo hard and swollen and scarred right now that it could be affecting the nerves. Dr. Lombard said it's not uncommon to have some temporary nerve issues in the arm after having lymph nodes removed, but that the numbness generally goes away. I hope so, because my poor right hand has taken a beating, getting bumped and scratched and nicked because I can't feel it very well. It's hard to be careful of.

CANCER—DAY 49 FRIDAY, JUNE 12, 2009

The usual—I was up at 5:30 a.m. Well, 2:30 a.m. really, but I finally got out of bed at 5:30 a.m. I do like the quiet of the early morning, but I'd still rather be sleeping until the sun is actually rising. After a busy morning of conference calls, with my back sore from sitting at the dining room table to work, I was glad to get out at lunch. We found a desk, well, a table really, today at IKEA. I'd never been to IKEA before Marco took me—it's crazy! Tons of people buying furniture in a row of checkout stands, like a huge Walmart on steroids or something. The "desk" I bought was really easy to put together, though, and now I have a workspace at the back of the house.

CANCER—DAY 50 SATURDAY, JUNE 13, 2009

Wow, 50 days since diagnosis. Still less than two months. That's so wild; it feels like it's been more like six months since this all started.

It's a relief to unexpectedly have had at least a couple more weeks post-surgery before treatments and stuff get started. And I'm pretty much not sick anymore with that nasty cold, so now it's as though I get back those two weeks that I thought I would get to have before chemo, after all. Today we ran errands for house stuff to make Marco's place more, umm, livable, for me. A toaster (toaster oven, actually, which is something I've never used in my life, but hey, as long as I can have toast with my eggs again, a toaster oven instead of a toaster is just fine with me), a fan for my office (wow, does it get hot at the back of the house), a wall mirror for the bedroom (guys obviously don't need to look in a full-length mirror to decide if a particular pair of shoes looks cute with a particular dress before they go out dancing), a laundry hamper . . .

"I need one too, right?" Marco looked puzzled then said, "No." Now I'm puzzled. I had considered just taking my dirty clothes home every week and doing my laundry there, but that didn't seem like something Marco would expect me to do. It's just the kind of thing I think about—little Miss Independent. "We only need one," he tells me. This had never occurred to me. Share a laundry basket? Wow, the things I am naïve about are truly astounding, eh? All the years I lived with Artie, I would throw his clothes in the machine with mine and vice versa, sure, but I always had my own laundry basket. (Then again, Artie had THE stinkiest feet on the planet—we had to put his socks inside a plastic bag inside his hamper inside the closet, otherwise they would have contaminated the entire bedroom! Before we lived together, Artie would put his socks outside of my apartment door at night, the smell was so bad. Right after he died, one of the few really good laughs his siblings and I had was remembering how stinky his feet would get in those old black sneakers, ruining all his socks.)

The idea of combining clothes in one laundry hamper at Marco's hadn't even occurred to me. So now I'm thinking in the store about how I have two baskets at home, one for whites and one for darks, and how I wash everything in cold and hang almost everything to dry rather than putting much in the dryer. I'm wondering how the heck I'm going to either let someone else wash my clothes, or else include theirs with mine. (I am notorious for only washing clothes every six weeks or so when I finally run out of underwear. It's a good thing I have two bedrooms in my house, because I always seem to have one bed buried in clean not-yet-folded laundry!) And it's not like we'd get our clothes confused by sharing the laundry basket, but it still felt weird to imagine throwing my clothes in with someone else's laundry. All this flashes through my mind in an instant and I ask Marco, "Can we have a separate one for lights and one for darks?" He laughs at me, shaking his head a little, "all right."

Not under the pressure of starting chemo immediately, now the whole preparing-to-live-at-Marco's-for-treatment thing suddenly has a different vibe. It feels more like a moving-in-with-Marco kind of vibe that I hadn't really paid any attention to before, if it was even there. I couldn't quite get my mind around that today. So much so, that tired as I was, I couldn't nap this afternoon because I was anxious about this "moving in together" feeling. I've managed to emotionally stay away from this kind of relationship for more than five years now.

I haven't brought it up with Marco in any detail, but this anxiety I was suddenly having was about it feeling like moving in together instead of just staying with him so he can care for me during treatment. I'm not quite sure how to bring it up with him. Either he's already comfortable with the idea of living together or he's thinking, like I had been all along, that it's temporary and that I'll go home to my old quiet life at my property when all this treatment stuff is over. But Marco doesn't act like that, like he expects me to leave after it's over. It's more the opposite—it's more like he's assumed me into his life, like, permanently. He's always using "we" and "us" in conversation with other people when making plans to do things now, instead of "I" this and "I" that. And this was fun because of how happy he seemed to be . . .last weekend he said that I'm growing on him, that he's getting used to having me around all the time. This was after some of the more difficult conversations we had a while back about relationship commitment. Back then he wanted to be my caregiver during treatment but he was supposedly still open to the possibility of meeting and dating someone else. He never says anything like that anymore, and he's acting like I am a permanent fixture in his life. The shift in his attitude was pretty sudden to me, and I am a little wary of it, afraid to trust him. Then again, I have a hard time trusting anyone other than my parents, period.

So anyway, I'm wondering about whether I should try to talk to Marco about these feelings, and how, but I'm also realizing that it doesn't have to be a big thing, that it's not really something that has to be "talked about" and a resolution found. Maybe I'll ask him tomorrow how he feels about it, but we already know we're doing this living arrangement during treatment, however long that is, and there will certainly be enough time to worry about the real *living together* side of things later after my cancer treatments are over. Meanwhile, the big picture is that I'm just lucky to have him and to be here, and once in a while I have to remind myself of that. Things could be worse.

You know, there are these times where I just have to get over myself, get out of my own way, and not think about everything so much. I've told my parents more than once about how my life always works itself out for the best if I just get out of my own way and let it happen, not try to "make" things happen. It's also kind of true of the way I analyze things. I ponder stuff and let it turn over and around in my mind, but the more I can let go of worrying about what it is or how it will turn out, the more enjoyable things are and the more they seem to work out for the best. Don't get me wrong, I still think it's important to make a concerted effort to be a good person: kind, generous, forgiving, patient (note, I didn't say that I *am* any of those things, but I do *try* to be). Still, much as my mind turns on and around these issues of what's going on in my life and my feelings on all of that, when it comes down to doing anything, I still try to tell myself to just try to be a good person, to experience the path life is leading, and to not create any more pain in this world where so many people say and do so many hurtful things in so many small ways all the time. Life isn't a problem to solve; it's a journey to experience.

CANCER—DAY 51 SUNDAY, JUNE 14, 2009

Marco's out in the garage doing "man stuff," rearranging things so he can set up his workshop. I went out running more errands to set up my office. I'd rather get some of this done on my own, rather than wasting Marco's time with it. And we shop differently; he's a lot more careful about scrutinizing his final selection to make sure it's as cost-effective as possible—no money wasted on features he may not need. I tend to find what I'm looking for, decide fairly quickly if I think the price is reasonable, and then get the hell out of the store with my purchase. I hate shopping! I find what I went into the store for, and get out again as quickly as possible; that's how I shop.

We went to a birthday party last night for Ryan, who is basically the instigator of the wine club that Marco is, no wait, that "we" are in, and so the birthday party was for a friend of "ours," to use Marco's vernacular. Anyway, besides the whole we're-a-couple-not-just-two-separate-individuals way of talking that I'm finding so amusing and heart-warming in Marco's conversational vocabulary, there are also a couple of neat little things or stories to write about. I was ready for the party in a summer party dress, but before we left, Marco said the party was casual and that I should change into jeans instead. I was bummed about it because this is a great festive little dress, not fancy at all just fun, but he knows the crowd better than I do, so I changed. And of course then I am the only girl in jeans, and everyone is wearing either dresses or skirts. Oh well. I get nervous about going to these things where the people are Marco's friends outside the tango community so I'm just meeting them socially as Marco's girlfriend, which I don't dislike per se, but it's hard to do. It's like business networking but trying to avoid my typical networking conversation questions "What do you do?" or "What got you interested in supply chain management?" Of course, in business networking you often know what it is you are trying to learn or create interest in, and I'm not seeing much translation to blind social networking there.

I got off to a fine start at the party . . . I was the first person to spill red wine. I wasn't the last, and luckily it was on the lawn instead of inside the house on the white carpet, but still! I was holding a plate and a glass of wine, and was trying to balance the plate and glass while trying to eat. This obviously required more dexterity than I am capable of at the moment. And of course I managed to spill my wine on the skirt of the woman I was talking to, Misha. Luckily it was a red dress! We went inside and rinsed it with cold water and used a blow dryer on it (cold blast only—stay away from using heat on wine stains), and after it was all dry later you couldn't even tell. What a relief; I felt terrible about that. So, that's how I met Misha, who was really interesting and fun to talk to, and now of course we'll never forget that we met at Ryan's birthday party.

I also had an interesting conversation with Lisa, who I remember meeting and dancing with at the last wine party a month ago. I didn't recognize a lot of people from the wine party to Ryan's birthday party, but Lisa was one of the ones I remembered (though admittedly Marco had to remind me of her name). We ended up having an interesting conversation about breast cancer (she's five-year survivor, almost), and she was very interested in the details of my treatment (she's also a doctor, a dermatologist) and she has a very supportive and caring personality (wouldn't it be great if all medical professionals had those characteristics?).

After it became dark, there was dancing. Mostly salsa, and some club music. At the beginning of the salsa dancing, I was standing a bit away from the patio with Marco, just enjoying the music and chatting a little, when Marco saw Lisa looking around from where she was dancing on the patio and, seeing Marco, waving and exclaiming "Where's my salsa partner?" So Marco gives my back a little nudge, and I go and lead Lisa for a salsa. Man, I have GOT to increase my repertoire of salsa moves. (Just like all of my students say!) I know a lot of salsa patterns, but I can't lead very many of them well while going full tempo! I need to practice leading someone slowly first, just like my students do, to get comfortable doing my more complicated moves out in public. But it was great fun anyway. Lisa gets such a kick out of a simple underarm turn; I think she was making the other girls want to do it too, because there weren't any guys there who led salsa (I would have loved to be led in a real salsa myself!). Then for the next song, Marco came out on the patio and we free styled together, which was tons of fun. He's so uninhibited in that kind of dancing; it's just a blast. He has no problem with doing something that other people would be self-conscious doing (in case they looked silly). He hams it up and has so much fun, which makes him so great to dance with regardless of whether he "knows" salsa or anything else. We mess around and do silly stuff, but we can also move together and "shake a tail feather" just having a great ol' time. I get a kick out of seeing him dancing with anyone and everyone, just this free, happy person. Misha (my new red wine red dress friend) commented on it later. She said something about how Marco and I have a good energy together on the dance floor. She seems pretty dialed in to that sort of thing, the energy stuff, and she and I got into some of that a little late in the evening. I was sitting with Marco on the couch (Marco was "trapping" people coming in the door by snapping photos from behind my shoulders), and Misha came to talk with me. We ended up talking about her husband, whom she's been separated from for a year and a half now but he's coming to Sacramento tomorrow, and we talked about some of the feelings she's having about that. We got into the same space somehow, just a great energy connection. Very interesting.

CANCER—DAY 52 MONDAY, JUNE 15, 2009

Good grief, what's wrong with me? Why am I awake six of eight hours in a night? And—this is rich—Marco was complaining about how he didn't sleep well either, that he kept waking up and being too hot because of me and then too cold with just the light blanket.

Sheesh, I could have knocked him upside the head. I was *there*, I know he slept well through the night, and I know it was only his own snoring that woke him up a little. I know that *he* was the one holding onto *me* so I couldn't get away to let the heat escape, and I know how soundly he was sleeping (and snoring) when I got up at 2 a.m. and when I came back at 5 a.m. And he's complaining to me about not getting enough sleep?

Partly, I just miss my cats, and my home, and my stuff. That's ironic. Here I am thinking that I have such a great attitude about not being stuck on "things" while complaining about missing them at the same time. Then again, Mizzou has been with me for more than ten years. I definitely miss him. After I've been in Sac four or five days (or longer) I start to feel like I've left an awful lot of myself behind, living out of a suitcase as it were. It will be different now, though, going in to treatment, I think. I've bought some stuff for the office, so I feel like there's a little space that's mine. And I like the idea of being within earshot and/or line of sight to Marco across the back of the house when I'm in treatment and also trying to work. If anything were to happen (the big worry being if I keel over from my heart condition if I have to do chemo and stop my heart medicine during that time), he would know right away. So, things are getting more settled for me at Marco's, but this week, now that I'm strong enough to lift things into Rubi (my bright green "electric lime" Jeep Rubicon), I need to box up some clothes to keep at Marco's for the summer.

In the meantime, I am really relieved to be home tonight, as well as all day and evening tomorrow. All day I'd been stressed somehow, wishing I were home instead of in Sac. So when I finally got through Placerville where the landscape starts looking like home, I stopped just past the river to do a trail walk and clear my head a little. I should have done that this morning down in Sac instead of trying to work through—a walk would probably have done me a lot of good, just to get me out of the office for twenty minutes. But anyway, after the walk down by Placerville, the rest of the drive home was more relaxed. Now that I'm finally really winding down I'm even feeling the lack-of-sleep tension easing.

But, let's face it. Waiting on this gene test . . . delayed on making a decision about chemo . . . I am getting more and more stressed. Sigh. What can you do? It is what it is.

CANCER—DAY 54 WEDNESDAY, JUNE 17, 2009

I've been up since 3:30 a.m., without hope for more sleep (it's about 6 a.m. now, so I have another ninety minutes before I need to go wake Marco up for work). For some reason, I couldn't sleep because my mind is circling around the "why me?" thing. The most positive "why me" could be considered altruistic . . . if it is me, then it's not someone else, and I'd rather suffer myself than make or see anyone else suffer.

Then there's the karmic perspective. Mom got me really thinking about it because in one of her difficult moments of frustration last week on the phone she got a little agitated and said, "But you just don't *deserve* this."

Well, the short "why me" answer to that, from a karmic view, is that, somehow, I do deserve this. I clearly have some things to learn, such as not sacrificing my heath to work and career. Sure, I had a skyrocketing early career, but I worked insanely hard to make that happen and keep it going, and my health suffered, if not as a result, then by correlation. Someone could definitely say there are some "just desserts" going on here if you look at the imbalance I generally have between work and life.

What I told my mom, when she said I don't deserve this, was: "Look at it this way. One in eight women are diagnosed with breast cancer in their life. If you line up the eight women in our immediate family—me, you, your sister, your mother, your sister in law, your daughter in law, and my two nieces—of this group of eight females in our family, who has the most inner strength and determination? Who would be the most likely to survive cancer? Of the eight of us, Mom, it can only be me. I don't think I deserve it any more than you do, I think, but the truth is that if I were forced to pick one of the eight of us to have cancer, I would choose me. I'm young, I'm strong, I'm determined, and I'm already a survivor. I survived the car crashes, I survived Artie's death, and I even survived multiple heart failures! Of the eight of us, I have the best prospect of survival. Besides, I would much rather suffer the worst cancer has to offer than to have someone else in our immediate family diagnosed with the disease. I would hate for someone else in our family to go through this." And I ended my little speech to Mom with "You know, it could always be worse."

For myself though, "why me" isn't necessarily about all that. I mean, it's true, if I could have cancer in place of another female in my family, I would take it. But my mind is focusing on another perspective for "why me"—to learn from it.

Mostly what I wonder about is how to be a good, kind, caring person, supportive of anyone around me who needs encouragement or support, even while going through this thing. I have been practicing kindness, compassion, and generosity for years and I've grown as a person but I know I can do more. And now I have this opportunity to take that to an entirely new level, one I never could have achieved without a severe life trial at this time in my life. It's one thing to try to be kind, compassionate, and giving simply because that's the person you want to be. But if there is a single ultra-positive "why me" to this whole thing, it is the personal growth that may occur if I can be kind, compassionate, and thoughtful of others when I'm suffering more than I thought imaginable.

There's a lot more to think about here. I have to keep reminding myself that I'm not just surviving, I am trying to survive and grow as a person. I'm still on the same three characteristics that have been my focus for the past several years—kindness, compassion, generosity—but now I have the opportunity to try to be those things while suffering physically. To be kind, generous and compassionate to others even when you're in severe pain, well, that's the kind of person I want to be. I don't know how to do that per se, but it's the goal, nonetheless.

CANCER—DAY 55 THURSDAY, JUNE 18, 2009

I noticed two pretty major failings in my personality this week, things that I know about myself and I think I'm improving on, but I'm far from actually having ingrained the desired behavioral change. Not that I only have two personality flaws, there are plenty . . . ridiculously independent, over-analytical, over-achiever, workaholic . . . the list goes on and on and on. Anyway, two are bothering me right now . . .

One problem is that I find it incredibly difficult to ask for favors or to specifically ask someone to do something for me. I was raised to keep an eye about, always looking for some little thing to do to make someone else feel special or to help them out a little. My mom is like that, to the extreme. The little things I see her do to make other people feel good are just phenomenal—never something that would have occurred to the person to ask her for. But I'm afraid to ask Marco the kinds of questions that will lead to him doing anything for me that isn't absolutely necessary, as that might inconvenience him in the least little bit.

The other area in which I continue to disappoint myself is the way I get in dating-type relationships. I always let the guy's life supersede my own. It will be very interesting to see how these two personal issues work themselves out over the next many months.

Oh, and—today's highlight! I can raise my right arm straight above my head again, with just a little pull in the scar tissue. But heck, a week ago I couldn't raise my arm higher than my shoulder. Finally! Not much pain anymore either, unless I accidentally try to press out of that arm to sit up or roll over in bed. No lifting yet, but it can hold some weight now, too. Uff da, I'd forgotten how nice it is to be able to stretch your arms when your back and neck hurt from working at the computer too long!

CANCER—DAY 57 SATURDAY, JUNE 20, 2009

I have this red dress. Well, OK, I have several red dresses, and admittedly, most of them are pretty sexy. I'm a dancer, what can I say? Then again, what red dress *isn't* sexy? But last night I wore the one that I know, from past experience in salsa clubs, well, this red dress has an effect. I didn't know if the milonga we were going to was casual or dressy, but this dress works either way. So . . . a couple funny red dress stories for you from the milonga last night . . .

One is about the woman apparently hitting on Marco. It was very close to the end of the night, around 1:45 a.m., and I don't know when she sat down, but there was this woman next to Marco while I was dancing. Sitting with her shoulder a little behind Marco so that she could sit really close to him, she was putting her head on his shoulder, etc., and it made me laugh out loud on the dance floor because of the look on Marco's face when she did that. I swear she looked like she was trying to find a way to hold his hand, or at least his leg! And Marco was sitting there, tired, ready to leave, stone-faced with his arms over his legs and his hands together, apparently not interested in the nonverbal situation she was going for. And not smiling, which *really* isn't like Marco at a milonga, unless it's late and past time to go home. Anyway, I saw this from the dance floor for a couple of songs, and when the tanda was over, I went to get my water bottle (which conveniently was right under Marco's chair) and I said something innocuous to him like, "How's it going?" Then I knelt at the other side of his chair to drink my water and watch the dance floor, and it was like she just evaporated or something, poof! I turned my head and she was gone. Marco patted the seat she had vacated for me to sit with him, and put his arm around me and held my hand, and, well, we sat together like that for the last tanda, tired and just enjoying the moment and watching the dancing. I'm sorry to be making fun of this woman, but it was just soooo funny how she just disappeared as soon as she saw me come close and realized that I was who Marco was with.

So, anyway, back to the outfit. I was wearing the sexy red dress, and my first tandas were with Marco and then Dave—for the rest of the night I only had one set of tandas with someone I know from Sacramento, and the rest were all guys I didn't know. They're all really different. Some lead snappy moves, some try to be, ummm . . . let's call it, "sensual" (one guy actually tried to lead me to grind—talk about tacky). Others actually get the meaning of tango and feel the music and move their bodies to it (those are the guys I can consider tangueros). So . . . the red dress has a flippy knee-length skirt that can flash, you know, a little more than knee, and with some guys it was like they were waving a red flag out there on the dance floor. Though I wasn't paying attention and didn't actually catch anyone doing this myself . . . I was apparently turning a lot of heads. Sarah told me on the way home that more than once between songs while she was chatting with a guy on the dance floor, he would actually turn his head to watch me walk by. She'd tease them for being, whatever . . . "guys," and they were like "Sorry, blond in a red dress, can't . . . not . . .look." And in telling me about it, she was like, "And it happened more than once!" We had a great laugh over that one after the milonga.

CANCER—DAY 58 SUNDAY, JUNE 21, 2009

Now THAT was cool! This was a side of Marco I haven't seen before, and he seemed to be in his element.

My new aquarium didn't come with the plumbing necessary to connect it to the aquarium. Lucky for me, unbelievably lucky for me, Marco is what you would call "handy." In this case "handy" is about the biggest understatement possible. The guy is amazing when it comes to this sort of thing. He was analyzing, working out all the different couplings and adaptors and valves and everything we needed (that I didn't have a clue about), and (I found this terribly amusing) when we went to Home Depot, he was like a kid in a candy store. Then we got home and sat down on the floor piecing it together. He was seriously in his game; he loves to tinker with stuff, and it was so neat to see him completely engaged and enjoying himself in this project! It makes me look forward to him finishing the setup of his workshop in the garage because it will be so good for him to go out there and tinker around. My dad has a workshop in the garage, and it's a similar thing. Dad just enjoys making stuff—mostly woodcarvings these days—but his workshop is the talk of the town because he has so many cool machines and "man stuff."

Oh, and here was my freak out, this-relationship-has-gone-too-far-too-fast moment of the weekend . . . after hours and hours of running around getting stuff for the aquarium (which also required a drive out to my house in Volcanoville to pick up the pump that had been mis-delivered) and doing other errands, we finally got back to Marco's. By the time we pulled into the driveway, I was sooo tired, and I caught myself in a thought that startled me. Marco noticed something in my body language and asked, "What?"Guess I'll tell him; what can it hurt to say it out loud . . ."I was just thinking that it's a relief to be home—which feels weird, because we're not at *my* home."

Ya gotta love these little gems from Marco . . . he replied, "Well, you have two homes now."

Chapter 9.
A New Rhythm

CANCER—DAY 59 MONDAY, JUNE 22, 2009

Ohmygodohmygodohmygod . . .two phone calls in the last hour . . .

1) adoption search agency—my biological aunt had breast cancer and my biological father died of lung cancer, so I do have some biological history of cancer, but it's not huge.

2) Dr. Lombard's office—the oncotype result won't be ready until July 7, two more weeks from now.

Two more weeks of waiting for chemo to start. . . or not. But—at least we'll know if it's going to help, and which cell-destroying chemo drugs will be most "effective" instead of just automatically doing the full standard chemo treatment that other oncologist, Dr. Sloe, was going to put me through.

In a sad workaholic kind of way, I'm relieved to get a little more time to work before chemo starts. This is just the worst darn month to leave off work.

CANCER—DAY 60 TUESDAY, JUNE 23, 2009

So I'm at Marco's, and it's a normal workday. OK, I'm a little slow after a long day and getting the draft report finished and sent out last night, but anyway we're both working in our little office rooms at the back of the house. It's late morning, and the doorbell rings. Not an especially common occurrence around here, not that I've noticed, anyway. Marco gets up to answer it, but then goes back in his office saying "Not expecting anyone." Apparently they get a few more solicitors down here than I do out in Volcanoville. I told him the only solicitors I've had were people trying to sell me Jesus, twice! I told them I went to Catholic school (not that that actually tells you a whit about my spirituality today, except that I apparently still have issues with anyone trying to tell me what to believe, given my attitude about people who push their belief systems onto others), and sticking to the point that I have read and heard plenty of the Bible and I just don't need someone else telling me how to interpret it, so that pretty much took care of the bible thumpers at my house. Except that they come back again once a year. Just in case I've lost my way and need to find Jesus, of course. So anyway, back to today's story, Marco didn't answer the door.

Then my phone rings. I'm too slow to pick it up, and it goes to voicemail. The message is from a florist saying they just tried to deliver flowers to me at Marco's address. Guess we'll have to start answering the door!!!

They left the flowers on the front porch bench, though, so we didn't have to go get them or reschedule delivery. They were from a friend of mine in Tennessee, who I see maybe once a year at a work QBR or something—how cool is that? I mean, if you have to get cancer, it might as well have this effect of bringing you more in touch with people you've always enjoyed and respected but have possibly lost touch with. And I've met lots of new people because of my illness, particularly breast cancer survivors who get referred to my blog by someone who knows me, and who want to share their experiences and empathy. I have at least one cyber friend now who I just have to make an effort to meet up with at a milonga sometime. We may never have met in person if I hadn't started the blog and she hadn't written to me after reading it.

A closing note on the flowers: at least here in Sac they don't have to be delivered in a box via FedEx or UPS like at my house in the forest, and they have a better chance of survival. (Mizzou and Seoul aren't here to eat them!)

CANCER—DAY 61 WEDNESDAY, JUNE 24, 2009

It's interesting that I find myself behaving somewhat differently in this relationship than in any other. Not really *acting* differently, so much as, well, reacting a little less to things that normally bother me in a relationship. I'm starting to think that the difference is in part because of the known or expected duration that we've already committed to regarding my living here for cancer treatment. And in the interest of not making the next several months an unbearably messy living situation, I think twice (usually) before reacting to something, or I give the benefit of the doubt more often, wait things out more, try to be more patient, and let things settle into their own rhythm before figuring out whether or not I can dance to that rhythm or if I really do need a slightly different tempo or beat. The old me would have been shaping things along the way, molding. Not that one way is necessarily better than another, but this definitely feels different—it's kind of an assumed in-it-for-the-long-haul commitment. And I started wondering . . . back when people made marriages work for a lifetime, did they have more of this attitude that I'm experiencing now?

Sometimes I think of my life as what it is at this moment, essentially an extended-but-can-still-be-considered-temporary living arrangement, and what it will be when I can "go home" after all the cancer treatments are over. Other times, I feel like we're assuming or treating this as more indefinite, to whatever point in the future it reaches. But, for example, before I bought the aquarium, I first measured where it would go in my house in Volcanoville, and I also made sure it would fit in my "office" at Marco's, which is really the place I bought it for, initially so I can hear the waterfall sound while I'm working during treatment. But it was important to me to be sure of where the aquarium would go, to make sure it would fit back at my own house, which is typical of my old way of not letting myself depend on anyone too much or count on anyone or anything as unending. A woman of the new millennium? Independent, self-sufficient . . . tenacious . . .

Marco and I were talking last weekend about relationships (I think it was about marriage or life-long relationships in particular) and how individuals change and grow over time. If you're looking at your marriage and trying to force your spouse to stay the same person as five or ten years ago, when you were married, I wonder how happy your spouse can be with that. People mature and grow over that time, but we expect them to still be who they were ten years ago. Marco and I agreed that long-term relationships can only work long-term if you allow each other to change and grow, and to still be individuals. I think that we should be supportive of and appreciate that change and growth in each other, too. Maybe then people wouldn't say they've "outgrown" each other, and loving someone could actually span a lifetime because you love who they become for what they are, rather than for what you wanted them to be (which they're not).

In general, I don't think we as people appreciate each other enough. Sure, people appreciate when you do what they want, but that's not really appreciation now, is it? One of the things I've tried to be especially cognizant of, in the last few years especially, is to appreciate people for who they are rather than thinking they should be something they're not. You know, like whenever you think a thought about someone that starts with "if only . . ." I try to stop myself right there and remember what it is that is appreciable in this person, instead of focusing on what's missing or lacking. I guess there could be a fine line between letting someone be who they are and letting them be something they shouldn't—for example, if you were in an abusive or otherwise dysfunctional relationship. Or being starved emotionally because you never tell the person that you desperately need to be held at night, or need to be thanked for doing something for them, or whatever. At some point, I guess we have to realize that the person he or she really is might not be good for us or isn't right for us.

Or maybe that's backwards. Maybe the fact that we change and grow is exactly why we can't be with the same person long-term, because we change in such a way that the person is no longer good for us. Or they change in such a way that we're no longer good for them. Hmmm, that wouldn't explain my parents, though. They've been married like 40 years and still have a fabulous relationship now that they're both retired. (They hold hands walking at the mall, how cute is that?)

Which sort of brings me back around to the original thought. It's hard to describe. I'm not *trying* harder in this relationship, exactly . . .but in a way I am. I'm trying to be more . . . pliable, more flexible, more accepting. Even without chemo, we know the radiation treatment will mean two months straight of Cancer Girl. And I know I'm a handful! Marco's really a hero and a saint throughout all of this cancer stuff, when you look at it a certain way.

Like Monday, when I received the two phone calls back to back—about the biological history of some cancer, and that the oncotype test won't be ready for another two weeks—so we still won't know if that reliability score puts me in the clear to not have chemo. Marco was busy with work and on the phone. I didn't want to interrupt him, but I couldn't keep in all the emotions brought on by the phone calls, so I blogged a tiny note on Monday and wrote something on my Facebook wall. Then I forced myself back to my report for work, because there was nothing else I could do. The report had to get done, Marco couldn't get away at the moment, and I honestly didn't want to talk about it, anyway. If my Mom had spontaneously called at that moment, I wouldn't have answered the phone. A simple hug would have been perfect, though. I was in a kind of state of shock after those two calls, and the only thing to do at that moment was to get back to work. A little while after Marco got off the phone, though, maybe half an hour later, he came over and hugged me from behind my chair, just that type of comforting hug that lets me know I'm not alone in this thing. Which of course put me over the edge, and then the tears came. He didn't say anything, just held me like that until I calmed down again, petted my arms reassuringly, and then he kissed me on the head and went back over to his office.

We didn't actually talk for quite a while after that, but in the early evening I turned to face him from my office, and when he looked over I said, "You know, I'm really glad I was here today. I'm glad that I wasn't home alone today." He nodded in understanding.

And now we have another two weeks of me being on edge and getting more anxious with each passing day, waiting for the day we find out about the oncotype reliance score thing, and chemo. There's no reason the unknowing should keep getting more burdensome, but I guess at the same time, why wouldn't it get more and more stressful? At any rate, that's what's going on. Marco still has a cold, and I'm so on edge that I can hardly stand myself sometimes. I don't sleep at night. I don't sleep during the day. I can't fall asleep. I can't nap. I start to feel like I'm assuming I won't have to do chemo; other times I find myself thinking I will, but I know that I can't plan either way—I have to just let it happen as it happens.

Talk about a life test! I've been through some very difficult times, but this situation definitely has some special trials for me. Life still has a LOT to teach me, that's for sure.

Quick side note . . .if you read my entry about the flowers delivery a couple days ago, you will appreciate how funny this is . . .

The doorbell just rang. Marco popped up from his desk, saying, "Flowers!" as he bustled to the front of the house to receive the new flowers for me.

But he came back chuckling and handed me a flyer and a little booklet. It had been a Jehovah's Witness at the door, selling him Jesus. Ach, the irony!!!

CANCER—DAY 62 THURSDAY, JUNE 25, 2009

This is cool . . . since the first biopsy in mid-April, more than two months ago, last night was the first relatively pain-free milonga I've had, and Jiminy Cricket, I had forgotten how much fun dancing is when you're not in pain or in fear of pain while doing it! And the longer I danced without the twinges of pain becoming more constant and severe (which is usually what happens), the less afraid I was of getting hurt by my partners and the more fun I had. Whew! I was starting to think that my dancing was just completely obliterated by all of this stress and pain and resultant lack of dancing, but I had a little glimpse of it again last night, a few moments of remembering what it's like to be dancing in my partner's music in the moment. I came home remembering that I was ridiculously relieved. It had started to seem like my dancing only got worse and worse each time I went, ever since the whole diagnosis thing, and I tell ya, it was to the point that I didn't even like going anymore. But I kept trying, hoping it would start to feel better again instead of getting worse and worse—I kept trying to remind myself how it felt, to not let myself forget that amazing kind of connection thing ("one heart, four legs") that we were having in those last few practices with Marco before my doctor found the lump and everything went crazy. Even just last Friday at SFTX (San Francisco Tango Exchange), I was still hurting enough that the fear of being led into sudden unexpected pain was keeping me incredibly stiff and resistant, completely unable to relax, which pretty much precludes anything akin to authentic Argentine Tango from taking place.

Now, don't go thinking that I'm suddenly my old self on the dance floor again, far from it, but at least last night I finally believed I'd get back there someday. The last month or so of milongas have been soooooo disappointing, I was getting really discouraged about dance altogether. I even had a period of time where I was like, "Well, who cares if there's no dancing in Nebraska where my parents live? It's not like I can dance anymore anyway." But, big sigh of relief, I will again someday. And if I'm really lucky, maybe I'll even get to Buenos Aires again for my birthday, if not this year, maybe next.

Chapter 10.
Chemo Limbo

Cancer—Day 63 Friday, June 26, 2009

You know, some days I just cannot pretend I'm fine. I wish I could, to make it easier on the people around me, but it's just not happening today. I finally gave up—I'm shutting down the computers, turning off the phone, and I am getting off the grid for a while. The underlying tension of this thing, of this cancer treatment *limbo* is just . . . sometimes . . . too much.

Cancer—Day 64 Saturday, June 27, 2009

Day 2 of waiting, and already the extended Cancer Treatment Limbo is creating tension that I do not know how to bear gracefully. You know who faces the brunt of my frustration . . . yet it's sadly comforting to me that Marco's frustrated by the wait, too. But his frustration is so . . . potent.

We had this "episode" tonight that started with me trying to tell him a couple things I'm having a little trouble with in the relationship, but the conversation turned into being all about *him*, and how I have too many "expectations" (like "expecting" him to come eat dinner with me when the food is ready, instead of staying at his video game for so long that I finish my dinner alone and then go for a walk to kill time). *I* have too many expectations, and *I* am the one taking it too personally when he's upset. It's hard to know whether he's directing his frustration at me, but he says he's not. Never mind that the very nature of the animosity behind his anger is what frightens me, regardless of where it's directed.

Somehow we're OK now, though, following a long walk after dinner and getting him to have some calm conversation while sitting on the front porch. Relationships can be so weird. Now he's playing World of Warcraft, and everything's apparently fine. Until the next blowup, at least.

Cancer—Day 65 Sunday, June 28, 2009

Well that worked out pretty well . . . Marco spent most of his afternoon and evening helping out some friends, and even though it's Sunday I needed to work—I didn't know when else I might have time to go home before our little weekend trip to Vegas (I'm taking Marco there for his birthday present) and I didn't want the cats to go more than a week without a refresh (and, and, and . . . yes, I am the queen of the run-on sentence, so sue me), so I went home to Volcanoville this afternoon.

I took the cats for a little walk partway down into my valley looking for cool dried wood and quartz stones for our aquariums, and that took all of five minutes . . . if there's something that's not lacking at my property, it's trees and rocks! I managed to drag that little task out to take half an hour though, then settled into my hammock to copy edit and verify numbers in the market report. Oy vey, those 80 pages all start looking the same, making it tough to cross-reference sums from Rick and me doing different analyses on the same (hopefully the same) data and then merging his pages back into the report.

On the upside, I may have been working all afternoon and evening on a Sunday, but it was more relaxing this way than in my little office room down in Sac. I was on the phone with my parents on the way out (hands-free, of course! It's not legal to hold a phone while you drive in California, you know, and I would never *ever* be caught doing something as reckless as texting while I drive). I told them I was going home to edit the report the old-fashioned way . . . lying in my hammock with the cats lounging around the back yard and coming over to get love when they felt like it. Hearing that made my parents happy.

Of course, when I went back inside with the cats and started cleaning up after them and getting stuff together to put in the car (I needed a suitcase for Vegas, and Mizzou knows the suitcase means travel), Mizzou went back to glaring at me from the top shelf of my desk. Mizzou used to bolt up the counter over the 'fridge and up to the top of the kitchen cabinets to lie behind my glass vases glaring at me because he didn't want to get in the cat carrier (he doesn't mind travel or the car per se—he lays in the back window regally surveying all that he commands—but he hates getting in the cat caddy to transfer from the house to the car).

Right now Mizzou seems to know that I'm not taking him with me, and that apparently has him pissed off. Sheesh, middle age doesn't suit Mizzou. Of course, he looks like he's put on a few pounds recently, which probably isn't helping his disposition, locked up in the house with annoying little Seoul always trying to play with him. Don't get me wrong, he definitely does better *with* her than *without* her (it only took three days of me being away when she was first here for Mizzou to realize that she was there to be a companion to him, not because I wanted him to share me with another cat after Kingsford died last year).

Anyway, the little escape today helped, and of course having an insanely busy workweek coming up will help distract me from the cancer-treatment-limbo annoyance. It also helped that we went for a walk after dinner last night and sat on the front porch for a while, talking about all this stuff. It was nice to be reminded that Marco believes we can handle this. When he's frustrated and it just projects outward from him in all directions, well, it's pretty discouraging.

CANCER—DAY 66 MONDAY, JUNE 29, 2009

You know, I haven't worked in the same "office" as other people in, gosh, more than five years. It's different! Not that I'm here every single day (well, OK, I was here every day last week), but I certainly work from here (Marco's house) more than from my Volcanoville home these days, and this office is now better equipped than my home office (due in large part to the fact that there's a cable modem here instead of satellite Internet). On the other hand, the view from my office window at home remains forever unrivaled . . . no view is as beautiful to me as my dense forest.

My workday habits haven't really changed except that I tend to eat more healthily. We haven't gone completely into the whole health food thing, but I'm already eating more whole foods and organics and such, and more regularly, and I don't think I'm even losing weight anymore. That was an unpleasant realization in May—that I'd lost 20-some pounds in a couple of months—but I remember one oncologist (the radiation guy, I think) telling me that weight loss is not altogether uncommon in newly diagnosed cancer patients. Heck, some days now I even eat breakfast because I'm hungry instead of having to remember to eat, and that's a huge improvement over my past habits of working at my desk without even standing up or getting dressed until after noon . . .

OK, but today I pretty much didn't do the healthy thing, except that we went for a walk at lunchtime. It didn't occur to me to have breakfast because it was such a busy day of model testing (ugh, now that'll make you cross-eyed, looking at spreadsheets full of data all day long, trying to QA and verify that the macros are calculating correctly). Dinner tonight was pizza, and other than those two breaks, I've been working all day and evening. About 9:30 p.m., I realized that I hadn't even gotten up from my desk to brush my teeth today! Embarrassing to admit, but true. I just get focused, lose track of time, and forget to take care of myself.

I got to talk to Artie's mom when she called today (she's like a mother-in-law to me, except that we're pretty close instead of the more classical antagonistic mother-in-law and daughter-in-law relationship). I usually seem to miss her calls, so it was good to talk to her. She reminded me again about how so many people are praying for me and sending me all their good intentions, and she firmly believes all that has contributed to my good recovery status so far and the possibility of not having to do chemo.

It's an amazing thing, the power of intention. I have this cool nine-hour DVD about quantum physics (OK, not everyone would agree with that statement, but it's cool to a geek like me), and part of it is about the power of intention, and there are these amazing photographs of water molecules and how different they are (beautiful, or ugly) after having some specific intention focused on them for some period of time. Interesting stuff. After seeing that the first time, I started putting the words "Love and Gratitude" on all my water containers and in my well house, to "bless" the water with good intention. Maybe it works, maybe not, but I feel good doing it.

Apparently a lot of people are reading my blog . . . I must have counted a dozen e-mails and text messages over the last couple of days from people telling me to hang in there and to call or write them if I needed to talk (not that there's much to talk about—we're waiting for the test results, and that's frustrating—not much discussion to be had. What I've really wanted was to just be alone and not hurt anyone by lashing out at them in frustration). My favorites were from Dietrich and Paul, though, just little messages saying things like, "Hang in there, kiddo, there's a lot of people rootin' for ya." Simple support, but it was just what I needed, you know?

Not that having so many people raising their hands to offer up a sympathetic ear for me to call is a bad thing; of course that's wonderful. I am pretty surprised at that, actually. Not because so many people want to be there for me (I can't even count how many people have done that in the past two months), but that so many people are reading my blog, and are really up to date! Heck, I can't even keep up with the blog, and I'm writing it! I've gotten a lot of e-mails from people offering up contacts of breast cancer survivors, too, and breast-cancer survivors themselves have written to me directly telling me their survival stories, which are really inspiring. Marco is always here of course . . . all these people are offering themselves up to talk to me whenever I need it, and here I don't really feel like I have anything to talk through. I mean, it's the wait itself that's frustrating and causing all this anxiety, and I don't really know what to talk about with people who offer for me to talk to them about the cancer or treatment or anything. Of course, if I'm journaling and blogging, obviously there must be some part of me that "needs to talk," if only to myself.

Ha. People must find it so amusing when I write myself in a circle like that.

Tomorrow is Marco's birthday. I left a little hallmark card on his desk this morning, sort of a cute it-doesn't-have-to-be-your-birthday-to-get-a-card kind of thing, and tomorrow . . . well, the world will have to wait to find out what's in the box that was delivered for him today from ThinkGeek (one of my favorite Web stores).

Oh, and we got my fish on Friday: Rerun, Opie, and Crystal. They're beautiful Ryukins. I'll have to write about them another day when I haven't been staring at the computer screen so long, though.

CANCER—DAY 67 TUESDAY, JUNE 30, 2009

So, I'm in the kitchen staring in the fridge, figuring out what the heck to make for lunch (we've been avoiding buying lots of groceries as we're leaving town for the weekend, so the pickin's are gettin' slim), and Marco scares the DAYLIGHTS out of me when he starts to come into the kitchen from around the corner behind the refrigerator. I was so startled and jumpy I actually scared him back! Then, after a good laugh he thanked me for the birthday card I'd left on his computer when he was taking Randy to the airport.

I hate buying cards in relationships, they're never quite right, you know? So instead, I'd written Marco a little note and a poem, and he thought it was really beautiful. I didn't quite expect such a reaction, I mean, it's not like I'm a good poet, but he really liked it and "beautiful" was his word. I debated whether to put what I wrote in my blog because it's a little weird to think of, like, my *dad* reading this, but the blog is for sharing this intimate journey, right? So, here it is:

A Moment

Escaped in sleep perfection lives
Only dreams such fullness give
When but a touch, a breath in turn
Can dance with fire and yet not burn

Woven, braided, threads entwined
A single life now fate divined
Perfection known in dreams so bright
The dreamer wakes to golden light

Still not sure of daylight's dawn
Knowing not whence darkness gone
Yet filled with warmth no fear of harm
The dreamer wakes in lover's arms

What dreamer's dream of dreams is this
So fully known in lover's bliss
A simple moment, to be sure
But in this moment, life is pure

Marco's birthday was a normal Tuesday, though; we both had a regular full work day, and Marco had to teach last night. I had talked to Debra (the studio owner), though, and she brought a card for all the students to sign; then I went over to the studio at the end of classes with an ice cream birthday cake for Marco to have with everyone. He was completely surprised, but he loved it. I can't remember the last time I dated someone who enjoyed birthdays so much! It was fun doing what I could to make his day special. Making other people feel good makes me feel good. Nice how that works, eh?

CANCER—DAY 68 WEDNESDAY, JULY 1, 2009

Marco and I got out for a pleasant Mexican lunch today, and had some really enjoyable conversation. He's almost glowing with excitement about flying off to Vegas to have fun this weekend! And he's getting a general glow of being happy with the relationship . . . I think we're both relieved that the test result is coming up soon and we'll know what treatment path we'll be on, in addition to everything else we've been talking about.

Marco says, "We communicate really well." I still have some reservations about that because I know there are quite a few little things that I have issues with that I haven't talked with him about yet, but maybe soon . . . on the upside, I am definitely learning how to talk about this kind of stuff with him.

For example, I said something about not planning my life too far beyond treatment in terms of me living with him in Sac, even though the relationship is fine now. He said a couple things that really got me, the better of which I don't remember, but in the car he said, "Well, yeah, I'm just assuming now that the relationship is working out indefinitely." Man, when Marco decides he's in, he is *all in.*

The other thing he said was something about how we are together as a couple, and that we have a really great relationship and something about how we're so much stronger than the average couple—something like that. Anyway, he *floored* me with that.

We even talked about my cats coming down here to live, that we'd have to figure it out—between giving them dander-prevention baths and keeping the house really clean of cat fur, and him getting better allergy medicine, he said we could work out the three of them all living together.

So when we went to bed and he turned out the light, I giggled a little and snuggled into his shoulder more and teased him: "So, that whole 'relationship commitment' thing back in May, are you all over that now?" He laughed, a happy belly laugh. "Oh yeah," he said, chuckling and hugging me.

So far in such a short time . . . yet right now it doesn't feel like a flash-in-the-pan relationship that will disappear as quickly as it arose. Then again, we made this commitment for the next many months regardless, so maybe that's why I want to believe it's all real and sincere. He certainly seems to mean it.

CANCER—DAY 69 THURSDAY, JULY 2, 2009

So, here's a new one . . . it definitely never occurred to me that I may have *this* dilemma for my cancer blog . . . of not being able to blog for a few days because of going on *vacation!* But I really don't want either of us taking our laptops to Vegas this weekend. We're just going to go and have fun!

CANCER—DAY 71 SATURDAY, JULY 4, 2009

We've had a great time wandering around in Las Vegas, and tonight we went to a Cirque du Soleil show that was, of course, amazing. I'd seen it before and knew Marco would be entranced. He was, in fact, mesmerized.

I wasn't thinking about the cancer thing too much, but it's never completely out of my mind. Every time I thought about how much fun we were having and how great it was that we could go on this little weekend trip for Marco's birthday, I would also recall that the reason I didn't book this birthday trip until a week ago was because I was supposed to have been in chemotherapy already. I guess waiting longer is better than being unnecessarily thrown into chemo, but the wait is wearing me down more and more all the time.

CANCER—DAY 72 SUNDAY, JULY 5, 2009

We're home, and (after, what, two hours?) I'm back to being so antsy and anxious that I can hardly sit still.

One of my fish, Crystal, was dead in the aquarium filter when we got home. Marco says she must have jumped over the edge of the tank. I drove out to Volcanoville to check on the cats. Mizzou is getting way too fat and apparently throwing up fairly regularly besides, and Seoul won't be held anymore, not for a moment. So I have (had) a suicidal fish, a bulimic cat, and a kitten that's reverting to being feral. The cats are starved for affection, and jumpy. Mizzou's foot slipped on my shoe and made a little noise that made Seoul jump about a foot, which in turn gave Mizzou a start, and they both just about bolted right out of their fur. The living situation with me being away and them being alone at my house is not good for them.

It's working out really well for me at Marco's, though. I had been thinking about staying in Volcanoville tonight when I went to take care of the cats, but drove back to Sac. I was getting so wound up inside that I didn't think it would be a good idea for me to be alone tomorrow, potentially spiraling up in that emotional/mental hurricane.

Tomorrow is the last day of this mess before we find out about chemotherapy—just one more day; I can do it. When you're a survivor, when you've lived through really, *really* difficult experiences and deaths in the past, it's not so hard to tell yourself that you can survive pretty much anything for just one day. Just one day, mind you, which is why taking it one day at a time can work. Of course, I would just as soon never have to survive another day like my surgery . . .

The biological-aunt-with-breast-cancer thing worries me.

I have this feeling. I'm slightly afraid to write it down, but any reader of this personal soap opera saga will want to know, before I go to find out, if I have a sense of whether or not I'll have to do chemo. I've been feeling that out for a while now, and I'm pretty sure that I am going to have to do it. This morning I asked the Runes if I was going to have to do chemo, and I drew *Nauthiz* upright (which means Yes). *Nauthiz* is the Rune of Constraint, Necessity, and Pain. It basically tells you that you have a lot to learn about the shadow side of yourself and that we learn most from adversity. All right, then, let's get this party started. Life, which you know as well as I do now, has a lot to teach me and apparently I'm not going to learn it the easy way.

CANCER—DAY 73 MONDAY, JULY 6, 2009

Strange, I'm not even sure Marco realizes how stressed out I am about this test result issue. I know he doesn't have time to read my blog, and last night he was sooooo into his game (World of Warcraft, which I've avoided trying out because I'm told that it is ridiculously addictive). He didn't seem to notice or care that after writing my blog post before dinner, I then spent the entire evening, like five or six hours solid, just reading more and more cancer stuff online. Marco seems blissfully unaware. This worries me in terms of care during treatment, but how much does he really need to do anyway, and how much should I be doing for myself? Why should I depend on him for my care anyway? Why not just think of him as backup support to me taking care of myself?

What's more likely true for him, now that I think about it more rationally, is that he doesn't want to talk about what we'll find out tomorrow morning because the possibility scares him, and he doesn't want to frighten me by letting me see that. But sitting ten feet apart all day at our computers and never talking about tomorrow, well, that gives my mind too much time to worry. I think that the mind, when allowed to run off with worrying thoughts, tends to get itself even more worked up and finds additional, likely imaginary, things to worry about.

So worry has been rolling around and building up in the back of my mind all day. But I still have to get through the whole day, so you, my dear readers, get to wait through the day with me and suffer through some of my thought wanderings.

One of my fish is sick. Well, one of my remaining two fish, anyway. Rerun had these spots starting to grow on two of his fins (he has seven fins, he's a big beautiful Ryukin). When we looked at him really, really closely today and then searched for a potential diagnosis for the spots online, we figured out that he has fish lice. So, get this: Marco held him in the aquarium and I used tweezers to pluck the two lice off, and then we went to three fish stores to find a fish lice medicine (it's not particularly rare, apparently, but not every fish place carries it). So early tomorrow morning, we're going to medicate Rerun and Opie's water (we're assuming Opie has been completely exposed to the lice, even if we can't see any on him yet). And get this: the treatment for fish lice is essentially . . . chemo for fish. Ironic that Cancer Girl is giving her fish chemo, isn't it?

I got an e-mail today from an old, old friend that I was on tour with in Europe years ago. What a trip, hearing from him. My "surgery" e-mail back in May had gone into his spam folder, and he just found the note a few days ago. But he didn't know how to reply right away; he said it took him some time to work up the nerve to write to me. It's really interesting, how this affects people. Older people seem to have had more exposure to knowing someone closely who has had (and, many times, survived) breast cancer, but they also often have this non-verbal reaction of OhMyGodYourRecoveryIsGoingToBeSoHorrible. The advances in technology for treatment are truly amazing, so even if I'm doing chemo, I'm hopeful that I won't have nearly as horrible an experience as a woman ten years or even five years ago would have had. But for younger people, friends my own age, hearing my diagnosis is often more of a shock and an eye-opener, realizing that even when we're young, life is fleeting. This wasn't the first person to tell me that hearing about my cancer has made them rethink their own life, and pointedly ask themselves some difficult life questions that they may have thought about in passing before but those questions were now poignantly sharpened by my medical news. My old friend ended his e-mail with this great Robert Frost quote: "The best way out is always through."

Marco's co-worker's step-mother and I (I think that's the right connection from her to me) have been trading e-mails (she's a breast cancer survivor, diagnosed at 40, the closest to my own age that I've met so far, but still significantly different in treatment and what the experience was like). She told me stuff that lots of other people have expressed to me about how the cancer made her really think about life and what it means to her or what she wants to get out of it, or that sort of thing.

Facing the fear of death: I empathize with everyone who's mentioned this to me, but it's odd because I feel like a counselor to them rather than the other way around. Yeah, OK, I don't want to die (who does?), but I'm not afraid of it because I've already died three times (according to my cardiologist and the machines in the ER), but they got me back, obviously. Because of my heart condition, which was diagnosed five years and five months ago (note the timing in relation to Artie's death, that's probably not a coincidence), and the emotional trauma of Artie dying when he was only 30 and having to deal with that, I basically resolved my issues with death a long time ago. It's just not something to be feared. It's part of life and part of our spiritual process. I can't tell you that there's a Heaven in exactly the way Religion teaches it, but I do know (from personal experience) that we each have a soul and that it's only the physical body that dies, not the soul. The physical death, to me, felt more like a transition; definitely not an ending.

With everything I've survived already (Mom and I figured out a while back, way before the cancer diagnosis, that I'm already on the ninth of my nine cat lives), and with a healthy dose of spirituality, it seems pretty obvious that I survived all of that because I still had a lot to learn and/or experience in this lifetime, and my spirit or soul wasn't ready to give up on this body yet. Practically from birth, my life seems to have had specific focus for me to learn about certain things, like trust. How could it be a coincidence for me to have been born and put up for adoption, to be in seven foster homes in six weeks and emotionally abused as a newborn, in order to end up with my parents, who got bumped up some 200 names in the list to adopt me because of their medical backgrounds and positions, and then for me to have such a wonderful childhood and upbringing? It was weird to hear that my biological mother later had more kids (multiple) who she kept, which means that I have biological brothers/sisters (Either? Both? No idea on the details—the adoption search woman mentioned it almost in passing, like it was information she thought I already knew). That was a little weird, but there's no question about whether anyone could have raised me better or in a more loving environment than my parents have. And given the situation of my birth and adoption, how can all that be a coincidence?

Now, Artie's death, I'm not going to blame that on my needed spiritual growth, though of course it had countless life-changing effects and did in fact make me grow as a person through learning how to live with such a loss. In that experience, I discovered that I have a much deeper reservoir of personal strength than I had ever realized. And then my heart condition diagnosis, after I collapsed while playing the flute in church . . . and the whole scare that they were going to put in a pacemaker that night in the ICU if I had another heart-stopping episode, before my parents could even fly out here, then not being allowed to drive for three months while they made sure the heart medication was working . . . now THAT gave me plenty of time and reason to consider the possibility/likelihood of my own death, to make my peace with it, and to know what the rest of my life was going to be about. It certainly isn't about my career, though I am still bound by the characteristics of my personality to care about doing a good job at what I do and not letting anyone down. My work ethic is both laudable and ridiculous. But a job is certainly NOT what life is about, and it certainly isn't reason enough for me to have survived what I already have in life.

All of this has made me a tougher survivor than I would have ever thought possible five or six years ago, and it has strengthened my tenacity for living to a degree that I didn't realize until very, very recently. I'm not one to easily give up on myself, and surviving cancer and the trials of treatment is no exception. OK, I might not always do it gracefully, but I'm working on that part! And I suspect I'll have plenty of opportunity to practice "surviving with grace" in the upcoming months.

OK, so tomorrow morning at 10 a.m., Marco is going with me to the medical oncologist to find out the reliance score result, and whether or not I have to do chemo. I'm expecting to hear "chemo." I haven't told Marco that, and I haven't even said it out loud, though I did let my blog followers know. I'm still hoping for the best, but I'm trying to prepare myself emotionally for the worst, so that I will handle the news as well as possible. We'll know very soon now. Finally. Maybe I'll even sleep tonight. Well, OK, maybe not. Maybe I'll sleep tomorrow night.

CANCER—DAY 74 TUESDAY, JULY 7, 2009

So! The news we've all been waiting a month for is here: the oncotype test showed my recurrence score is a 25, so we're going to do chemo. No Adriamyacin though, which is great because that's the one that's damaging to the heart, the one that freaked out my cardiologist. We will have another test to see if I have the genetic BRCA genes that indicate higher breast cancer risk, which may make him add in Herceptin with the Tamoxifen—I think that was how that went, anyway. But that won't matter until after radiation.

So I start chemo on July 21. Before that, on July 17, I'll have surgery to get a port receptor put in, which is this little reservoir type thing with a long tube that goes into the heart through a vein so that they don't have to dig into my arm to find my veins every time they draw blood and give me chemo. I hate needles and blood.

The chemo is going to be just four months long; that's the *really* good news. And it's going to be just two drugs: Taxol/Taxotere, and Cyclophosphamide. Then a month after chemo is done, I start radiation (anticipated at 6-1/2 weeks) and Tamoxifen (5 years+). Basically all this stuff is going to make me menopausal, and Dr. Lombard kept asking if I want to have kids, because this is pretty much going to damage my body to the point that there is only about a 50/50 chance that I could conceive. But I don't care about that; if the time comes when I want to raise children (which, no offense to parents, becomes less and less likely every year), I'll just adopt like my parents did. No big deal—who needs ovaries anyway. Well, except for all the reasons women need estrogen in their body, that is. Uck, I am not looking forward to having menopausal side effects at 32; everything I've read/heard about that is just plain awful as far as I'm concerned. That's probably going to be the worst thing for me. I'm not concerned at all about losing all my hair, and all the treatments are just something I have to bear, but the drug-induced menopause is the thing I dread most.

At least the month of waiting is finally over, and I have something to take action on again. All this time I've just been reading more and more stuff on cancer, and it's pretty depressing when you think about it. It was getting to a point where it wasn't healthy for me to be doing cancer research almost every night, and it's really good that we're finally moving forward. I have a whole list of things that I need to get done now in order to coordinate and help things go as smoothly as possible.

You wouldn't believe the list of drugs they're giving me—five different drugs to start with—for helping with chemo side effects like nausea. And one of them causes insomnia; that's just great. The nurse, Heddi, said I should up my Ambien prescription, because I'm going to need it more than once every three nights during chemo. Let's hope not—one of the other drugs causes some people drowsiness, so maybe the two will cancel each other out. Let's hope for that.

They're having those meds all delivered rather than me having to go pick them up at a pharmacy, which is cool. But when I was reading through those pages in detail tonight, it looks like they switched my other medications over to Dr. Lombard too, and switched them to generics in the process. That's not good because with two of them I know from past side effects I can't take generics for those two meds. So, another phone call back to Dr. Lombard's office tomorrow to make sure that's not happening. You really have to stay on top of this stuff, you know? It may seem like a little thing, generics versus original prescriptions, but why allow their habitual way of handling prescriptions put me in a situation of reliving old side effects and having to deal with all that again, on top of everything else?

The last problem is my cats. Well, not really, there's also the problem of this sudden trip to Phoenix for Marco's work that I might take with him, but basically the fundamental problem there is simply avoiding infection. Heddi said if I'm going in an airplane, I should wear a surgical mask over my nose and mouth. Ugh, I don't want to deal with that; maybe I'll stay home instead of going with Marco to Phoenix, like we had originally hoped I could do.

But the cats . . .because I'm going to be so susceptible to infection, we have to be exceedingly careful about what I come into contact with. Like, I need to remind Marco to wash his hands a lot when teaching, between classes and before he comes home, and he has to be careful that *he* doesn't catch a cold or something and bring that in the house and infect me. And I'm not supposed to clean a litter box. Well, how the heck am I going to manage that one? Marco can't even enter my house in Volcanoville because his allergies are so bad, and I'm certainly not going to ask him to go in there and clean up the litter box and their mess every weekend (though at some point he is going to have to see an allergist so he can coexist with my cats, some day). And the cats seem so unhappy all alone up there; Mizzou is gaining weight daily, I swear. He's blimping up big time. Seoul's not getting fat, not yet, but she's getting more and more skittish; she'll go completely feral eventually. I teased my mom today about sending my cats out for them to take care of in Sidney, but I don't want to ship the cats to Nebraska and back. So I've been thinking about it, and I think I'm going to try to find a kennel nearby Marco's place (*our* place, I mean . . . I am so bad at talking couple-speak!). There's a cat place not too far away where I took them for Christmas while I was in Hawaii; it's a cat "bed and breakfast." They had two-story kennels (cages) next to each other with their own litter box in the bottom and a shelf with a sleeping pad for the upper story, and the kennel people let Mizzou and Seoul out together in the play room (lots of cat trees to climb and toys to play with) more than once a day. The cats weren't thrilled to be there; they were actually happy to get in the car when I picked them up. But I think they did better there than they're doing alone at my house out in Volcanoville. Plus, now that chemo is for sure, and we know I'm really going to be living at Marco's for the next six months (by the time radiation is over), I don't want to leave the cats alone up there that whole time. Anyway, this cat bed and breakfast is only about ten minutes from Marco's place, I think. And I've seen several vet/kennel places here in the neighborhood, in case I want the cats even closer. Maybe the place will give me an extra discount because the cats are being boarded fairly long term for my cancer treatment. Hey, I haven't used the don't-you-want-to-help-me-just-because-I-have-cancer thing; maybe this is the time to play that card and see if it helps.

So, all in all, both a good day and a bad day. Good to finally know, but that first half hour or so back at the house after the appointment . . . I was pretty lost in my mind, in a bit of shock, even though this was the treatment I expected. It even happened the way I suspected, which was that the recurrence score is technically in the "gray area," though very much at the high end (25 is the cutoff). I suspected my score wouldn't absolutely put me in chemo, but that I would have to choose to do it. Well, with a score of 25, my oncologist recommended chemo, so I didn't really have to make the decision, but still, it's weird that I had a feeling about what range the score would be in. Dr. Lombard (the oncologist) thought that was pretty interesting and said that it's women's intuition.

FINALLY! I am thrilled to finally be able to take action and move forward. No wait, not forward, think Robert Frost . . . *through.*

Chapter 11.
The "Caregiver"

CANCER—DAY 76 THURSDAY, JULY 9, 2009

It's strange. I feel relieved to be done with Chemo Limbo, but Marco seems even more stressed out now. And annoyed, or maybe just crabby. He's been stressed and generally annoyed since the day we found out the chemo decision was being delayed another two weeks. I thought the strain of Chemo Limbo was making him tense and irritable, but that doesn't explain anything now. Is it me?

All the cancer literature tells you to expect the patient to be moody. But what does that mean exactly?

How do you know if it's just moodiness versus something actually being wrong? I don't know if I'm being moody or not, but little things definitely bother me, just not all the time, and I can't seem to remember enough of what I was like before the cancer stress to know if the same things would have bothered me pre-cancer or not. It concerns me. My dad told me once about a friend of his whose wife had cancer and after all her treatment (chemo in particular) she was never the same again. Given that the guy didn't give my dad any other consoling details, I'm assuming that she didn't change in a good way.

So . . . what if I'm changing into a "less good" person because I can't manage the moodiness? I feel like I'm supposed to cover everything up and pretend I'm fine, that nothing is bothering me. I feel really uncomfortable trying to mention little things to Marco that I would prefer to be different, because I don't know that they really are little things or not, to him. Like, I don't understand why Marco piles up dirty dishes in the sink and on the counter when there is a dishwasher right there to put the dishes in, and then the kitchen won't smell like rotten food or moldy water. I'm really nervous about touching on something that, to me, seems it shouldn't matter much, but in reality it turns out to be a real issue for Marco.

Over time, in dealing with people, I've developed this habit of testing the waters by going around a point and feeling it out before deciding to go ahead and touch directly, yet lightly, on the subject, if the person seems sensitive to it. Every time I do that with Marco, though, he seems to react as though I'm attacking him when I haven't even gotten to the heart of the matter yet. And if that's how he reacts to me getting on the edge of something that he has issues with, what's he going to do if I have to directly ask him to change something?

I've never asked Marco to change anything. Nothing. Not how he acts or what he does or how he lives, not a thing. For the last several years I've been making a serious effort to appreciate people for who they are. It is not my place to change people. There's a reason it never works, trying to change someone else. The only person that can make you change is *you*. But when do you know you've reached the breaking point? How far do you let it go before you admit that who that person is, well, that just isn't the right kind of person for you to be with, or vice versa?

And how much of my fretfulness is just me being a moody cancer patient? Or is Marco the one being moody?

CANCER—DAY 77 FRIDAY, JULY 10, 2009

Marco finally told me why he has been so tense all week. There is a complication for my care during chemo. Marco's company is moving offices in Phoenix. His job is as offsite IT support, and he wasn't expecting or planning to be out there for the move because he's committed here as my caregiver—and they know exactly what he is committed to here because he made it explicitly clear to his company. Right after *The Decision* of him becoming my caregiver, he told his company he could not travel during my chemo. The office move, though, will happen during the week after my first chemo, so basically week two of the chemo cycle.

Turns out, his company is insistent that he must be there—for a week, possibly a week plus two weekends. Sheesh. We just found out chemo starts Monday, three days from now, and already we're having caregiver complications.

CANCER—DAY 78 SATURDAY, JULY 11, 2009

No sleep again last night—worried about this Marco-being-gone-for-a-week for work thing. When we talked this morning, Marco said it only has to be three or four days really, not a whole week, and that it's not even confirmed yet. So, who knows how it's going to work out. Worst case, I know my parents would come out if I asked them to, and then I can stay at home with the cats, which would be really nice. I miss them. I really need to call the pet spa place Monday to find out just how pricey it would be to have the cats there for a month or more. I did the math on what I paid for them to be there at Christmas time, and it's prohibitively expensive to have them there for months. Maybe they can board the cats together (make them share a kitty condo) or something to give me a lower "monthly" rate. I have to try, at least. I'm going to go see the cats tonight, which I know will help settle down my thoughts.

It will be good to give Marco some time to think, too. This week has been weird—it's like he's suddenly mad at me for having cancer and putting him in this awful situation or something. He's glad I'm going home so he will have some time alone. I think it is a good thing that we will both have some time alone with our own thoughts.

CANCER—DAY 79 SUNDAY, JULY 12, 2009

I think the whole Marco-leaving-town thing bothered me because I had been relying on the thought of Marco as my caretaker too much in making myself believe I can get through this. It's as though I've been counting on the last bit of strength that I thought I needed to get through this as coming from believing in him. He was supposed to be my extra strength for getting through treatment or something. So this little business trip hit me as a shocker, because I couldn't believe he would even consider leaving while I'm in chemo. If it were the other way around, even if I barely knew the person, if I had committed to being a caregiver for anyone with cancer I wouldn't leave town even overnight during their treatment; it just seems wrong to me. And no job is worth that. At the end of my life I wouldn't think back and say, "Oh, darn, I really wish I had left that cancer patient with other people for a week so I could go to Phoenix for that company whose name I can't even remember; I made the wrong decision to stay and fulfill my commitment to her care rather than leaving for work."

But it's easy for me to say that. I know what it's like to look back on your life and see where you made the mistake of putting work first only to have it cost you dearly in your personal life, and I know it's not worth it. Not everyone has had those experiences. Marco definitely has not.

Saturday morning before I left to go out to my house for the weekend, Marco tried to justify his leaving by saying he cares about his company like I care about my company, and I was like, "Sure, I absolutely care about my company, the people there are long-time friends and amazing colleagues, and I often put my work ahead of my own best interests (nine times out of ten). But I would never put work ahead of family or something like this." So, our conversation before I left ended with some heavy stress for him, and pretty heavy disappointment on my side. Instead of staying and getting into a big fight about it, I came home to my place of peace and tranquility to calm my nerves.

But then . . . there is more to the story about this "work thing" that didn't make the blog, yet it is important to include in my journal.

Saturday afternoon at home was not good, in terms of communications between Marco and me. While I was home (in the hammock with my laptop), Marco instant messaged me and said "I told them I can't come, but I'm getting pressured to be there for at least a few days, probably Friday, Saturday, Sunday. And Monday." Given how our last conversation on this topic ended just a few hours earlier, I was still a little snippy, and I typed back "Look, just do what you think is right. Maybe you'll salvage something, maybe not, but all you can do is what you think is best, then the world has no choice but to live with that." His next message was that he was having them book his flights for Thursday through Monday. "Let's be honest," I snapped back, "and as for Cynthia's trust in your care?" Then Marco hit me with a zinger.

"I will not be held emotionally hostage. You need to quit being so self absorbed and work though this with me." Shocked, I replied, "That was a hurtful thing to say." "How truthful is it?" he asked. I replied: "Well, I guess that depends on your perspective. If you consider it self-absorbed for me to be focused on being engaged and knowledgeable regarding cancer treatment and what I may have to deal with, then you are alone in that opinion. I can list a hundred people who would tell you that caring about your cancer treatment and trying to manage it is not self-absorption; it's survival. It is not selfish for a cancer patient to pay attention to her own care. And if you think you are being 'held emotionally hostage,' well, that is completely a yoke you put on your own neck. I never ask a thing of you. I never ask a thing of you because I'm afraid that if I do, you're going to get upset, and you are frightening and mean when you are upset."

Some time passes, and then he comes back online to type: "I'm concerned about your care. I wouldn't do this if I didn't think it was important, and my commitment is unchanged." Unbelievable. I write back: "I am having a very hard time believing that, Marco." I went on, "You have these moments where I feel very lucky to be with you, but you also make me feel really bad about myself sometimes."

This goes back and forth a bit more, and finally I say, "It doesn't matter if I stay with you. My parents will come if I need them, and LOTS of people have offered to come be my caregiver. One wants to drive in from San Francisco, another wants to fly out from Atlanta, just to make sure there is someone with me when you're out of town. I've had friends offer to quit their jobs to take your place. You do not have to do this if you don't want to." He bickered a bit saying other people can afford to offer that because they make more money than him or have more freedom than he does with his job, so I said it again: "As I said, you do not have to do this. You don't ever have to see me again, for that matter. I'm ready to make the calls that will completely change my caregiver situation to one that would be less stressful for me and lets you off the hook entirely." "Stop exaggerating," he snaps. He didn't seem to get it, so I summarized. "What I'm saying is that I will do whatever you want. I am NOT forcing you into anything, treatment, relationship, or otherwise." To which he replied, "I know that."

The conversation then turned to how he deals with stress, which is basically to vehemently vent it out, and we talked about how awful that negativity feels to me even if it's not directed at me. It's hard to be around that kind of energy, grungy green-yellow-black waves just emanate from him in every direction when he's frustrated or mad, and there's no way for me to know if it's supposed to be directed at me or not, because either way it's definitely coming my direction, intentional or not.

We messaged for several pages about things we each do and could change to make the situation more amenable for us both. But I thought he was skirting the real issue, so I brought it up bluntly again. "Are you absolutely sure you want to do this chemo thing? There is still time for me to put alternative options in play if you have the slightest hesitation. Seriously. I don't want to be with you for this if every time I'm scared and worried about my health or care you tell me I'm being self-absorbed." He changed the subject.

We had cleared *some* things up, though, and I messaged him later in the evening: "You feel better?" He replied, "Starting to miss you." LOL! I bounced back, "Isn't that what you said you want, alone time?" He chose to ignore that, and started asking about the schedule for Thursday, my first chemo infusion. He was planning to take an hour off work to be with me, and I was like, "What? This is going to take all afternoon, and I have an appointment with the oncologist prior to that. Just drop me off and pick me up." He said, "You shouldn't have to sit in there by yourself." "There's no reason I can't," I replied. "I know," he says, "but I would rather be there." This comment finally set me off after all this back and forth mess—*now* he's making an effort? I lashed out.

"Your suddenly very active participation in my actual treatments seems like a really inappropriate conversation to me right now. I'm basically trying to plan how to get through my treatment process *alone*, only depending on you when absolutely necessary and then preferably with planned backup already in place. While you may not agree with or understand how I feel about this, the things you have said have done a lot of damage to our relationship and my trust in you. I am *NOT* OK with that. I want to give you a chance at this, but it seems unwise to actually trust you with it." And then I added, "If you think this is an appropriate way to speak to someone you supposedly care about *"You need to quit being so self absorbed and work thru this with me. It's not my fault you chose to hide in the mountains for years and don't have any friends to turn to now,"* then I need to think very carefully about being around you." I added: "The mean-spirited nature of your criticisms are hurtful and damaging." He started talking about the building move and told me, "I wouldn't go if it wasn't important." I had to explain to him: "This is not about you being away for a few days, though admittedly staying would have been a more positive resolution than going. The issue though, is how you handled it, how it's made me feel, and the fact that how it's made me feel didn't seem to matter to you. Unfortunate all around."

Marco and I are very different people. I've had little creeping doubts about just how much Marco can handle, but I want to give him the benefit of the doubt because this is such an enormous opportunity for him to do that "something important" in life that he told me he's never really done. Giving him the opportunity to do that by being my caregiver was definitely a point I considered when making the caregiver decision. It may sound strange, but giving him the opportunity to do "something important" that would make him feel better about himself as a person even if meant treatment would be harder for me to get through, that was a point counted on the list of reasons to stay, not the list of reasons to leave.

I didn't sleep much this weekend, thinking about Marco's away-for-work thing. But then I found my strength, and thusly, my calm, because I remembered why I decided I could give him this growth opportunity even if I wasn't sure he could achieve it.

I came to the conclusion that I do know one person right here that I can count on without fail: myself. So now I think that I need to take that approach with this thing, rather than trusting that someone else is truly willing and fully capable of managing what may become an enormous life trial in so many ways. That's just too much to ask of any one person.

But I know I can do it for myself. I am capable of managing enormous life trials, I know how awful this can get and I know how to survive emotionally when you think you've sunk below rock-bottom. I was a survivor long before I was diagnosed with cancer, and I know I have the internal fortitude to survive this. Marco doesn't have to be there *all* the time. Soooo many people want to help, there's no question I can easily find a dozen or more people to check in on me or stay with me for a meal or just visit for a while. I can get through a week with Marco out of town even if I'm ill with the chemo drugs. It's not like I'll be alone just because Marco isn't there.

CANCER—DAY 80 MONDAY, JULY 13, 2009

A new day. Sometimes it seems like a new day will never come. But it did. This new day brought mutual apologies and some new planning for the port surgery on Thursday, and things were pretty much smoothed over . . . so, onward . . . through.

CANCER—DAY 83 THURSDAY, JULY 16, 2009

Dr. Thatcher told Marco that the surgery went well this morning. Now I have this lump an inch or two below my left collar bone, and a tube from the port going all the way into my heart, as I understand it. It's called a port-a-cath (portable catheter), and this port is where they'll give me all my chemo treatments and do all the blood draws and stuff, which is really good because I was feeling beat up from all the needles during the two weeks of biopsies and tests back in April and May. I get really queasy about blood now, ever since Artie's motorcycle wreck. Gory movies and stuff never bothered me before he died, but now when something gross or bloody starts to happen in a movie, I turn away. By the way, anyone who can't stand needles should be careful about seeing *The Incredible Hulk*: there's a scene where a guy gets a nasty injection into his spine. I didn't see it; I happened to be wearing a cap and when I realized what was coming I quickly lowered my head and didn't watch it happen. Which, apparently, was a good thing, because even Marco made grossed-out noises during that part of the movie. Anyway, how did I get on that subject? Oh yeah, the port-a-cath . . . surgery today.

Well, I did really well immediately after the surgery this time. Post-op went a lot more smoothly in terms of them controlling the pain much better (this wasn't nearly as invasive a procedure as the lumpectomy and reconstructive surgery of course, and I wasn't in pain beforehand this time, which I think helped a lot!). I was also chatting with the nurses and asking questions and stuff. Last time, I was a lump of pain—it was awful.

So after maybe 30 minutes in there with the nurse, they took me back to the surgery ward and let Marco come in. He sat with me for an hour or so while they made sure I was stable and the pain was still controlled, and by 1:30 p.m. we were back in the car heading home. We stopped and had burgers for lunch, then I dozed all afternoon in my office across from Marco while he worked. I tell ya, from my perspective as someone who's worked from home a long time and also someone who's starting chemotherapy and afraid of what that will be like, this is about the best home office set up for two work-from-home professionals (doubling as cancer patient and caregiver) that I could ever have dreamed up. I'm far enough away that we don't bother each other or interrupt our work, we both have doorways but not doors, and he can easily keep an eye on me when I'm resting on the LoveSac beanbag chair thing that we put in my office. Around 5 p.m., Marco came over and sat with me for a while, and I swear it was about the best (deepest sleeping) nap I've had in, like, forever.

I was even well enough that we went over to Corti Brothers and got some advice for the wine club party tomorrow night. They have this goofy wine guy who looks like my cousin Dane, but wears a bow tie with a plaid shirt, and he's only in his twenties! But the guy definitely knows a heck of a lot about wines, and they have a ton of them, so that was a fun little excursion. We followed that with dinner at home. I made a chicken fiesta salad, but I couldn't eat much of it.

All in all, I was doing pretty well until about 8:30 p.m., when I started heaving and lost my dinner and my lunch. Uck. Wow, I've never heard Marco hustle quite that fast before, I think. First, he rushed to the bathroom when he heard me, but I told him it was OK—I was being sick but I was OK. Then, he rushed off and wet a washcloth, and sat with me on the floor for a minute while I caught my breath. After that, he dusted me off when I was OK to get up. (Yeah, um, we're going to have to clean the bathroom floors a little more frequently and thoroughly during chemo, especially if I'm going to be getting nauseated like this!)

Uff da. I got sick from anesthesia once before. I told the anesthesiologist that before the surgery today, and he said that they'd give me some anti-nausea stuff before they woke me up so I wouldn't get sick. Apparently, it either didn't last or it didn't work, because this was the same kind of nausea I had the other time I got sick after surgery. Hopefully that's it, just the one bout so far. Now I'm having a slice of dry toast so I can take the pain medicine, because all of that heaving really pulled on the muscles around the new port-a-cath. Sheesh, just when you think I'm going to have a simple surgery recovery, eh? Still, I'll take this over the last surgery's pain levels any day.

Kinda worries me a little though . . . if I'm getting nauseated now, how am I going to be next week after getting a chemo treatment? Oh well, I'll just have to get through it. They gave me all kinds of medicines, so hopefully we'll be able to keep the nausea manageable so that I'm not throwing up all the time!

Marco's gaming now in *World of Warcraft* while I'm journaling, but before I got sick he was online looking at chemo/cancer cookbooks and found a couple that he says he wants to get. One of my friends in Illinois who is a five-year breast cancer survivor told me that we absolutely had to get *The Cancer Patient's Cookbook*, which she said really improved her nausea and I think even helped with fatigue once they started using it to prepare her foods during her chemo. I swear though, the biggest food issue we're going to have during chemo, if we try to have meals together, is that we don't' seem to have any common tastes in vegetables! Too funny. The ones I like raw he only likes cooked. The ones I like cooked (steamed is actually my preference), he only likes cooked and doused in sauces because he doesn't like the vegetables' flavors that much. All this fuss about organic this and healthy that, and the guy hardly eats any vegetables!

All in all, this was a much better surgery day than the one a couple months ago. Of course, it wasn't nearly as stressful either, as there weren't any unknowns coming out of it. Last time, there was so much stress and worry through it all, not knowing yet if the cancer had spread; today was totally relaxed in comparison.

CANCER—DAY 84 FRIDAY, JULY 17, 2009

Ugh, I spoke too soon last night journaling . . . I ended up throwing up two more "series." Man, oh man, do I hate that kind where you're heaving and nothing comes out, but your body's all locked up, heave through heave, so you can't take a breath . . . ugh, last night was awful. Of course I threw up all the pain medicine and couldn't keep anything down at all, so the surgical site was hurting, and all the heaving made the incision ooze, but not enough to warrant a trip to the hospital.

Finally, around midnight or 1 a.m. I was like, "Oh come *on*, we have all these anti-nausea medicines for Monday, let's figure them out and try something." Marco smiled a little through the worry lines on his brow, saying "There's my Tenacious C." We sat down on the floor with the bag of meds and read everything and decided to try the Ondansetron (Zofran). That got me through the night, but today I was still feeling awful, so I started the day with one Zofran and then tried a Prochlorperazine (Compazine) around midday. I cooked over-easy eggs and bread (barely toasted) for us for lunch, and I was able to keep that down. I didn't do much of anything else all day, just read a few articles in a journal, and checked e-mail but didn't reply to anything. We still went to the wine club party. I wasn't too nauseated, although giving hugs did hurt quite a bit. The wine club party was still fun. Lisa, the two-year breast cancer survivor in the wine club, complimented me on selecting a summer outfit that didn't show or exaggerate the port. That was really nice, actually, because I must have spent an hour trying to figure out the right thing to wear given the port. The part of the port that presses my skin out is round, maybe the size of a third of a golf ball. This round lump just below my left collarbone pretty close to my neck. That's a tough spot to cover with a summer dress!

CANCER—DAY 85 SATURDAY, JULY 18, 2009

Wasn't too bad this morning—we went for a tandem bicycle ride and got a new seat for me. Then I got car sick this afternoon, couldn't nap to get over it, and now I'm still feeling icky. We tried a little tango embrace and ten seconds of tango in Marco's office, and figured out that I can't take a guy's shoulder or chest against my port-a-cath, so no Firehouse 9 for me tonight. I could probably dance with Marco because of our heights and body fit, but I'd be so nervous about the other guys inadvertently hurting me, that it wouldn't be an enjoyable evening for me. I told Marco that I would be fine by myself, and that he was welcome to go without me, but he said he wasn't sure he felt like it, anyway. Then I started watching movie trailers on my computer, thinking maybe I'd go to a movie, and he couldn't resist coming into my office to watch some, and now we've decided to go see *Hancock* tonight (the Will Smith super-hero movie).

One more day before chemo, and there's still so much to be done. Cleaning, buying proper groceries . . . and I have to admit I'm scared. I know I just have to do it and I'll get through whatever I must. Worrying won't change anything for the better at this point—it is what it is—but I'm scared anyway. I mean, come on, it's cancer. It's chemo. Wouldn't it be more worrisome if I had *no* fear right now?

CANCER—DAY 86 SUNDAY, JULY 19, 2009

I feel crummy, and chemo doesn't even start until tomorrow. I made us breakfast and washed all the dishes (why Marco thinks washing an entire sink full of dishes by hand with water running the whole time conserves water, I'll never understand). Then I checked on my aquarium because it was getting low on water. I was on the floor under the desk to look in the aquarium door, and then I was just too tired to get up, so I reached for the chemo book off my desk and stayed on the floor under my desk to read more of it. This is not normal Cynthia Swan behavior, just in case you're wondering.

Halfway through the book, Marco came in from whatever he was doing in the garage and yard. He saw me on the floor, and asked how I was doing. He didn't hear my quiet response because he had already turned away to walk into his office, so he asked again from over there and walked back into my office. On the floor with his feet, I was too tired to turn my head to look up to find his face. And in a flat, worn out voice I tell his feet, "My stomach hurts and I'm tired." I have no idea what he thought of that because he didn't say anything, but after a moment he left again and went back outside doing yard stuff. Why the yard matters now, today, is beyond me. Shouldn't we be getting stuff for my treatment, cleaning the house, and stuff like that? Who cares if the leaves that were on the driveway yesterday (and every day of the last two weeks) are still there tonight?

This whole caregiver thing is weird. I'm too tired to care what happens to me at the moment. I'm alone on the floor, half under my desk, with my blackberry and my chemo book, and I know we don't have any groceries or a lot of the things I've read about to make the cancer patient more comfortable during chemo. Yet, he seems to think he's taking care of me, when I feel like I might as well be alone at my property in Volcanoville for all the "care" I'm getting. In a few minutes I think I'm going to nap right here on this dirty floor (he's lived here three months with carpet that was dirty before he moved in, and there's never been a vacuum cleaner run through the house, nor does it appear high on the priority list to purchase one). I can barely keep my eyes open, even though I'm such a bundle of nerves I'm trembling, which I have been since seven o'clock this morning. Actually I think I've had a little tremble since lunch yesterday, now that I think about it.

Later . . . I managed to get off the floor, and got dressed in street clothes to go run errands by myself. As I was about to go out the door, Marco was coming in, coughing from all the gunk he was kicking up in the yard. We had a brief conversation where I said that I'm going to the post office and to see the cats, and I left, no goodbye.

I went to the pet spa to hang out with Mizzou and Seoul. I think they're better off at the spa than left alone in Volcanoville. They were both sleeping but happy to see me and get out of their condo cages to roam around the play room some more. Mizzou clearly knows the way to the top of the cabinets, just like in my kitchen at home. And Seoul's becoming a sniffer, checking each little smell along the way, wondering what the heck makes that kind of smell. Very different from the smells in the woods at home, that's for sure.

Mizzou needed some serious hands-on love (constant petting) for the first ten or fifteen minutes. I'm really glad I went down there; I think it was good for them and for me too. Then, driving back, I didn't know what to do. A couple hours had passed, but I didn't want to go back to Marco's. There was a park near the river, so I pulled off the road and went for a little walk in the shade in the park. I called my parents—we talked about a bit about what's going on here but they also had some interesting things going on at home that was fun to hear about. It was nice to just talk with them for a while, regardless of the subject. Toward the end of the call, I felt a little bad about venting to them about the situation at the house with Marco, and what seems like such a lack of emotional support. I haven't told them most of the disturbing issues going on with Marco, because I know that would make them worry even more than they already are.

Mom's told me more than once that I just need good emotional support and I'll get through treatment just fine. But that's exactly what seems to be lacking here, and it's making me even more nervous than I would be about chemo if I were going through treatment on my own instead of with Marco as my caregiver. While it may be good to talk about these things, I hate putting that negativity out on other people. And when it's something about Marco, I don't want to say anything negative to my parents because it may upset them, you know? But our conversation ended with me telling them that I was going to talk with Marco about the whole caregiver thing tonight and make sure we understood what we are doing together before we go to the first chemo treatment tomorrow.

After that I had some voicemail to check, and I decided that I wanted to go to a movie rather than go right back to Marco's after a trip to the grocery store. But that would mean I wouldn't get back until seven or eight o'clock, and by that time my "caregiver" should be concerned by my extended absence. I went for a five-minute walk without telling him several weeks ago, and he flipped out, telling me how worried he'd been and all that, and I promised not to do that again. I promised to tell him where I was going if I was leaving.

So I sent him a quick text. "I think I'd like to go to Kung Fu Panda @ 4:40. Want to go with me? Else, just a head's up so you don't worry about where I am." He doesn't always reply to my text messages anymore, but lo and behold, in less than sixty seconds, the surprising response was "Yes!"

So I drove to the house to pick him up, and tried to be really nice and hug him and not make him feel like there was anything terribly wrong. There wasn't anything terribly wrong, but I knew we were going to have to have a difficult conversation later in the evening, and I also knew that this wasn't the time to stir that up.

We went to the movie, which was great fun, and then went to Safeway for "chemo-nausea" foods. On the way into the store I said something like, "We need to get some foods that I'll eat even when I don't want to eat." And then, "I can be belligerent" (that made him chuckle) so we need to make this food thing as easy as possible for you so you're not running off to the store searching for some certain food that I think I can keep down if I'm not eating because of chemo nausea."

Lately, I've been doing a lot more of the cooking than I would have expected, but hey, if it means I get to eat foods I know I'll eat, then right now that makes it worth the partnership being lopsided regarding me cooking everything. Cooking isn't something I particularly enjoy doing, mostly because I never seem to have enough time to do it justice. Cooking and eating just aren't high on my priority list, especially at times like this, when I'm stressed and my stomach is tied in knots and the last thing I want to do is put food in it. Marco gets cranky when he doesn't eat for a while (something he openly admits), so I knew that he needed to eat if we were going to have an amicable conversation about his caregiving later. I went into the kitchen and chopped up the stuff and grilled the chicken and made dinner. It was a 20-minute job—not the least bit fancy or anything, but decent.

After we had eaten, I still hadn't brought up the caregiver thing, and I couldn't finish my dinner so I had to seal it up and put it in the 'fridge. He stayed in his seat at the counter and started playing with the remote control helicopters I had given him for his birthday. It was cool, because he's getting good at flying them, so his "flying" got us both laughing and in good spirits. I was at the sink doing the dishes from dinner (no, he's not yet acknowledging the hints I drop about using the dishwasher instead of washing by hand; he's shockingly good at not hearing what he doesn't want to hear). So the mood was light, I've just finished the dishes, and it's now or never.

"We need to talk about the caregiver thing." He agreed. "Yes, we do." I went on, "I know I can be difficult, but I can easily teach you how to deal with me if you want to learn it. I know how you feel about people having expectations of you and I really try not to have any expectations and just appreciate you for who you are, but in a situation like this the patient has to know what to expect of the caregiver, to know what care will be given . . . I don't want to impose patient expectations on you like that . . . so I guess what I'm saying is . . . you have an opportunity here to set expectations so that I won't expect more than you can do and I will know what I need to cover myself." No pause. He starts right in telling me that what he needs me to do as a patient is tell him right away when I need something and what it is . . ."No." I interrupt. "While I agree that we need to talk about my role and behavior as a patient later, that is not what this question is about. First we need to talk about you as a caregiver. What do you plan on doing as a caregiver? What are you expecting of yourself as my caregiver?" Now we have the pause I had anticipated, as the response to the actual question formed in his mind.

He listed a lot of important stuff: going with me to appointments and making sure I'm comfortable when it matters; making sure I eat, rest, take my meds, do what the doctors tell me to, and that I am doing OK dealing with the side effects and stuff; and being there in case something goes wrong and we have to call the doctor or take a trip to the hospital. I tell you, this was just tearing my heart out to hear these as the only things he saw as his responsibility, that it was so sterile and lacking in recognition of what may be the single most important thing of all—emotional support. But I managed to swallow it down to reply to him downright calmly.

"Those are all good and important things, but I'm even more worried now, because what my mom and lots of people are telling me is that I just need good emotional support, and with that I'll get through the rest just fine." My voice started doing that wavery I'm-really-scared-and-can't-quite-control-my-voice thing . . . "But the one thing that seems to be completely lacking in this relationship is emotional support. I'm really trying to be a good patient and be thoughtful of your needs as a caregiver who needs time for himself as well. I figured today that the unexpected self-excommunicated afternoon of yard work was in some part your way of dealing with the stress of what you're facing tomorrow and this week." He nodded in agreement to that, said something that kind of sounded like he hadn't thought about it like that but he realized it was at least in part true. But there's more to be said, and here came the damn tears . . . "And I am just an emotional *wreck* right now. I really needed to *not* be alone today, but you took off—even after knowing something was wrong, even if you weren't sure what it was—you still left me alone on the floor to deal with it on my own, and that was why I left. And the sad part is that you could have defused the entire situation with just a few kind words before anything ever happened. And that's where your learning how to deal with me will help us both tremendously, if you want to learn it."

And then—this kind of shocked me—we got into a good healthy discussion about that, as well as the topic of what I know I am like as a patient (from having mom try to take care of me when I've been sick before) and how he can deal with me during the times when I'm being difficult. Let's face it, I know how difficult and belligerent I can be, but I also know how someone can defuse that or take action to redirect it and get me to do what they know they need me to do for my own good. I mean, come on, I've been dealing with me for more than 30 years. If I can't tell him how to do it, certainly no one else can!

He had come around the table while we were talking, and we hugged and he held me a while. We talked some more, standing in the kitchen, and I jumped up on the counter. He continued to hold me while we kept talking, and it all went everywhere it needed to without degrading into the defensiveness that has frightened me off from telling him so many things that were bothering me in the past.

Then we got the bathroom scrubbed up to make sure there wasn't any bacteria that's going to get me sick with my weakened chemo immune system, and he came into my office to lie on the LoveSac while I fed myself a little reward mint chocolate chip ice cream. He thought he wasn't going to be able to relax to sleep tonight because he'd slept late this morning, and, well, there's a lot on our minds. I sat with him a little petting his hair like we do, and just, you know, gave him some love just like I'd done for Mizzou this afternoon. He became completely relaxed and said, "Well, maybe I could fall asleep." I was still petting his hair, and his eyes closed. "Yeah, I can definitely go to sleep. Time for bed."

So, even though things between us are totally "fine" now and I have no huge worries about my caregiver or our relationship at the moment, I'm still nervous about tomorrow and what my body is going to feel like. That's blocking me from sleep. After an hour or so of trying to do a Sudoku puzzle, I finally whispered to Marco that I couldn't sleep and I was going to go back to my office so he could sleep. He wanted to know that I was OK, and I really sincerely was, but unfortunately here I am five hours later (wow: have Internet—will kill time) still awake . . . but at least yawning. Let's hope getting in the bed will do the rest. Then again, I can always sleep all afternoon after chemo, if that's what my body needs. I am so relieved that I took medical leave from work for chemo week. My brain is beyond fried, and in the region of next to useless, from what I can tell right now.

But my caregiver is committed, at least to the mechanical stuff, and he said he understands how important emotional support is too, so I guess we're in the best state we can be given the situation. Ach—Chemo—Tomorrow. It's still scary, but I'm getting to tired to care. I just want to get it over with. When the first chemo is over, I will be less afraid because I'll know what's coming up, instead of trying to see into this ominous cloud of potential side effects and issues, not knowing which side effects (if any, besides nausea) are going to drop down from that cloud and whack me on the head.

I have to chuckle at a thought that just popped into my head.

It's kind of like going out on the dance floor to tango with someone you've never seen before. There is absolutely no telling what the experience will be like until the music starts and you actually touch your partner to sense his movement and intent. OK, Cancer Dancer, now it's *really* time to tango.

~ Act II ~
Treatment

Chapter 12.
First Chemo

CANCER—DAY 87 MONDAY, JULY 20, 2009

No major problems during the first chemotherapy treatment, though we were a little surprised that I was getting chemo for more than four hours today, and I was at the infusion center a total of six hours. Marco took the afternoon off from work and patiently stayed with me the whole time . . . he started reading a book to me (I'm hoping we'll find a more interesting book for future readings, but it was a nice gesture nonetheless).

We actually had a rather nice quiet afternoon "together" amidst the hustle and bustle of the chemo ward. We had a little three sided room almost across from the nursing station so it was easy for them to keep an eye on me but it was also nice to have a little room like that rather than being lined up in a row of chairs of chemo patients, which is what I've seen at two other facilities now. Ucky. I am very glad I went with my instincts and found a different oncologist and got Dr. Lombard and the Marshall Cancer Center. This facility is new, and much more patient-friendly. It's less creepy and scary than the other infusion centers I've seen, with patients lined up in chairs, each alone.

Today I had some discomfort and I definitely got woozy and a bit nauseous when we got home, so I figured out which nausea medicine to take and had a little nap.

The night was amazing in a way, though. It was a long, scary day, but tonight we snuggled together to watch *Little Miss Sunshine* which I'm pretty sure I saw with my dad already, but it's a good quirky film that can be seen more than once. Afterward, during the credits (Marco always watches all of the credits because of his theater arts background), I leaned more toward Marco and absentmindedly pet his hair a little while thinking about what we experienced together today.

After enjoying getting his hair played with a moment he asked me, "What do you think?" I said, "Altogether not too bad, really." He clarified: "The movie?" Whoops! I said, "Oh no, I liked the movie and its quirks. But I meant that, as a whole, the first day of chemo wasn't so bad. Thank you so much for being there all day, it really helped a lot." And we hugged. Then he caught me completely off guard when I looked in his eyes and saw that he had tears running down his cheeks. I tucked his head under my chin and pet his hair and hugged him, and when we leaned our heads away a little, he said "I don't want you to hurt." He clutched me in a bear hug and let more tears fall. Eventually he calmed down in our embrace.

Maybe it's the drugs, but now that the first infusion is in, I'm not as scared. I'm not afraid of being sick or hurting, that's just stuff you have to deal with as it comes. I was touched that Marco would be emotional and sensitive about this now, because if I remember the past few weeks correctly, he's been pretty sterile about the treatment stuff. Kind of like my surgeon—concerned, but focused on the medical treatment and not emotional or mental health. The "Caregiver Talk" I had with Marco yesterday seems to have helped.

One of the difficulties I brought up in conversation yesterday was that I wake up early in the morning (2 a.m., 3 a.m.) worrying about things or scared but I'm afraid to wake him for comfort and thus bother him because he gets cranky and annoyed if he wakes during the night or doesn't get enough sleep. Instead of waking him, I get out of bed and go try to nap on the big cushy LoveSac in my office. I rarely fall back asleep because I can't stop worrying, so I end up being awake most of the night. By the time Marco gets up for work many hours later, I'm pretty much a wreck of stress and worry, and it takes most of the sunlit morning for me to smooth out my mind. Tonight, as we snuggled in our usual pre-sleeping snuggle embrace at the end of my first day of chemo, Marco made a point of telling me to wake him if I'm hurting or if I need anything or I'm scared and I need to be held. I let the goodness of that hang on the air a moment, my head tucked under his chin, then I asked him, "Can I wake you to tell that you I love you?" That got a BIG grin. He said, "Yes, of course you can do that" and he gave me a bunch of little kisses so I went on lightheartedly "Because, you know, that could happen." He didn't say I love you back and I hadn't expected that, this had just been an unanticipated perfect moment for me to be able to tell him verbally that I do love him without pressuring him into a verbal I-love-you response, and I'm so glad the opportunity arose for it to happen that way. The first I-love-you can be so awkward, you know? But this was nice.

I didn't rouse him from his slumber when I got out of bed an hour later. There wasn't anything wrong and I didn't need anything from him and I'm not scared. I'm just thinking about the day and I wanted to write. When I started writing this little story, I was thinking it was strange that my first day of chemo brought us closer together, but as I look back on it, maybe that's not such a surprise. Marco spent all afternoon essentially demonstrating his love and concern for me, worrying about me and making sure I was OK during the chemo infusion, and I was deeply grateful. When I think about it that way, there's no surprise at all that today was one of those intense shared experiences that can strengthen a relationship.

CANCER—DAY 88 TUESDAY, JULY 21, 2009

Wow, people are so amazing. Brian baby-sat me while Marco taught tonight, which was both heart-warming and fun. When Marco got back after class he told us it had been amazing, that soooo many of the students were asking about me and how I'm doing and telling Marco to tell me they're thinking about me and sending their love and good intentions and on and on. Soooo nice. Heck, I practically cried when he told me about it and both Marco and Brian were misty-eyed, too.

CANCER—DAY 90 THURSDAY, JULY 23, 2009

"Stress Relief Mineral Bath Salts." Hmmm, RrreEEaaly? Well now, let's see if they work! Not that I'm feeling any particular stress that needs relief at the moment, but after all that tub-scrubbing Sunday night to get it cleaned up before chemo, I *had* to give the tub a try. Aside from a minor ant problem and some sorely needed re-grouting for the tile, you could say the bath area is sufficiently calming. And yes, it is possible that if I were not in the bath blackberrying it could be even more relaxing, but as I said, I'm not feeling stressed per se, and blackberry journaling really works for me sometimes.

I say I'm not particularly stressed, but I am frustrated. I can't think. Literally. I can't think. I repeat myself. I repeat other people. I wonder that there's not a single unique thought in my head, and yet still I can't seem to keep track of which food is for being constipated or what time I took the med that's on an 8-hour cycle versus the two meds on 6-hour cycles and which one is the one that makes me so drowsy I sleep the day away. Here's what my week has been:

Tuesday: Sleep, call prep, sleep, work conference call, have evening babysitter, day gone.

Wednesday; Get up, nap. Eat some yogurt, nap. Look for wigs online, sleep, day gone.

Thursday: Ah now, here we have a busy one! Wake up, eat banana *and* pudding, nap, go wig shopping and buy a cute everyday wig. (Whoohoo! Big accomplishment!) Nap. Try to eat, feel extra nauseous from getting car sick going to the wig store. Ride tandem bike to Trader Joe's for fresh fruit and veggies, make a nice dinner for Marco. I didn't feel like eating, but I did have some dinner with him. That's probably what's killing my stomach now, though. The Stress Relief Mineral Bath Salts haven't done much for my physical discomforts. Chemo is definitely not fun. Ach, I think it's time for more sleep. Goodnight, Thursday.

CANCER—DAY 92 SATURDAY, JUL 25, 2009

You know, I was just trying to be nice, but it backfired. We had plans for the day, but this morning I offered to Marco that I could get someone else to be with me a while if he wants to go to the tango workshops this afternoon and tomorrow (being so last-minute, this would require some effort, but I could surely work it out with several phone calls). The offer was really just a gesture though, you know? I didn't expect him to jump on it like he did. Marco went on the studio website, reviewed all the workshop sessions in detail, and pointed out that there is also a performance workshop on Wednesday night, right before his Phoenix trip next weekend. I feel like an idiot for drawing his attention to any of the workshop stuff now, because instead of him saying something like "Oh, that's thoughtful Honey, but we already have plans," now he's all up in his head thinking about himself instead of thinking like a caregiver. If he does that performance workshop that will make it seven nights in a row that he's not here for me during my first chemo cycle. A whole week sounds like a lot. Maybe I should let my parents come after all . . .

On the chemo side . . . it's my fifth day since my first infusion, and physically I feel awful. The first night wasn't so bad, but now it's like my insides are a firefight in the War in the Pacific and the generals are willing to sacrifice every soul on the island to put a flag on top of it. Every pilot in the Battle of Cynthia Island is a kamikaze, crashing and burning inside my guts, while battleships fire missiles onto the island and hundreds of troops pour on machine gun fire trying to capture Cynthia Island. So, which med do I take for *that*?

CANCER—DAY 93 SUNDAY, JULY 26, 2009

I went for something a little more upbeat today, both to cheer myself up and to give Marco another break from me. I visited my cats at the pet spa and now I'm blackberry journaling while hanging out with them in the cat play room.

I should remember to bring my camera with me the next time I come here. Mizzou of course is, as always, the nonplussed patriarch of every situation whether he's been through it before or not. Everyone here laughs as I walk in and points to the top of the cabinets where he likes to hang out. Lord of all he surveys, that's my big black cat Mizzou. Mizzou is a smart and stubborn King of the Castle though. When he's misbehaving, he makes sure you're watching and he gives you the evil eye while he does it, to make sure you understand that he's behaving badly because you pissed him off, not because he doesn't know any better!

My kitten Seoul, on the other hand, was fascinated by the sink for like, twenty minutes after I used it to refresh their water bowls. The sink is a good fifteen inches deep, and Seoul is still very small . . . she sits upright like a squirrel in the sink and only her eyes and ears show as she playfully peeks just over the edge. Too cute! And her coloring is so pretty too, she has white outlines around her eyes and these black Cleopatra lines back from the corners of her eyes that just make her very pretty and exotic. Her purebred Siamese show cat mother shows through the wild tomcat that completes her lineage. The bright explorative expression in her eyes is vastly different from the world-wise piercing green of Mizzou's orbs surrounded by all that rich black fur. Mizzou was born on a farm in Missouri (the local university is MSSU, and the football team is called the "Mizzou Wildcats" so it was the perfect name for this little guy when I got him. Apparently only three out of nine kittens in his litter managed to consistently escape the wolves that circled the barn at night, snipping away what they could. Mizzou's a survivor, definitely, and a very strong one at that, which makes him perfect for me, and Seoul's an explorer and a believer, and that makes her perfect for me, too. There's a brightness about her that's hard to describe but undeniably buoyant.

Ah, there is a special comforting balance in the world when I get to come visit my cats at the pet spa. So, disregarding all the physical stuff today has been a good day.

CANCER—DAY 94 MONDAY, JULY 27, 2009

I spent thirty minutes on the phone with the nurse this morning, after a night completely void of sleep and wreaked with discomfort, a rash that seems to be progressing rather than receding, constant gut pains, and some severe central chest pains if I slouch or lower my head. Altogether this seemed much more severe than anyone had anticipated, and it was time to talk to a medical professional. I needed to know whether or not the near-hell I was suffering was of side effects that they are—or are not—surprised that I am having. Turns out, no surprises, except that I apparently have *already* experienced practically every side effect known to chemo, some much more severe than anticipated, especially given that it was my very first week.

Friday night we finally decided we should call the doctor about my pain and discomfort, to make sure there wasn't anything wrong and that what's happening is within some kind of norm for chemo side effects. Marco called in and left a message for the on-call doctor to call him back on his cell phone (Dr. Lombard wasn't on call Friday night, unfortunately). When the on-call doc called back though, Marco just handed his phone to me. Ugh, I can hardly think, let alone re-explain what the heck I just spent fifteen minutes trying to describe to Marco and then hearing him succinctly summarize in twenty seconds to the message service when he explained why he wanted a return call. Anyway, I don't even remember the whole conversation with the on-call doc now (that's what I get for not journaling about it right away or at least the next day, eh?). But I do remember the guy had a strong accent and talked really fast, tough combo for Chemo Girl's brain to process and converse at the level the guy apparently expected, since at one point the doctor even said "Are you still there?" Next time, I'm not letting Marco give me the phone in a situation like that unless the doctor insists. The outcome of my conversation with the on-call doc Friday night was that he was going to send a message to the emergency room at Marshall telling them to expect me and to get me attention right away when I showed up. The possibility of a hospital visit was because of the constant central chest pain I have if I curl forward (unlike heartburn, which I guess is a temporary flare up and has nothing to do with your body position). But by then it was getting on midnight and I was so exhausted, and the pain hadn't gotten any worse in the hour it took to have all those conversations and phone calls, so we decided to wait just a little bit longer and if it didn't get worse, give it the night to see how I felt in the morning. It's not like I had a fever or anything suggesting an infection (which is apparently what scares the bejeebbers out of oncologists), and it was conceivable that everything I was feeling inside my body could be considered "normal" though somewhat extreme side-effects . . . the side effects seem to be more severe and much earlier than anyone expected for me at this early stage in my first chemo cycle.

I didn't go to the hospital this weekend, but I did speak with the on-call oncology nurse, Michael, early this morning. I was on the phone with Michael about 30 minutes, ticking off all my side effects and being told what to do about each. Then Marco had to take me to the drugstore to ring up the additional things Michael suggested, and now I am *literally* a walking pharmacy.

I have this lunch bag sort of thing chock full of meds and directions as well as my calendar charting of my meds, food, and liquid intake. For my calendar charting, I keep a printed copy of my Google cancer treatment calendar of appointments and scheduled meds, and then I write in everything else as I go. Like: last Monday I had two pre-chemo meds to take at certain times before the infusion, and I had to put Lidocaine on the port at a certain time in preparation for the infusion. That was all pre-printed on my calendar, and I checked off each item as it was completed. Then I hand-wrote in everything else as the day went after the chemo session: what time I took what additional meds, how much fluid I had to drink, what food I ate at what time. Going into next week, I definitely need to start charting the side effects too, not just the meds I'm taking (though it is obvious that taking Compazine means I was having nausea and Midol means I was having bone pain, and so on). Maybe the side effects charting should be separate from the treatment charting. My treatment chart is already in a tiny font and hard to read as it is.

CANCER—DAY 95 TUESDAY, JULY 28, 2009

Did I mention I seem to have a consistently low temperature? By like an entire degree or more below the "normal" 98.6 degrees Fahrenheit. I've been in the 97's pretty much every day since the infusion, and I was under temp when they took it there too. Strange.

One week in and my body is a mess. I don't want to think about it. Thinking about it, even just long enough to explain to the on-call medical people, makes it feel worse in a way, more intense because I'm focusing on it to figure out exactly what it feels like so I describe it fully to the medicos. In the interest of not making the side effects feel worse, I need to distract my mind with other, more positive thoughts, otherwise this is going to get very depressing very quickly.

Chapter 13.
Kindness

CANCER—DAY 96 WEDNESDAY, JULY 29, 2009

The "Cynthia-Sitters Needed" Blog Post:

OK all you Sacramento-based Cynthia-sitter wanna-be's, here's your first big chance to put your feet where your e-mail is! =D

Marco (my primary caregiver, as I'm sure everyone knows) is leaving town tomorrow afternoon after my day 10 blood draw. He's going to gone from Thursday afternoon through Monday night. My secondary caregiver, Brian, is going to be out of the country until Sunday afternoon.

So!!! I'm at a pretty good point in the chemo cycle in terms of being able to take care of myself, but they say days 10 through 14 of the chemo cycle are when my immune system is weakest, and we don't really know what to expect since it's only my first round of chemo, so Marco and I would both feel better while he's in Phoenix knowing there are some people stopping in to check on me or that I'll be spending some time with this weekend so I'm not all alone at the house the whole time. Just in case, ya know? (Wow, I am totally the Queen of the Run-On Sentence! Sheesh!)

Many people have sent me e-mails previously offering time to hang out with me during chemo when Marco has other commitments or just needs a break, and I'll go back through my inbox to find those e-mails if I can, but if you are someone who has a little free time this weekend and would like to hang out a while, have a lunch or a dinner or a simple cup of tea, or if you have time to stop by the house sometime this weekend to check in on me, please let me know via e-mail (preferably soon of course, Heaven forbid I plan anything too far in advance during chemo, eh?).

If you would like to be a volunteer Cynthia-sitter or do a drive-by this weekend, let me know.

Thanks!!!

P.S. If you have even the slightest hint of a summer cold, that does unfortunately disqualify you from being an active participant in the Cynthia-sitters weekend. It's really important that I not get too close to anyone who is sick this weekend. Sorry.

CANCER—DAY 97 THURSDAY, JULY 30, 2009

OK, this is not going on my blog because I don't want Marco to hear about it, but I'm very happy about this so I'm certainly going to journal on it for myself. Right after Marco left for Phoenix, I went and sprung the cats out of pet spa jail for the weekend!

I also stopped to buy a vacuum cleaner for the house. The carpets here have *never* been vacuumed! Uck. Marco doesn't own a vacuum cleaner and my hinting that it may be a good idea to purchase one hit a brick wall because Marco only wants some kind of super-vacuum (Dysen?) and they're really expensive so he doesn't want to spend the money on that right now, yet neither is he willing to "waste" money on a cheaper one in the meantime. (Seriously, sometimes I really do not get his thought process.) So, in the entire time he's lived here, the carpets have *never* been vacuumed. Hence, at my first opportunity when Marco could not argue with me not to do so, I went and bought a vacuum cleaner for the house. I figure I'll just leave it here when I move back home later, since I already have a good vacuum cleaner at home. Marco can keep it or sell it to buy his fancier vacuum cleaner or whatever after treatment.

So anyway, that was a side-track from why I am excited today. The cats are here! I have an anti-allergen machine filtering the air, throw sheets over all the furniture, and a tall dog gate blocking the doorway to Marco's office. Mizzou looked through the gate a moment, decided Marco's office was completely uninspiring of mischief, and came back into my office to supervise Seoul's discover of my new aquarium and fish. Too bad that series of photos, *Cats Meet* Fish, can't go on my Facebook—at least not until well after Marco's back and I'm sure the cats being here didn't miserably aggravate his allergies. I hope that the air filter and furniture covers will suppress any indication that I brought my cats here, since Marco says he is so ridiculously allergic and is no longer interested in the possibility of taking medicine for it. Man, the shifts and changes in relationships happen so fast. Or maybe this is normal and I just don't remember what it's like to be in a new relationship because I haven't done it in forever. Or maybe the shifts just feel sudden to me because I'm in a weird mental state, you know, being Chemo Girl and all that.

Holy cow, it is absolutely insane how many people, in just 24 hours, responded to my "Babysitters" blog post. I have some logistical planning to do!

Sunday, when Brian is here, I'm going to have to put him to work vacuuming. Well, after her gets the boxed-up vacuum out of Yoda's back seat and assembles the vacuum (Yoda is my car, a Toyota Camry I bought from my parents for a dollar so I wouldn't have to commute four hours to Sacramento in my Jeep to teach dance lessons). Brian's an engineer too, with a great happy personality, so more likely than not he'll actually have great fun doing it. As for me, after taking the cats back to the pet spa/cat jail, I'll be spending my Sunday afternoon giving the kitchen a very, VERY serious scrub-down! I am really looking forward to having a clean kitchen for once, even if the cleaning and scrubbing process completely exhausts me.

CANCER—DAY 98 FRIDAY, JULY 31, 2009

Blog Post for *Cynthia-Sitters Weekend Extravaganza*
THE SCHEDULE

Thank you, thank you, thank you to the many people who have volunteered their time to visit me in person or check on me via phone this weekend! So many offered that I had to beg off several visits to see people at the milonga instead in order to make sure I still rest a lot the weekend!

Here's how the weekend is playing out:
Friday, July 31st

- *6:30PM–8:00PM Emmy White*

Saturday, August 1st

- *12:00PM–1:30PM Joe & Donna DeLang, Marie Mason*
- *8:30PM–9:30PM Mice Gonzalez*
- *9:30PM–11:00PM Firehouse 9 Milonga*

Sunday, August 2nd

- *11:00AM–12:30PM Brenda Tate, Jenny Tate*
- *3:00PM–8:00PM Brian Bradford*

Monday, August 3rd

- *Randy Westfield in and out all day*
- *Marco comes home at 10PM, yay!!!*

This is great because I still get plenty of rest time, but I'm also going to have a fun weekend! Meanwhile, I also promise to get the regular blog caught up by Monday!

If anyone wants to call to check on me (I've already had calls from Debra Wellington and Jen Barston, besides Marco and my parents, of course), feel free. I turn my phone and computer volumes to mute when I'm resting, so you won't disturb me by calling and leaving a voicemail if I don't answer during a nap.

Thanks Everyone!!!

CANCER—DAY 99 SATURDAY, AUGUST 1, 2009

I had THE nicest lunch with my old friends from San Jose today! They were going to Oregon to visit some friends and go wine-tasting. When they saw on my blog that I needed babysitters this weekend while Marco and Brian are gone, they offered to visit me today. Actually, Donna offered to drive up by herself on Friday night to make me dinner Friday night and stay at her sister's then come make me breakfast and take care of me Saturday until Joe and Marie and Stewart got here and then they all could stop in again Monday on their way back, to make sure I'm still doing OK.

I continue to be just dumbfounded by the unbelievable kindness in people and how much they're willing to do to help me and what they're volunteering of themselves for me. I mean, come on, these old friends live in San Jose for Pete's sake! They certainly don't have to drive to Sacramento to help out this weekend, but here they are. And tonight I have another Bay Area babysitter, Mice (how's that for an awesome avatar name?), coming out from Castro Valley (near San Jose) just to visit with me before the milonga. Unbelievable. I don't even know how to thank so many people for so much kindness. I should throw a big party, maybe when chemo is over.

CANCER—DAY 100 SUNDAY, AUGUST 2, 2009

Too tired from cleaning to think, but the day must be recognized.

Day 100. We're in the triple digits now. To quote my Norwegian Grandma Inez . . . Uff da!

CANCER—DAY 101 MONDAY, AUGUST 3, 2009

OK, OK, I concede. I am definitely more emotional now than I used to be. Mostly because it's so easy to make me cry now. Not so much the physically difficult stuff like pain, discomfort, and new unexpected side effects that are really bad but the doctors mention in a list as something simple like, "fingertips tingling." That physical stuff has to get REALLY bad to make me cry. Don't get me wrong, the pain has made me cry, like the first time I had bone pain . . . it was sooo deep in my spine and so utterly unexpected that I was practically knocked down the first time bone pain exploded me. At the same time, I was also so nauseous from the smells of cooking dinner that I had to go sit outside in the back yard while Marco threw out the casserole I'd been baking, and instead cooked some plain rice for me to eat and opened all the windows to air the house out. More easily than pain, though–what makes me cry ridiculously easily now are all the little kindnesses I get from so many people, every day.

I've spent the last several years of my life with a personal focus on being kind, and trying to be kind to everyone regardless of how they treat me or others, and I've had a lifetime of examples of generally unnoticed kindnesses from my mom (who incidentally is an R.N., and was just *loved* by her patients for her kindness and caring, as well as being smart and efficient). When she has guests, even just my brother's family and me at holidays, Mom somehow anticipates everyone's needs so they don't even have to ask for something because she brings it in the room at just the moment they would think to want it. And out in Sidney, Nebraska, she's been unequivocally classified "the nicest lady in town."

It was about four years ago now that I felt like everywhere I looked I saw people treating each other badly for no reason. Even though weather delays are not the gate agent's fault, for example, how many times have you seen someone take their frustration out on the gate agent at the airport? How often have you heard someone speak sarcastically "down" to a waiter, like he's some lower class person just because he's working nights as a waiter (or dance instructor)? For some reason, many years ago I started being really sensitive to the insensitivity we treat each other with. It felt like darkness to me. It reminds me of the tearful Tinkerbell line in *Peter Pan*: "Every time a child stops believing in fairies, somewhere, a fairy dies." Something like that. I was traveling a lot for work then, and it just seemed like everywhere I turned I caught humanity at its worst.

As a result, I've been trying to be kind for what seems like a very long time now to me but really is no time at all in the big scheme of things and how long life is. But aside from trying to think of little ways to be kind like my Mom is, without recognition or realization by the receiver, I've never "thought" about how to spread kindness per se. Nor had I noticed much effect one little person such as myself had on the world, if any. But I feel better when I manage to catch and stop myself from contributing to the negativity in the world.

Now I'm starting to really believe in the saying that "what goes around comes around." At least, I hope that's why I'm on the receiving end of so much kindness now. I am at a loss for words to express my gratitude for the countless kindnesses of others since I was diagnosed. And so, lacking words but full of emotion, tears come. Usually I manage to keep them to myself, meaning, alone in my office in the very early morning, or like a lot of the last few days with Marco out of town, any time of day when I have downtime from all the activity of being "baby-sat." (Babysitting Cynthia basically involves entertaining me with conversation during a walk or while getting calories into me, though Marco has the singular privilege of also babysitting me while I nap and when I'm throwing up or other awful stuff.)

There were tears today while I talked with Terry (my current VP and also an old friend) for the first time in two weeks (versus texting or e-mail) and had to tell him I don't think I should be working during the third week of my chemo cycle because the side effects have been so debilitating and I honestly have such a hard time thinking or getting anything done that I just can't imagine trying to do my job during this. I didn't want to tell Terry I can't handle it. I wanted to be the dedicated and reliable Cynthia everyone knows professionally, the Cynthia who always delivers top-quality projects even through sickness, adversity, grief . . . but that's just not true of this. I don't know if it was in my voice or not, but as Terry was telling me not to worry about it, that my company will be OK, telling me to just make sure he knows what has to happen and they'll get it covered and I should just take care of myself and my health through this, well, it wasn't a long conversation with Terry but here's emotional me afterward with tears streaming down my cheeks and being so thankful that I've known Terry and John and so many of my colleagues for so many years through multiple companies so that I feel like they're my personal friends in additional to professional associates. If this had happened while I worked for any of my previous companies, well, I'm sure I would not be the recipient of such unwavering support.

There were more tears while I was talking to Debra, who's called me every day while Marco's been away, just to check on me and see how I'm feeling. She even wanted me to go stay at their house Thursday night but I begged off telling her I was OK to stay here alone at night. She had to be behind that card I got from everyone at the tango studio, filled with notes from more than 45 people wishing me well. And this evening here I was, tears streaming again, while Debra so politely asked me if it was OK for her to put my name on the prayer list at her church. She didn't even have to ask my permission to do that, but she didn't want to do it if it made me uncomfortable. I've read a lot about the power of intention and I think there's a lot to be said for "wishing" someone well, and I know there have been a lot of people doing their darndest to intend or pray me back to health. Maybe that's the reason chemo is only four months instead of six. Could be, you never know.

The kindness that put the tears over the top and stopped me in my tracks tonight was a card from a couple whom I've only met once or twice; they're good friends of my parents out in Sidney (you know, the little town in Nebraska I chose not to go stay in for six months of chemo back when I had that crummy medical oncologist who said to give me the generic 6-month chemo treatment including the drug that's bad for my heart without any additional testing to confirm that chemo would or would not be helpful, and which drugs were or were not needed). Just seeing the Sidney, Nebraska return address on the envelope stopped me in my tracks right there in the kitchen, I didn't even get all the way back to my office. I froze in place, a couple tears slipping out in my disbelief that people I've only met once or twice in my life would take the time to send me a card in the mail. Who sends cards in the mail anymore? I didn't even open it at the time, I set it aside to open later tonight when I was "less emotional." Yeah right.

How can you not bawl your eyes out when someone writes a letter to tell you what good friends and people your parents are, and how much they talk about what you're going through and worry about you, and that "your folks have their bags packed ready to roll if you ever need them. . ."

I have a good friend in Atlanta, Georgia who just had a baby last week and she texted me one day a couple months ago saying I should have a warning message on my website to caution pregnant women to read my blog with tissues handy because it will make them cry. I think at the time the blog was that whole emotional story about Marco deciding he wanted to be my caregiver. It seems like forever ago. And now she has a baby!! But I remember her texting about reading my story with tissues handy now because I don't think I could read what I've written tonight and not cry again. So I'll not read it again, maybe not for a long, long time, not until all of this is over.

CANCER—DAY 102 TUESDAY, AUGUST 4, 2009

I'm shedding hair faster than my cats, I swear, and we buzzed my hair off completely last night so as I shed now it's just all these little short hairs getting all over my shirt like pet fur. But, not for long, I'm starting to have bald patches, tiny little areas so far, none grown together to make any great big bald patches yet. At this point, I'd just as soon get it over with and be completely bald, rather than having to brush the little fallen-out hairs off myself all the time.

Then again, I'm glad to be brushing off these little pieces of hair rather than clumps of the 18+ inches of hair I had before diagnosis. I really didn't realize how long my hair was until I started cutting it shorter and shorter as chemo made it more and more ucky. I cut off about ten inches the first time, in anticipation of chemo, (remember the notary guy asking when I had cut my hair?), then I cut at least another five inches off, then a few more. Marco buzzed off what was left last night. So that's something to be thankful for, I guess. I'm thankful that it's just these little stubby pieces of hair all over my clothes, instead of clumps of super long hair that would be depressing to pull off my shirt or pillow.

It's not that I mind being bald for some period of time. Actually, I think it's going to be kind of fun getting to change wigs and looks between huge extremes as frequently as I want without having to dye my hair or cut it or grow it out. It's the professional dancer in me, the Cynthia Swan that does performances and shows and competitions, always looking the role for whatever the show is. I went shopping online on Saturday and found this great wig website (www.wigs.com, how's that for a no brainer?). I ordered a couple more wigs and hairpieces for the bald phase of my treatment. It should be entertaining to change my profile pic every few days with a completely new look, long, short, blonde, red, black, brunette, blue-streaked . . . you name it, I can probably wig it!

I have lots of different wigs now . . . long, short, golden blonde, platinum blonde, brunette, bright red, dark auburn, black . . . and I wear a different wig every time I go anywhere. On Sunday, to "babysit" me over lunch, I met Brenda Tate at Sephora wearing my latest and greatest short hair wig, a bright but deep cherry red. I've never really done the red hair thing much, so we went for makeovers and to hang out at the mall for a while. The make-up artist was superb. The colorings looked great with my skin while complimenting the colors in the wig and still being shades I can use with other wigs as well. At the beginning she asked if we were also interested in skin care products, so I showed her the little red rash bumps on my neck and asked if they have anything that might cover it up. (Brenda had already told the girl I was a chemo patient, and, I think, told the girl to be very nice to me or Brenda would have words with the management. Brenda is a nurse, and she was not going to tolerate anyone making me uncomfortable about my wig even if it was an inadvertent slip of not knowing I had on a wig.) After I showed her the rash, she said "I have just the thing, be right back!" She came back with a skin cleanser and moisturizer called Kinerase and told me that it had been particularly helpful for people having chemotherapy and these rash bumps. So, all in all that was a useful trip, and fun to go to a real make-up artist to see what an expert would do for make-up with this sassy dark cherry wig!

I don't know if I wrote about this earlier, my head is generally fuzzy now and I forget my own thoughts, but today I keep thinking about a comment someone made to me . . . that maybe it's a good thing that I'm having so many side effects, because maybe that means my body really is very healthy and is fighting the chemo drugs like mad just like the body should. That's the most positive perspective on chemo side effects that I've ever heard. I wonder if there's been any medical research about *that*?

Here's something else pretty cool . . . my niece Nicki, who is nine, decided many months ago, well before my cancer diagnosis, to grow her hair out to have it cut and donate her hair to Locks of Love so someone somewhere can have a human hair wig. She got the cut just a few days ago, and my dad e-mailed a photo of her and one of both she and my nephew, Eric, today. Nicki looks so cute with her fashionable short cut, and her hair still reaches her chin, so it's certainly much, much longer than my hair is today! Gotta say, my brother has adorable and good-hearted kids.

I've been wearing my favorite pink cap most of the time so far, primarily to keep myself from constantly itching at my head. And wow, does it ever itch! At least now with the hair really, really short, it doesn't feel so icky to touch anymore. It felt like there was Elmer's White School Glue coagulating on top of my head. Before "the buzz," my hair felt all gross and dirty, even while I was washing it. It had a four-days-camping-without-water kind of grime feel to it, with the glue mucking in the grime on top. Ever heard of "grunge" as a style? I was there, baby, and I definitely could not do grunge on purpose just to be trendy.

While I honestly like the convenience of the buzz cut, all I can really say is . . . I am not butch enough to pull off this look!

CANCER—DAY 103 WEDNESDAY, AUGUST 5, 2009

Well, here's an unanticipated twist for you . . . we're probably going to move sometime in October, hopefully during the couple extra weeks recovery I have between the end of chemo and the start of radiation. Apparently the house we're living in now is going to go into foreclosure or something in a couple months. It will get listed in the market soon, and though foreclosures don't sell quickly, we'd just as soon get out of here and not have the stress or worry about moving during my treatments of either chemo or radiation. So, Marco's starting to look for a new place, and my full-time occupation now is managing the cancer stuff and taking care of myself (with Marco's caregiving support secondary to his work and house-hunting).

We had an appointment with a nutritionist today and learned a few things that we can do to help with the nausea and mouth sores. Marco took some other notes down too, things we're supposed to look for at the store. One of them was certain kinds of fruit juices. Water, even really clean filtered water from the co-op, tastes just terrible to me. Water has an awful rusty-metal salty-blood taste to it now, so I've been drinking a ton of juice, and Cool-Aid. Apple juice is my drink of choice, but we ran out last night so today all I had was Cool-Aid, and WOW was I hyped up on the sugar from drinking my own Cool-Aid (haha). I was so jittery I couldn't nap this afternoon, and I'm feeling pretty worn out now from working a few hours later than I was planning on, trying to tie up loose ends before taking off from work completely.

Tomorrow we're going to pick up the tandem bike (Marco was having some welding done on it while he was in Phoenix), so hopefully we'll start bike riding again. That's turned out to be a lot of fun, and the tandem isn't as tiring for me as riding a bike alone. I imagine if I were really wiped out I could just let Marco do all the work to pedal us home, right? Not that it's really in my personality to let him do that, I'm stubborn that way. Tenacious C, that's what Marco calls me.

Marco and I finally talked about some serious stuff on the way home from my appointment with the nutritionist today. Things haven't been going very well in the caregiver-patient relationship. I told him I was disappointed in my caregiver and don't feel cared about let alone cared for, and he told me he doesn't like being made to feel guilty when I'm disappointed. Basically we're both going to try harder, and he wants me to tell him right away when I need something, so we'll see how that goes. I'm terrible at asking for help, and it seems to me that my caregiver should maybe, like, you know, keep an eye out for me or at least consider that if he's thirsty I may be too. I'm certainly not going to bother him every time I need a glass of juice, you know?

The conversation ended in the kitchen with Marco getting more emotional and shedding tears while he held me and told me "I do love you, I really do love you." He was adamant and sincere, emphatic really, and it was nice to hear.

I have to say, it is really hard to give a relationship the attention it needs and deserves when you're constantly distracted by cancer treatment and side effects.

CANCER—DAY 104 THURSDAY, AUGUST 6, 2009

I didn't know how lovey Marco would stay after finally saying he loved me yesterday, but last night as we were going to sleep I was giving him a kiss and he said "love you." So I was the responder: "I love you, too." I think the shock registered pretty clearly on my face as I replied, but I'm glad he said it again. I love having that be the last thing said at night. There's just something comforting and peaceful about it for me, probably because my parents would say that before I went to bed at night as a kid, and as an adult every phone call with my parents still ends with "I love you." That's just how I was raised.

I had maybe 30 minutes worth of work to do this morning, which took me two or three hours to actually do, then I was posting files they might need with me out, and by then it was time for a nap, or at least a little rest, so I settled into the LoveSac and watched my fish swim for a while.

My fish are funny. I have this cool special aquarium called a ZeroEdge, and water flows over the top of the tank, down into a reservoir in the cabinet below, then it's pumped back up from inside the middle of the tank. It's kind of artistic and beautiful in and of itself, and the quiet waterfall noise it makes all the time is really peaceful. I actually had it running for two weeks before I bought any fish, to get the water ready to have fish, and I love the sound of it. But it creates a really strong current, so it's lucky that I like the chubby Ryukins, a "fancy" goldfish (did you know there's an AGA–American Goldfish Association? I kid you not!). The Ryukin goldfish are chubby-wide with huge fluffy tails, seven flowy fins in all, and they're not as likely as some other fish to jump. And given that the water itself runs over the edge of the aquarium, well, we didn't want to get any jumpy fish! Ryukins are not the strongest swimmers which is good because they probably won't go swimming over the edge (though Crystal, my Ryukin who was mostly white, did commit fish-suicide by going over the edge while we were in Vegas for Marco's birthday in July). Even with slow-moving fish, I can't have the pump on full-speed because it seems like too much current for them to swim against all day long. And in order to feed the fish, I have to turn the pump off so the fish food doesn't go over the edge before they can get to it.

Rerun is pretty smart. He's an older fish, and he's figured out that when I turn the pump off, chances are they're going to be fed, so he gets all twitchy and hyper when I stop the pump. I named him Rerun because he was the biggest Ryukin in the store, and one of the most beautiful, but he was just as cheap as the smaller, not-as-pretty Ryukins. I asked why he was so inexpensive, and the fish guy told me that he had been given to the store by someone who couldn't keep him anymore, probably because he got too big or they had to move or something. So Rerun is, well, a "previously-owned" fish, and I am his second home, so it's, well, like a rerun on TV. Then Mario told me there was a character named Rerun on some old television comedy, so apparently the name is both logical and humorous.

Opie's name is more obvious, I think. He's completely bright orange in the body and the color fades out in his tail. His solid bright orange immediately made me think of Opie on the *Andy Griffith* show, which aired in reruns a zillion times when I was a little kid. Ah, the good ol' days, when television was more wholesome and trustworthy of not damaging a child's psyche! Or maybe I just think that, when it was actually my parents exercising television "parental control." Who knows.

The newest fish, Snow, hasn't even gone into the ZeroEdge aquarium yet. She's been in a separate "quarantine" tank for almost two weeks now, and on Sunday she'll get to move over to the ZeroEdge aquarium with Rerun and Opie. Apparently it's better for the fish if you isolate the new one for a couple weeks to make sure it doesn't have any fish illnesses that it would give to your existing fish. I'm just learning all this stuff since I just bought my first aquarium a month ago. (Holy cow, a *month* ago? Cancer Time is seriously warped!) Snow is completely white in the body with an orange shock of color on her forehead and some flecks in her tail. Another beautiful fish. We couldn't decide at first whether to call her Snowflake, or Snow White, or just Snow. We had just seen that kung fu movie with the female assassin named Snow in it, and we ended up calling the new fish Snow all the time before I officially named her that. She's sparkly like a new snowflake on a cold snowy day.

As for how I know the gender of each fish, well, I don't. I just gave them names I liked and now I refer to them as him or her based on their name. How do you tell what gender a fish is, anyway? Never mind, I don't really want to know.

All in all I've had a quiet day. I managed to cut my finger while slicing cheese for a snack tonight, so Marco took over. Luckily it was a very small cut and stopped bleeding quickly. Last week I had scratched one of the chemo-reaction rash spots and it bled for ten minutes or something ridiculous like that. With my immune system jumping around and my platelets being low from chemo, I bruise more easily and it takes longer for cuts to stop bleeding, so I have to be extra careful. I *was* being really careful with the knife tonight, but my hands fumble somehow, and next thing you know I have a bloody finger. Marco is starting to dictate new house rules for me. "No more excessive cleaning" [like on the Sunday he was gone when I scrubbed the kitchen]. And "No more of *that* either" [anything with knives].

One of the weirdest chemo side effects has been with my hands. They feel crazy dry, especially the tips of my fingers. So much so that most of the time everything I touch with my fingertips feels like it's made of insulation and the asbestos fibers are catching on and slicing into my fingertips. Sometimes my fingertips get numb (which people have reported as a side effect of chemo—it's called neuropathy), which makes it really hard to type quickly and correctly!!! It is also making me generally a bit more clumsy than normal, and I can't open anything with ridges in the top (like pill bottles, or the apple juice bottle) because the lines in the cap hurt my hands too much. It's wild.

I was ridiculously tired today, probably because I worked most of last evening, but I feel so much better about leaving off my job now that it was worth it to work late. It's as organized as I can get it now, and I trust the people taking over my projects, so it's been an enormous relief today, knowing work will be fine and no one is assuming I'll be able to work during the rest of chemo. I can help out on stuff when I'm feeling well enough though, which is cool. No pressure to work, but if my brain gets really bored and my body can muddle through, I can always jump back in to help out and work a few days here and there. Did I say how lucky I am to be with this particular company when the cancer hit the fan?

Oh, and by the way, Rerun will also flick water at you with his tail over the edge of the aquarium. He has a gargantuan tail, so he can flick a LOT of water at you if you're within a foot of the aquarium! Right when I'm settling into a nice relaxed state listening to the waterfall sound of my aquarium, ReRun suddenly flops out all this water on me. It's ridiculous!

CANCER—DAY 105 FRIDAY, AUGUST 7, 2009

Uff da! (As my Norwegian grandmother would say.)

We'd just gotten back from the blood draw and Marco decides to make himself something to eat. He doesn't ask if I'm hungry or if I want any of what he's making. Turns out he was making a cheese quesadilla with Randy's jalapeño tortillas, which smell bad to me even cold, so I started making a plain dry peanut butter sandwich for myself.

Then Marco put the bad-smelling tortilla in the toaster oven, and the whole house filled almost immediately with what seemed to me to be a noxious fume of jalapeño nastiness, instantly permeating every room in the house. I honestly think I would feel better right now if I HAD thrown up. But I had taken a Compazine for the car ride to the blood draw earlier, so there was just the deep nausea and *wishing* I could throw up from this nasty cooking jalapeño smell.

I bolted to the back yard and cried with the ache of it for a few minutes until the gut pain subsided a little bit, then I took my sandwich in and asked Marco to put it in a Tupperware for me to eat later. And ugh, in those few minutes I was outside the smell had gotten even stronger and I couldn't be in the house. I grabbed the receipts Marco was supposed to scan for me and took off to walk to FedEx to make the copies for work. That only took a few minutes, so I walked a block out of the way to come to the new crepes place for a strawberry blintz for lunch. They have an outdoor patio, and it's not too hot today, so the smells here aren't bothering me. I wonder if the house still reeks?

I have a feeling I'll be eating a few more mushy not-too-smelly meals here at the crepes place before all this is over. Oh well, there are definitely worse things in life than having to eat delectable cold strawberry crepes for lunch because the house smells bad!

CANCER—DAY 106 SATURDAY, AUGUST 8, 2009

I'll start with the not-so-good story for my journal, but end on a positive note I can put out on the blog . . . I keep almost all of the relationship stuff off the blog now, for two reasons. First, I don't want to worry my family and friends with concerns that, besides all the physical issues, I'm having relationship issues that may be impeding my care and recovery. Second, I don't want to blog anything bad about Marco. Most of his friends read my online *Cielem'el Cancer Journal*, and out in public he really puts on a good game face in terms of projecting for others that our relationship is still wonderful. Everyone in the tango community seems to think highly of Marco. When people talk with him at milongas, he definitely comes across as a nice guy with a good laugh. The thing is, Marco just plain doesn't go anywhere when he's in a bad mood, so no one ever sees anything but the Happy Marco. I don't want to put anything negative about him out on the blog because I don't want to tarnish his reputation. But here in my private journal, I think I have to be real with myself. Even if all that accomplishes is getting the negativity out of my head and into the pages, well, that's definitely an improvement versus stewing this kind of thing around and around in my head.

Getting on with today's stories . . .

Marco doesn't seem to want me around today. He's generally ignoring me, which I've discovered is actually the best way for things to be when he's not in a good mood. I'd rather be ignored than have anger or even discontent directed at me for no discernable reason.

I'm getting more and more worn out, and I'm preoccupied. I really don't want to start another round of chemo already, even though it's been three weeks since the first one. The side effects are already much, much worse than anticipated. Will another chemo treatment make the current side effects more severe? Will I have new side effects? My second dose of chemo is still two days away, I've only had one chemo treatment before, but I am absolutely dreading Monday anyway.

Debra just called and asked Marco to teach with her tonight. He never teaches on the weekend, usually Dietrick subs in if Debra needs a Saturday night teacher. Marco and I had plans to go out for dinner before the milonga tonight, you know, like, on a date. There's nothing wrong with Marco changing his (our) plans really, but in my new, more sensitive emotional state, it actually made me feel bad somehow, unwanted, for Marco to suddenly cancel our "date." Of course, when you're living with someone, going out for dinner doesn't seem to count as a date anymore. So, I was already oversensitive to feeling unwanted today because he's been ignoring me, and that is pretty much what was on my mind when Marco leaned back in his chair to look across the hall and ask me if I was OK with going to the studio early and sitting around while he taught, or if he should come back and pick me up for the milonga later that night, or if I would just drive myself to the milonga later or stay home alone, or what. I was kind of speechless, strangely too tired to care but somehow not really OK with it, so I said "I don't know." He pressed it though, asking if I had any issues with him going to teach the class. Ha! Like he's going to let me have a say anything like that. Marco does what Marco wants to do, that's how life works for him, and if I have any issues with that, he gets upset with me. If I told Marco I didn't want him to go teach tonight because I wanted to go on our planned "date," that would really send him off into Mean-Marco land, chastising me for being so selfish and who knows what else. I quietly said "Even if I did have an issue with it, I wouldn't tell you. I'm not that dumb." And I turned back to my computer. He told Debra it was fine for him to teach tonight, and he hasn't spoken to me since, he's just playing World of Warcraft.

I wish I could go home.

On the brighter side . . . I do have a blog-able story for today so I don't have to publicly write anything about what today has really been like.

I got the *nicest* handwritten note in the mail today, from the CEO at my company. He was my first boss at k2 back in the day, some ten years ago or so. Wow, ten years? Anyway, this note is so nice, I just had to include it in the blog for my family to see . . .

Cynthia,

I started to drop you an e-mail but I thought it would be too impersonal for what is a very significant personal challenge that you are facing. I want you to know that all of us are thinking of you and are eager to offer support in any way that we can. You have always proven yourself to be a strong individual and the tone of your message to the team demonstrates the strength and courage you are applying to this fight. I want to personally offer you my prayers and support. Please to do not hesitate to reach out to me if there is anything I can do. I know you will be victorious and this will be an experience that strengthens your spirit and your bonds with friends and family.

Sincerely,
John

Uff da, talk about nice! Then I started wondering . . . what the heck did I write in my chemo message to the company that "demonstrates my strength and courage?" Well, at any rate, I thought it was incredibly kind and thoughtful of my CEO to send me a handwritten note like that.

Have I mentioned how continually awestruck I am by all the kindness I receive?

Chapter 14. Every Side Effect Known to Chemo

CANCER—DAY 107 SUNDAY, AUGUST 9, 2009

You know, I don't feel bald. Well, until I rub my head. But when I don't have a wig, hat, or scarf on, my head feels like I still have my old long hair and it's just pulled back in a French knot. I wore it that way every day for years teaching dance, and without anything swishing around my face or down my back, I just feel like I'm wearing a French knot.

Until my head gets cold.

For more than 100 days now, I've read everything I can get my hands on about breast cancer. Though I tend not to use the aphorism "knowledge is power" because I don't like the power overtone, it is definitely true for me that knowledge can dissipate fear. The more I research and learn about what breast cancer is and what other people have gone through, the more prepared I am and the less afraid I am when something I've read about happens to me. Knowledge doesn't make it any easier, but for me knowledge does help me be less fearful.

I've read dozens upon dozens of lists of side effects in chemo books and online, and as far as I can tell even the most comprehensive lists do not include *everything*. It could be that a thorough list would just be too scary and daunting, but it's more likely that no one puts out a truly comprehensive list because that would surely include rare side effects that are actually uncommon in cancer treatment. Every cancer patient is different. In addition, though no one seems to talk about this in any detail, there are side effects to the meds they give you to counter your side effects to chemo and radiation. Besides all the cancer treatment side effects, you could also have a litany of additional side effects if your body reacts negatively, or is simply sensitive to, the additional medications they give you to help counter the side effects of chemo. There are side effects to treating your side effects. How messed up is that?

I'm not any kind of expert or medical professional that can explain exactly what med or combination of meds caused each side effect that I'm experiencing. I am simply a cancer patient trying to comprehend the experience.

First I need to just compile the list, my personal comprehensive list of potential breast cancer chemotherapy side effects, including potential side effects of the medications they're using to counter my chemotherapy side effects. Then I can use the list so I don't forget anything when I make my notes on the details of what side effects I've been having so far, so I can discuss everything with Dr. Lombard tomorrow.

Chemotherapy Side Effects and Side Effects of Medications Used to Mitigate Chemo Side Effects:

- Anemia
- Appetite changes
- Being clumsy and losing your balance
- Bleeding
- Body aches
- Bone pain
- Changes in taste and smell
- Chills
- Confusion and memory problems
- Constipation
- Decreased bone marrow function
- Dental problems
- Depression
- Diarrhea
- Dizziness
- Dry mouth
- Early menopause
- Easy bruising
- Eye changes
- Fatigue
- Feeling light-headed, fainting
- Feeling weak or tired
- Fever
- Fingernail or toenail changes
- Hair loss
- Headache
- Hearing loss
- Hiccups
- Hot flashes
- Infection
- Infertility
- Irritability
- Itching
- Low blood pressure
- Mouth sores
- Muscles and joints weak, sore, tired, or achy
- Nausea
- Numbness, burning, pain, or tingly feeling
- Pain when walking
- Secondary cancers
- Sensitivity to hot/cold foods
- Shaking or trembling
- Shortness of breath even with mild exertion
- Skin rash
- Stomach pain and cramps or heartburn
- Sun sensitivity
- Trouble picking up objects or buttoning your clothes
- Urinary burning or pain
- Vaginal dryness
- Vomiting
- Weight gain

Now that I'm compiling a complete list of side effects from my chemotherapy drugs *and* the drugs they're giving me to counteract the side effects of the chemotherapy drugs, it's no wonder any given cancer booklet can't list all of them. There are soooo many possible side effects, it's mind-boggling.

The medical people at Marshall said that I must be more sensitive than most people to the medications because I seem to have had about every side effect they have ever run into. Marco agrees with them, that I seem to be fairly sensitive in general to any medications and things they do to my body. Like, it REALLY hurt during the first biopsy and I described the pain to the doctor as feeling like little chunks of me were being plucked and torn away from inside my body and he said something like, "Wow, that's actually exactly what's happening, we'll give you more numbing medication then." Duh. That was an awful experience. The day I had five biopsies was worse though.

Compiling my comprehensive list of potential side effects, I'm relieved to say that I actually have NOT had *every* side effect, at least not yet (of course, I've only had one round of chemo so far). I want to share my personal detailed descriptions of the side effects I've experienced, for any young women reading this before they start chemotherapy. I say young women because in general all of this cancer side effect stuff is much more intense in women under 40, and so, being in my early thirties, my experience may be more relevant to younger women than older women. Not that older women don't have it just as bad, or worse in some cases, I'm sure some do. However, I've come across studies showing that older women don't usually have as much difficulty with the multitude of side effects of cancer treatment as younger women do. I also get that impression first-hand from older women I've met in breast cancer support group meetings or online. So, anyway . . .

Get this, though. I have definitely had additional side effects that are atypical or at least never mentioned as potential side effects to the various medications and the specific chemo drugs they're using on me. Would that equate to side effects of the side effects of the side effects? I'm sure these symptoms are documented somewhere on the Internet on in an academic journal; I just haven't found them in relation to the medications they're using on me. So my list includes additional side effects that I have had, even if they aren't described as chemo-related side effects in the literature I've found in my cancer research. This is the whole kit and caboodle for my side effects in the first three weeks of my first chemotherapy treatment.

Anemia. It's hard to say if I've had anemia, exactly. I've definitely had some of the side effects known to be caused by anemia (heart pounding, weakness, dizziness, faintness, and fatigue), but as far as I know my red blood cell counts are still fine in my blood draws, otherwise the cancer center would have called to tell me. The side effects I've had that could be attributed to anemia can also be caused by other meds for chemo side effects and even the cancer treatment experience in general.

Appetite changes. It is such a bummer to suddenly despise foods I know I actually love to eat. The most annoying "appetite change" has been becoming lactose intolerant, and not being able to tolerate milk or ice cream. It's not really an appetite change though, so much as some other GI side effect. Tomatoes too, I can't eat them anymore, they make my stomach cramp. I've had unexpected cravings though. Like, red licorice is suddenly one of my favorite foods, I keep it on my desk and eat some every day. Some calories are better than no calories when you're too drowsy to walk to the kitchen, I figure.

Being clumsy and losing your balance. In addition to being clumsy and losing my balance easily (not good for a dancer!), I've also become very jumpy. For the last week or so anything sudden in movement or suddenly high-volume has not just startled me, it's scared me right out of my skin. Tonight Marco was walking back to our offices from the kitchen as I was walking from the offices out to the kitchen and he was just suddenly there in front of me in the doorway. I jumped so far that I slipped on the linoleum and almost fell down. My feet were literally skidding back and forth like in a cartoon, my socks were so slippery on the floor!

Bleeding. This is definitely annoying. Any time I itch I have to try sooooo hard not to scratch. I scratched one of the rash bumps the other day and it seemed to bleed forever. You may recall that I'm not allowed to use knives anymore, since I cut my finger a few days ago. I have to be very careful not to get any cuts or scratches because I bleed profusely for an inordinate length of time.

Bone pain. Oh yeah, this is a *bad* one, and they were not expecting me to have bone pain with the combo of chemo drugs and other medications I'm on. But girlfriends, let me tell you, this one hits you like a Mack truck, it comes out of nowhere, and it is so intense that it hits a 9 on the pain scale pretty much the moment it strikes. The first time it happened to me was deep in my lower spine. This cannot possibly be categorized as muscular ache or pain; it was absolutely in my spine and sharp. Unfortunately this was the night of the caramelized onions episode of nausea that sent me flying to the back yard to recover, but we did have one good discovery from that experience . . . Marco was petting me on my upper back to be supportive when I was feeling so awful, and the warmth felt good so I put his hand over my lower spine where the pain was and I swear the heat from his hand helped ease the bone pain. Now I have a heating pad in my office and often use it on my lower back when I'm at the computer or even lying down.

Changes in taste. A lot of things just taste different. Water in particular tastes unbelievably awful now. I finally figured out during the day 10 blood draw that the nausea doesn't just put a metallic taste in my mouth, it tastes salty and metallic, like rusty blood. Thus water, having no flavor, now tastes like I'm drinking blood. Nasty. I would never make it as a vampire, which is too bad because Edward Cullen is just yummy! Apple juice substitutes for water in my diet now, which is also good because you get some vitamins out of it as well. When you can't eat, apple juice is a good way to go, or at least it has been for me.

Changes in smell. Oh yeah, baby, this one is definitely more than a little annoying, though at least it's not physically painful per se. There were certain things I was already hyper-sensitive to in terms of smell (cigarettes, onions), but just tonight Marco had to do all the prep work to make the buffalo patties and season them before putting them on the grill. Usually I do all the indoor stuff, prep the meat, make salad, and cook vegetables, and he does the outdoor stuff, the actual grilling part. But the smell of the raw meat in my hands was just too much and I knew it would only get more unbearable if I kept working the raw buffalo meat in my hands to form the burgers patties. I was OK sitting away across the room describing to Marco how I do it and he made a great dinner, which was kind of fun to do together that way, actually. Other raw stuff I usually don't dislike that has bothered my sniffer lately include Randy's spicy jalapeño tortillas and, get ready this one is strange, I hate the smell of a closed bedroom with an unmade bed in the morning. Weird, I know. I call it "sleeping people smell." I've noticed it before with minor disgust, but now it's an unbearably strong odor that can prohibit me from entering the bedroom, so Marco had to learn to pull the covers back up over the bed when he gets up, rather than me going back in to make the bed mid-morning after he's awake, per our usual pre-chemo daily routine.

Chills. Yep, definitely. But for me it probably hasn't been that bad, at least, not compared to what I've seen in movies. Yes, I get freakishly cold sometimes, so much so that it has a seriously detrimental effect on my mood, but I haven't shuddered uncontrollably with cold really (except maybe the day my temperature was 100 degrees and we almost went to the emergency room).

Confusion and memory problems. Don't laugh! I know I started whining and complaining about similar sleep-deprivation symptoms before chemo even started. But these issues are a common known side effect of one of my chemo meds. Now I'm so confused and mixed up memory-wise that I'm afraid to make decisions because I can't think straight. I'm pretty sure I've completely bumbled my finances in Quicken trying to figure out if I can afford to pay my mortgage and base living expenses on disability income. I also cannot remember whom I have told what, so I think I repeat myself a lot. My head is befuddled. What drives me nuts and even scares me a little though is knowing I'm in the middle of a thought and have suddenly forgotten what I was thinking about. At least when I write I can go back a paragraph or two to remember what story I had begun telling, and find my way back to the point. When I just think without making any notes, my brain seems to revolve in a constant merry-go-round rife with tangents pulling me away from the central idea like the centripetal force that pulls you away from reaching the center on a spinning merry-go-round.

Constipation. Lawsy, Miss Daisy, is this one a doosy! My first five days after chemo found me completely constipated, then I had one day of near-normalcy before going into several days of diarrhea. Apparently with the two chemo drugs I'm on, patients have the joy of having both constipation and diarrhea in the same cycle, as opposed to just one or the other. Joy of joys, I know, right? Not.

Dental problems. I wasn't prepared for how bad the chemo-induced dental problems can get. My gums started bleeding on day two of chemo, so I stopped flossing. Not long after that, I also started having gum bleeding while brushing my teeth, but now that I have a super-soft ultra-sensitive toothbrush, the bleeding hasn't been as bad, and I don't floss anymore. I couldn't stand the way my teeth felt tonight and I just had to floss, very carefully, after we had corn on the cob with our grilled buffalo burgers. I still had some bleeding, gentle as I was about the flossing. Sheesh. Other dental problems . . . well, my jaw gets sore. I think I'm clenching my teeth a lot without realizing

I do it which contributes to my jaw soreness. Clenching my teeth, *hard*, seems to go along with trying to overcome pain. I also get a little scrunch line between my eyebrows from constantly squinting my eyes trying to block out pain.

Depression. I don't think I'm depressed, but I have definitely seen how to get there. This is something where being with Marco and around people a lot is probably making a big difference. I see my best friend Brian frequently to give Marco caregiver breaks and because Brian is so upbeat it's pretty much impossible to be depressed in his presence. I think depression would surely kick in if I didn't have to keep my chin up for interaction with other people. I am adamant with myself that I will do everything possible to *not* bring down the people around me no matter how sick I get. A wig and a smile, genuine or not, go a long way to helping people think you're doing better than you really are. I learned a long time ago to put on a pleasant engaging expression (generally necessary for work) regardless of my personal situation, but chemo is really putting me to the test to stay upbeat. I think I've done an OK job of psyching myself away from any severe depression. So far.

Diarrhea. Yeah, it's not fun to find yourself swapping from constipation to diarrhea and back, but the nutritionist told me it's common with many chemo drugs, so this is just one more thing that has to be dealt with each day. I can tell you though, if you've ever had a colonoscopy, this diarrhea isn't as bad as what you get when you drink the stuff that cleanses out your system the night before a colonoscopy. Or an enema . . . this isn't nearly as bad as having an enema in my opinion.

Dizziness. Yes, this has happened, and once so severely it was suspiciously like one of my heart episodes (wow, did that freak Marco out, he's probably more afraid of me having a heart failure episode than anything else in these four months of chemo when I can't take my heart medication). I get up very slowly now, and I am careful to increase any exertion (particularly tango) only gradually so that I don't get dizzy. I still have dizzy spells, though.

Dry mouth. I was getting dehydrated the first week when water tasted so awful but we didn't have much else in the house that I could drink except a few herbal teas. That was before I got on the apple juice kick. Now I sip on apple juice any time my mouth is dry. I read that it's better for me to stay away from caffeine, so I'm not having tea much anymore, only herbal teas like mint leaf without caffeine. But a week after my first chemo, starting on the day of my day 10 blood draw, just when I thought I was getting enough fluids again, my mouth got so dry I started getting sores on my tongue. More on that below, under "mouth sores."

Eye changes. I saw this mentioned in a generic NCI (National Cancer Institute) chemotherapy booklet. It's not noted as a side effect for my specific medications, but my recent eyesight changes have definitely been bothersome. It didn't really occur to me at first that it could be another chemo side effect, but after my first chemo treatment I realized that I couldn't see the small fonts on my laptop screen, or even on the big 20" screen, without squinting my eyes. I've had to change the system settings on both to make all the font sizes 125% instead of just 100%, and I'm switching to Firefox instead of Internet Explorer because it has a zoom in feature that I seem to need now. I've joked with Marco because it feels like I turned forty in four or five days instead of eight years. (I've heard that a lot of people don't need glasses until just after turning forty.) The dip my eyesight has taken has made it all but impossible to read street signs, but I haven't gone to an eye doctor yet. We'll see what Dr. Lombard has to say about this one, but I suspect it's another problem they'll expect to go away when chemo is over, so I've been hesitant to pay for an eye exam and buy new glasses/contacts when I may only need them for two or three months.

Early menopause. The more annoying thing I've had here so far is the vaginal dryness thing, which I'm not going into any detail on because it's just too personal for someone of my "prudish" Midwest upbringing to write for public consumption. I've also had hot flashes at night, being suddenly woken up with my pillow and pajamas drenched in sweat. One of my cancer-survivor friends in Chicago told me about these little cool packs to keep with you for instances of hot flashes that come up at awkward moments. She said most people don't really know you're having a hot flash, it's just something you have to deal with. So far this has only happened to me at night, so instead of hot flashes it's more like night sweats except for the suddenness of the heat.

Easy bruising. I was already like this because of my blood pressure medicine, and I don't think it's gotten any more severe since chemo, so I'm inclined to think it's still just a blood pressure medicine side effect rather than a chemo-related one. But yes, I can bump my shin on the edge of the mattress and get a bruise.

Fatigue. Absolutely, every day including now, and a severe episode just last night which was the next-to-last day of my "recovery week" when I was supposed to not really have any side effects and just be recovering my strength for the next chemo infusion. The fatigue can get so severe that I can barely move, my eyes glaze over, I struggle to talk, and even exhausted as all that I still can't sleep. I lie down to nap and end up watching the fish for 30 minutes because I'm just not sleepy. I'm exhausted physically and mentally, but not sleepy. It's weird. Last night I sent Marco off to the milonga by himself because I just couldn't fathom putting forth the energy it takes to go to a dance and be social last night. I stayed home and watched a movie on the computer instead. I hated it, because dancing tango is without doubt my favorite social activity and to know there was a milonga but I just couldn't go was emotionally agonizing. I didn't want Marco to miss it because of me, but let me tell you, it was really hard to keep a positive encouraging demeanor for him beforehand so he wouldn't feel guilty for leaving me alone to go dance. It was sure to happen sometime in chemo. We know he needs time and space to recover from the stress of being a caregiver. (Like tonight, he's been in World of Warcraft for several hours, which seems like a very addictive game and I'm not too upset that none of my laptops have the graphics capabilities needed to join the game because I would surely lose countless unproductive hours wandering around in the WoW worlds.)

Feeling weak or tired. Absolutely, definitely, no doubt. I expected to be tired, I expected to be fatigued, but I didn't really get what it would mean to feel "weak." That's literally what it is, though. I'm suddenly weak. I can't vacuum the house (though I can sweep the kitchen and bathrooms since they're smaller). I can't do much of anything for long unless my personal drive keeps me going because I've committed to getting something done. I did that to myself last Sunday with the kitchen scrubbing thing, and every day that I worked this week (just Monday—Wednesday, well, actually, Thursday too, though I didn't claim that as a work day). I loathe not completing something I have committed myself to.

Fever. I tend to be low, so when my temperature went from 98.4 degrees to 99.6 degrees in a few hours (was that last week? or earlier? I don't remember, these days I mix up timelines like there's no tomorrow, I swear) we were getting ready to take a trip to the emergency room, which would have been a real pain because it was Tuesday and Marco was supposed to teach that night. I felt sick for a few days before and the day after that, so I'm inclined to think I had a slight cold or flu, maybe caught at the milonga about three days earlier.

Flu-like symptoms. Speak of the devil. Yes, I had a few days during my first round of chemo when I felt like I was getting the flu with a sore throat, headache and fever. It's possibly a reaction to the drugs, which explains another reason (besides a potential infection) why they told us to go to the emergency room if my temperature goes over 100 degrees.

Fingernail or toenail changes. I'm keeping my nails really, really short so that if they get brittle they won't get caught on anything and tear off like some people have reported. Uff da, now there's pain for you. Get a fingernail tear into the quick of your finger and tell me how tolerable you think it is. That's definitely something I am being very careful to avoid by keeping my nails really short. No more long manicured dancer fingernails for me until chemo is over.

Hair loss. Yep, absolutely. I should be completely void of any remaining fuzz in the next couple days I think. All I have right now is a thin bit of fuzziness of the short hairs we buzzed my head to a week ago. It was falling out every time I touched my head, so I started running my hands along my head in the shower and trying to let as much hair as possible stick to my fingers to get rid of my locks, rather than have them constantly on my pillow, my clothes, my desk and keyboard, or Marco. I hear varying guidelines regarding when the hair grows back. The shortest I've heard for re-growth is starting four weeks after chemo. Re-growth may not start until three months after chemo, though, and even then it can be spotty so I may need to keep using wigs and shaving my head until I start growing hair all over my head again around Christmas or so. I seriously like doing the wig thing, though. Whenever someone comments on awful it must feel to have lost all my long blonde hair, I say "No way! Being bald is the only good thing about chemo. I love it!" And I mean it. Still, I probably won't shave my head to remain bald forever after treatment is over.

Headache. This was a later one for me, I've had a headache for the last three days now and Ibuprofen helps but doesn't stop it. It's not a migraine though, in the past I've had those to the point of not being able to look outside because of the bright light, and this chemo headache is just annoyingly persistent, definitely not a migraine.

Shutting the blinds and taking a nap can usually rid me of the headaches I get nowadays.

Hearing loss. You know, I have wondered about this, but I'd never seen it as a possible side effect until last night when I mired through the fine print lists of side effects, word by word, for the medications they're giving me to counter the side effects of chemo. I didn't think of this as hearing loss before . . . basically, it's just harder to make out the differences in the words when someone is speaking to me. It seems like everyone is speaking with poor enunciation and it's hard to understand what they're saying. Heaven help me when someone talks fast with an accent I don't know well, then I'm just lost. It's frustrating though, to have to ask Marco to repeat himself three times because I just can't make out what he was saying. I didn't really think of hearing loss as a possible side effect, but that could explain (to some degree) why I've had to keep asking Marco to repeat himself. Too bad I don't know how to read lips, that would be a very valuable skill to have these days.

Irritability. Ya think? Man oh man, this is no joke. There are certain things that have put me waayyy past the edge business-wise and I've let my agitated response sit in my e-mail Drafts folder overnight before NOT sending it in the morning after reading it again. It's sort of like e-mailing or blogging while on Ambien . . . e-mailing while irritated is simply not a good idea and should be avoided whenever possible. Ditto to Ambien – never *ever* e-mail on Ambien because you won't remember you wrote or sent anything. I guess if you're just experiencing irritability you will at least remember what you wrote, but I'd wager highly that you'd also regret it. Other Ambien suggestions, btw, include not talking to anyone on the phone (again, because you won't remember doing it), not reading at your kitchen table (a certain someone I know had to go to the hospital because his face lost a battle with a clay flower pot when his chair fell over backwards because he was knocked out on Ambien, and falling over backwards hitting the flower pot with his head didn't even wake him up!), and, of course, avoid e-mail, Facebook, MySpace, IM (instant messaging), texting . . . if you've taken an Ambien, avoid any and all interaction with other people. Ambien works really, really well by basically shutting down your brain, and even after someone describes the entire conversation you still won't remember having had the conversation with the person after you took an Ambien, so, better not to have those kind of conversations I think. On the other hand, when I *have* had to be reminded of conversations I completely lost to Ambien, it was funny because I kept saying, "yeah, that sounds like me, yep, I would say that." I guess if you lie a lot things would probably get messy when you can't remember anything after taking an Ambien.

Itching. Oh heck yeah, and this is an annoying one because I'm supposed to be so careful about not getting cuts and scratches. These little rash bumps, and now my almost bald head, itch so badly that I'm sure I could scratch them to bleeding even with my stubbly little fingernails. We used cortisone on the rash bumps, but I've put off trying it all over my head. I have to get some of those head-protector caps they make for wearing under wigs . . . I think wigs are pretty scratchy and surely are causing some of the itchiness on my head. I itch under scarves and hats too, though.

Low blood pressure. This is an interesting one. I've been on blood pressure medication for years, and even with medication my blood pressure was still always something like 130 over 90, which is higher than doctors like. Since my first chemo three weeks ago, my blood pressure seems to be dropping to even better levels than on blood pressure medication, like 120 over 80 or even 78. It will be interesting to see how this plays out over time. For me, lower blood pressure as a chemo side effect is an unexpected bonus.

Mouth sores. I started getting sores on day 10 following my first chemo infusion. These sores started as little white dots that felt like an unskilled acupuncturist had been practicing on the tip of my tongue. Ugh. I had two days of liquid diet using straws until I got that situation under control. The mouth goo they gave me does numb my tongue, but it doesn't last very long, it doesn't stay on just the spot I put it on in my mouth, nor does it taste good. Maybe we'll hit the pharmacy again tomorrow to find better mouth goo (man, that place is getting a lot of money from me these days). The nutritionist gave me some mouthwashes and stuff for dry mouth when I met with her last week, so I'll see if any of that helps during the second round of chemo.

Muscles and joints weak, sore, tired, or achy. The worst of this has been in my knees, neck, and around my shoulder blades, especially my right shoulder and right knee where I have scar tissue from a car wreck years ago. The neck soreness could easily be from sitting at the computer too much early in the week, but that wouldn't explain neck pain on, say, Saturday when I pretty much stayed away from my laptops.

Nausea. This one has been worse than I anticipated. I expected to feel sick to my stomach and not feel like eating, but I wasn't prepared for the massive carsickness I developed. It was absolutely awful at the beginning of my first chemo cycle but has been getting the tiniest bit better each day. It still surges up if Marco hit the brakes too quickly or takes a turn too quickly in the car, though he's generally driving more gently for me now, I think. Carsickness was not a common thing for me in the past. I did get carsick a few times as a kid, but it was rare. This, in comparison, has been insanely bad. Just braking the car while backing out of the driveway can make me want to throw up. The other insanely bad nausea has been with the smells of certain foods, especially when foods are cooking and stink up the entirety of this little house. Usually the aroma of a good meal cooking is a very pleasant house smell, but boy oh boy, not anymore. I've been able to tolerate some cooked food smells, but even when I like the smell it can be overwhelming and turn my stomach. We don't seem to have gotten to a good med solution for this, though they gave me like four different nausea meds. I've heard there's one more that we can ask to try, so maybe they'll prescribe that too, who knows. Or maybe they'll take up my aphorism that "it is what it is" and I just have to keep suffering through.

Neuropathy—numbness, burning, pain, or tingly feeling. This has been most noticeable in my fingertips. I would think there would be a tingly feeling first (like the prickling you get when you try to get up after your foot falls asleep), but with me it went straight to being painful, not just prickly. My fingertips started feeling scratchy (maybe that's what they're calling a tingly feeling). A couple days after chemo started it began to feel like everything I touched with my fingertips was made of asbestos (you know, those slicing fiberglass threads in insulation?). Everything I touched with my fingertips felt like it was making these tiny glass slicings in my fingertips. Ugh, not fun when your work and at least some of your entertainment involves typing. About halfway through week 3 the fingertip pain lessened, but now I have these numb spots in my fingertips, and typing has become nearly impossible. My fingers are clumsy with the numb spots and I mistype all the time. Now the fiberglass-cuts pain is also in the finger joints, especially the joint closest to my fingertip, and in my thumb. And my hands in general are really sensitive and feel, well, thin-skinned. The little ridges in pill bottle caps kill my hands. Can tops are even worse. I can't open any kind of can or bottle with my hands. My thumbs have gotten the worst of this one, though, because of all the pill bottles and how frequently I have to take different medicines. Last week my thumb tips felt like they were burning and bruised all the time. Now I keep my pill bottles open inside Ziploc baggies, but now even those are getting hard to open, so I think I'm going to look for some of those plastic baggies with actual zippers you just slide. My hands have bothered me a lot and it's been a very frustrating side effect.

Sensitivity to hot/cold foods. This is definitely a side effect I am having, but we've been pretty careful not to give me anything steaming hot, and I drink refrigerated juices but I never use ice cubes because they seem to burn like frostbite in my mouth. The only really cold thing I've had is a fruit popsicle and some sherbet. This hasn't been too bad, though, really. It's like that old joke about the guy who goes to the doctor, sticks his arm up in the air and says "Doc, it hurts when I do this." And the doctor replies "Then don't do that!" I'm staying away from anything hot and anything cold.

Shaking or trembling. Hmm, no shaking so far, but I do have a tremble in my hands that isn't quite constant but is generally there. The only time my whole body has shaken or trembled has been when I'm crying, but that's just what happens when I cry, I don't think it's because of my chemo drugs.

Skin rash. Uck, this is not a fun one. I got a rash that was all red and bumpy on my neck the first several days, and then it spread out over my torso as well as my face, scalp, and back. I even found a few rash bumps down on my legs, these little red and white bumps that itch so irritably it's nearly impossible to not touch or scratch at them. We bought some cortisone cream to put on the rash spots at night, and gradually the rash has been going away, though I still have a lot of little bumps up both sides of my neck. I managed to get rid of most of the ones on my face with some better face scrub and lotion stuff when I got the makeover for my red wig last weekend. The only bumps that are still blooming radiantly right now, as I'm about to go to my second chemo infusion, are close to my port where I've been really afraid to itch because I don't want to create any possibility for infection near that still-healing surgical scar. A couple of the rash bumps right next to my port-a-cath scar are still big bumps with white in the center and deepening red around the edges. Not pretty, not fun. But hey, is anything about any of this pretty or fun? Actually, I take it back. Getting to play around with completely different lengths and colors of hair has been fun. Yesterday I was chatting for maybe half an hour with a friend and her fiancé, and the fiancé (who I don't think knew I was in chemo) didn't know I was wearing a wig or that I'd drawn my eyebrows on, he thought I'd just colored it from blonde to dark red/brown since he first met me. That was neat; to know someone genuinely did not realize I was wearing a wig. I like that!

Stomach pain and cramps or heartburn. OMG, this one was awful too. It started while they were giving me the infusion and lasted two weeks, with varying degrees of pain. At its worst, this GI pain was from the top of my neck to the bottom of my bowels, a constant ache with small piercing burning pains inside, all up and down my middle. The best way I have to describe that pain is to liken it to a film I've seen on quantum physics and how our biology of neurons in the brain function and connect for us to learn. The movie showed the neurons all separated but with these little flashes going off inside and between them like a fireworks show, and those little electrical charges shooting between neurons and gradually connecting them are how we "learn" or develop motor skills (and probably other things that we do by habit over time). That's the best visualization I have for it. Well, that and the Battle of Cynthia Island description that seemed to make more sense to Marco. I felt like there were little fireworks exploding in me all the time, sometimes everywhere in my entire middle from top to bottom, everywhere I have esophagus or stomach or intestines in my body. Marco said someone else told him it felt like mice were crawling around inside her, but for me the pain was much more piercing and bright than some little prickle from mouse claws. I could almost see this stuff sparking off inside me if I closed my eyes, that's how intense it was. I think this side effect may be what I'm dreading most about going back for my second chemotherapy infusion. That, and the bone pain in my spine. Well, and the carsickness and nausea. Oh yeah, and this mess with my hands. Well, OK, let's face it, I'm dreading all of it.

Sun sensitivity. Definitely, I burn easily now and I am very, very careful to try to stay out of the sun completely. I also put on sunscreen every morning just in case I go outside, because it is always sunny in California. I haven't gotten any bad sunburns yet though, so this hasn't been too big of a problem for me other than remembering to be preventative about it.

Trouble picking up objects or buttoning your clothes. Big time!!! Between the clumsiness of my fingers and hands, and general weakness, I can't even open simple juice bottles or pill bottles anymore, and buttons are a serious problem. I have a blouse that has a tight row of little round pearl buttons down the front and I couldn't undo them, so I ended up pulling the blouse off over my head and almost tearing it because I couldn't undo the buttons to take it off. Now I pretty much wear stretchy stuff all the time, which is much easier in terms of dressing and undressing. Even my dresses for milongas are mostly one-piece stretchy things so I don't have to do a lot of work to get them on.

Urinary burning or pain. This feels the same as a urinary tract infection (UTI), and if you know the burning pain of a UTI, I am truly sorry, because it is not fun. The best thing to do for it is drink a ton of liquids, which of course makes you need to go to the bathroom really frequently which of course you dread because doing so increases the burning, but that's how it is. With chemo, UTI burning seems to come and go. I haven't found this to be linked to anything in particular, some days it burns, other days it doesn't. Weird science.

Vomiting. The only times I actually threw up were when I had reactions to anesthesia used for the surgeries. The night after getting the port put in, I threw up so viciously for such a long time that I felt like I was going to suffocate from not being able to take a breath between surges. But once I had my first chemo and was on *four* anti-nausea anti-vomiting medicines, I didn't throw up again. I still get nauseas, but I can't vomit now. Whether that is an improvement or not is debatable.

Weight gain. Everyone thinks cancer patients are going to lose weight, but the medical reality is that at least half of breast cancer patients actually gain weight during chemo. I've been careful to make sure I still got calories even when I was on a liquid diet, but I've also been careful, especially in week 3 when I've had a much stronger appetite, not to overdo it too much. I haven't lost a single pound, even with a vastly reduced appetite in chemo weeks 1 and 2. The reality is that I get absolutely NO actual exercise whatsoever, especially compared to my life just four months ago when I was teaching a lot of dance classes and lessons and practicing for pro performances and so on. Now I'm lucky if I go for one six-block walk in a day. So, I'm expending zero calories in exercise, and I just don't need to ingest as many calories as I used to. I know my body is supposed to be burning a lot of calories to fight the chemo drugs and kill the cancer cells, but it must be a far cry from how many calories I needed to maintain my weight as a professional competitive dancer several months ago. They don't want me to lose any weight, and they don't want me to gain any weight. So one of my jobs right now is to manage my weight, and make sure I get more calories if I start to drop, and make sure I back off the higher calorie stuff if I start to go up. Mostly, I just barely eat.

Secondary cancers. This is horrible to think about, but in some patients the Cyclophosphamide chemo drug actually causes secondary cancers later. Repeat mammograms starting as a young woman can also cause cancer, as can radiation. Let's keep praying THAT doesn't happen.

So, that's what's been happening with me with side effects. It's a lot of detail, but I wanted to note everything before we go to see Dr. Lombard in the morning, no wait, it's just a few hours from now because I seemed to have spent most of the night documenting my side effects. Well, at least everything will be fresh in my mind so I don't forget to tell Dr. Lombard about any side effects that he may determine are important to address. I wonder if they can do anything about this stuff, or if I just have to bear up and live with it to get through chemo?

Chapter 15.
Second Chemo

CANCER—DAY 108 MONDAY, AUGUST 10, 2009

This afternoon we go to start it all over again. It's my second chemo infusion today. I've been dreading it since I woke up Saturday. But I'll go, I have to do it no matter how awful all this side effect stuff gets. It would be like letting down my parents and Marco and everyone who's sending so many good intentions my way, to let the side effects defeat me from completing chemo as scheduled.

When it's really, *really* bad, when it's so bad I just don't care about my body anymore and just want it to be over (as in, I don't care if I live or die, and dying would definitely be easier), when it's so bad that I don't think I can force myself to try anymore . . . instead of letting those depressing thoughts ensnarl my entire brain, I change my mind set to suffering through it for them, for the people who love me and who more than deserve for me to do everything and anything to survive cancer, and cancer treatment. I cannot abandon them by succumbing to the disease. When it's too difficult to bear it for my own health and well-being, I make myself bear it for everyone else. And of course I'm also trying to be kind and thoughtful of others as much as possible too, not focusing on myself, and hopefully not worrying anyone. Mentally, that's how I got through the first three weeks.

Ugh. Three more treatment cycles. Three more months, and then it's time for radiation treatment. Uff da.

CANCER—DAY 109 TUESDAY, AUGUST 11, 2009

They gave me more anti-nausea medicine during the infusion yesterday, and I was pretty groggy once they started. I dozed off quite a bit while we were there. Back at the house after the infusion, I slept right through bedtime and all day today, except that Marco and I went to these group support sessions at the cancer center this evening. Mine was for cancer patients and his was for family and caregivers. Marco said he had to leave the family and caregivers session early and go straight to the studio to teach, so Brian picked me up from my support group meeting and took me to his house where I rested for a while.

Brian had a friend visiting him from Germany, and she went out to get us all some take-out chicken. It was good, I enjoyed the company. I know I had fun because I remember laughing, but I couldn't for the life of me tell you want we talked about, I was so tired. Brian got me back to Marco's just as Marco was getting home from teaching, and I pretty much fell into bed with my eyes already closed.

Wow, this chemo round has really wiped me out. Then again, we're being more aggressive on the anti-nausea meds, which of course have me much more woozy but at least not on the constant verge of hurling or disgusted by every little smell.

CANCER—DAY 110 WEDNESDAY, AUGUST 12, 2009

I'm still sleeping almost constantly, but I want to make a note about how Marco is handling this second round of chemo. He's been so good, so concerned, so carefully watchful the last couple days, wanting so much to do everything right when neither of us really know what the heck either of us are actually supposed to be doing or how to communicate about it. Communication is definitely an issue in our caregiver/patient relationship, but how can you not appreciate his effort and want to trust in him completely when he has days like this?

Can't say that I do, though. Trust him completely, that is. My underlying sense of it is that, although he may be worried about me, he doesn't know what to do and he doesn't spend any time learning what to do by reading about it on the Internet, or simply asking what I need or if I need anything. (Nor has he read my blog that I know of . . . there's a wry irony in all this in that soooo many people read my blog every single day and infer quite a bit more about how I'm feeling than the guy closest to the action knows).

My first line of defense against cancer is myself. It's not like this is new news. I've known this for a while now. Getting through cancer treatment is my responsibility, not Marco's. I can do it.

CANCER—DAY 111 THURSDAY, AUGUST 13, 2009

I am in shock. I had to ask Marco: "Is it really Thursday?" The last few days just haven't existed, I slept them away.

The Internet is down at the house. Actually, it's not really down, the router is putting out a weak signal, but none of our computers are working on it. Every time something goes wrong in this house where it could be related to a utility, I get antsy that we're going to start having problems with the owners not paying the utilities and suddenly one day we won't have electricity, or water, can you imagine? But Marco said that Randy (the spouse in the ownership of the house) is moving out by September and then we can put the utilities in our own names so at least we know those bills are getting paid correctly. Apparently in order to be protected by CA state laws regarding tenancy, we have to keep paying the rent even when the house goes into foreclosure around us.

On the up side, there is a new law for foreclosures that requires 60 days notice to tenants in a foreclosure property. We've been looking, and we think we can find a place before October (when we think will be the easiest time to move between chemo and radiation), and once the utilities are in our names we'll pretty much be as set as we can be until we actually move out. I wonder where we'll end up?

CANCER—DAY 112 FRIDAY, AUGUST 14, 2009

I can't believe how much I've slept this week. And when I am awake . . . it's not pretty. This pain from my esophagus all the way down through my guts is just hellish. My latest description is that it's like there's submarine warfare going on in there, heat-seeking missiles being launched, countermeasures firing to draw the heat seekers, torpedoes firing back and forth, some connecting and blowing up enemy submarines . . . that's what it feels like is happening inside me when the chemo is doing its thing and the meds for the chemo side effects are not.

CANCER—DAY 113 SATURDAY, AUGUST 15, 2009

I had been complaining to Marco for a while about my eyesight getting worse and worse, almost since the first chemo day, now that I think about it. I finally gave in and changed both my laptops to first 125 percent and then 150 percent greater font sizes in order to be able to read what was on the screen. It was so frustrating those last few days trying to work, and this week my eyesight finally got bad enough that I wouldn't dare drive a car.

I asked Dr. Lombard about it on Monday before my chemo session and he said that they've heard this complaint from other patients on Taxol. It's a known side effect. He also said that my eyesight should return to the level it was at prior to chemo within a few months of completing chemo. Which of course does me no good whatsoever right now except as a bit of peace of mind that I'm not going blind (at least not for good). He said I could consider getting a temporary eyeglass prescription if it really seemed necessary, and that I probably wouldn't need it anymore around the time I finish radiation.

I've been constantly noting headaches on my cancer calendar every day this week, and taking Ibuprofen hasn't helped with the headaches much. Maybe the headaches are from straining my eyes to see? Marco and I finally decided that it would be worth a trip to the eye doctor to get my eyes checked out to at least make sure my eyes are still healthy, and to see how badly my current vision may be compared to what it was just a few months ago when I had my last eye exam. So we went in, and lo and behold my vision has drastically changed for the worse, so I bought new contact lenses. My actual eye health was wonderful, though. So now I have these super-power contact lenses. It's hard to wear my glasses with the wigs anyway, so I do pretty much go through the effort of putting in contacts every day. I wonder how hard it will be to put in contacts if I lose all my eyelash hairs too? Wild. What a strange thing to worry about.

Anyway, joy of joys, I can see my computer screens again, so I can go on Facebook to see how my friends are doing and I can read again without giving myself a splitting headache. Leave it to medical science to develop a medical treatment (chemo) that basically destroys your body in the process of hopefully saving your life.

Dr. Lombard did say that there is a known correlation of the intensity of side effects being greater in women 36 and younger. In general I have to admit I'd rather be a common statistic than an outlier, but ugh, I have yet to hear of any perks to getting breast cancer in your early thirties. Everything is more severe, and everything is more aggressive, both the disease and the treatment.

I need more sleep.

CANCER—DAY 114 SUNDAY, AUGUST 16, 2009

Anyone see that beautiful huge orange moon low on the horizon tonight? I didn't notice it sitting at my computer, but when Marco got back from picking up Randy at the airport he took me in the back yard to show me this huge orange moon. Wow. Beautiful.

It was actually also a beautiful moment in and of itself. Before Marco had to leave for the airport, we'd been sitting together on a lounge chair on the back patio, just looking up at the wind blowing in the trees trying to huff up a storm (yeah, right, like there'd ever be an actual STORM in Sacramento with thunder and lightning like we get in the Midwest) and we were just enjoying a few moments together. When he came back and took me out to see the moon, the mood was still like that. We were talking a little while looking at that big orange moon, but really we were just being there together. I honestly got lost in that moment and managed to forget for a little while all the life stuff and complications and big issues we're facing together right now. Maybe that was how I was able to forget, because I feel like we are facing things more together with this second round of chemo. We've settled into a shared rhythm of sorts. Marco says we're going through it together, good and bad, cancer and life, and I have to agree that we seem to get just a little bit better at it each day, a little more settled into it. More . . . well . . . *together*.

Wow. All it takes is one big beautiful moon to get me all romantic and flowery? At least some of the new side effect drugs are working!

CANCER—DAY 115 MONDAY, AUGUST 17, 2009

Ach, there are all these events coming up that require more driving and I'm dying to go home to my own house and here I am always getting so carsick it's pathetic. At least it's better when I drive myself, because I drive really slow and go on the gas gradually and lightly coast into the stops. Avoiding sudden jerking movements makes the car ride more tolerable, that's for sure. I'm on so much medication, though, I really, really should not be behind the wheel of a car. I went to a fish store and then thought I'd go visit the cats after, but I ended up getting lost and totally confused about where I was or where I thought I was going. They even have a term for this kind of confusion in chemo patients, it's called "chemo brain." I ended up taking some unknown highway to come in from the other direction to another fish store closer to the house, and bought another head scarf at the store next door. I never did find my way to the cats, and I kind of forgot my original intent today was to go visit them.

Marco was texting to ask where in the world I went (I should have been back already), then he asked me to pick something up at another store for him. I knew my way home from that place really well, so no worries about me getting lost on the way home. Actually, there shouldn't be any serious worries about me getting lost *period*, thanks to the GPS in my blackberry. Of course, I have to remember that I have the GPS, which never occurred to me today while I was lost. SHEESH! I should not be driving.

CANCER—DAY 116 TUESDAY, AUGUST 18, 2009

I have to admit, I have wondered what it would be like to have some little thing go wrong, get an infection or whatever and have to go to the emergency room. Not a bad emergency, but I wonder what it would be like to go in there saying I'm Dr. Lombard's cancer patient and my temperature is 102 degrees and I don't feel good, so now what do we do? Can a little infection really be life-threatening? Or like, if I just had a simple cold/flu kind of fever but everything else is fine, what would they make of that? Tell me go to home and have chicken noodle soup, just like my mom would tell me to do?

Tomorrow is the 19th. It is always a hard day for me, no matter what month it is, because my boyfriend Artie died on October 19th. I don't even have to know the date . . . in the evening after a crummy day I'll realize the date was the 19th and suddenly know why the day was as difficult as it was. But especially now as there are just two months between now and October 19th, my mind goes there a lot. I remember conversations Artie and I had the last couple of months before he died, and emotions and experiences we had, a certain look of love and longing that was only in his eyes when he looked at me, and then . . . loss. The 19th is often a difficult day for me, sometimes with a hefty dose of depression.

Marco's talking at me about Halloween costumes, and all I can think about is getting down to L.A., to Rancho Palos Verdes, to that cemetery where I need to be for October 19th and nothing else in October matters much to me. I'm certainly not worrying about what I'm going to be for Halloween. Oh right, and we have to find somewhere else to live and move in October, because the foreclosure on this house should be going through by then and we'll be evicted. So we should be thinking about that a bit, which hopefully is ranked higher in importance than what we're going to be for Halloween. Jeez Louise. Halloween? Who in the world plans what to wear for Halloween in August? Marco, apparently.

Chapter 16.
Take Care of Your Caregiver

CANCER—DAY 117 WEDNESDAY, AUGUST 19, 2009

Great. Marco came home from teaching last night saying he feels like he's getting sick. He spent the day grousing around his office and I pretty much steered clear of him. Staying out of the line of fire is about all you can do when he's in a bad mood that isn't your fault but you certainly feel like it's your fault when the frustration is directed at you simply because you happen to be nearby. So, I lay low and keep to myself when he's like that. I think I finally had a decent nap today, if I remember right. Or was that on Monday? I get so confused with the whole chemo brain thing. Tonight Marco's been pretty harsh all evening, snapping at me for no reason I knew of. I was relieved to get out of the house for my first yoga class by myself, though the sour mood wasn't any better when I got back so I quietly scrounged around the kitchen for leftovers and eventually put a pizza in the oven for myself. Not exactly healthy Chemo Girl fare, but apparently my caregiver took the night off from even tolerating me. I hope he's feeling better tomorrow.

CANCER—DAY 118 THURSDAY, AUGUST 20, 2009

No such luck, on the whole let's-hope-Marco-feels-better-so-he's-nicer front. Keep crossing your fingers for Friday. We seem to both have the stuffy head thing going on, so I've been keeping pretty close tabs on my temperature and, though it shifts quite a bit, I haven't gone over 99 degrees this time.

I spent the entire morning filling out forms for this genetic counseling thing which I suspect is a waste of time because the genetic counselor (now *there's* a job title, it sounds like someone who counsels genetically mutated sheep or something) said she is going to go though the forms for me and then make a determination whether genetic testing is appropriate. I already know that Dr. Lombard wants the genetic testing done, period, so it's not like the genetic counselor actually has any say regardless of what she reads in all these forms. So, here I am all morning filling out forms so they can "determine" that I need genetics blood testing when in reality it's a given, already ordered by my medical oncologist.

Ah, bureaucratic paperwork. Far be it for me to buck the system and not fill out their forms, asking them to just do the blood draws, run the tests, and let my doctor and I know the results. That would an over-the-top "Tenacious C," not putting up with unnecessary time-wasting paperwork. But Chemo Girl is much more docile than Tenacious C, until you do something that actually gets in the way of her care. Then look out because that sort of behavior gets zero tolerance even from Chemo Girl, and brings her alter-ego Tenacious C to the surface in a flash. Guess I have my own little Jekyll & Hyde thing going. Chemo Girl is the quiet one you can practically walk all over, while Tenacious C is the one who's not taking any B.S. in any way, shape, or form. Tenacious C is the one managing her illness with or without support.

That explains a lot actually, about things I'm tolerating now that had no place in my prior life. I wonder how tolerant I'll be after treatment. Then again, I won't be "done" with "treatment" until January, 2015, after five years of Tamoxifen. Who knows what kind of person I'll be at that point?

The fatigue thing is weird. I'm exhausted tired, and I mean *exhausted* as in too tired to reach down to the bottom dresser drawer so I now I keep my socks in my beside table drawer because it's hand height and requires less effort. I slept practically the whole first week of this second chemo infusion. Now, in the second week, I'm not sleeping but still ridiculously tired. Everything takes me ages to do, but somehow I still do things. It's the old me in me. Monday I did laundry. Tuesday I went nuts trying to reorder prescription refills, chasing down why I haven't gotten any disability payments from CA yet, and searching for the genetics forms I seemed to have filed too smartly for myself to find again. Now that was an exhausting day, because I was stressed too. But Tuesday night I went to have this thing called Reike, which is sort of a massage/energy thing that a couple of my friends practice, and they wanted to work with me on it. The bummer is that we were hoping it would help me be more relaxed and sleep better at night, but exactly the opposite happened. It was like I was jazzed up on caffeine and I couldn't sleep to save my life Tuesday night. Wednesday either. It took two Ambiens to get three hours of sleep Wednesday night. Not good.

Wednesday I managed to slow down a little in the pace of my day, and went to my second-ever yoga session. I liked it, and I am going to have to do more of it. I'm hoping to get both the body calmness and quietness of mind that I'm under the impression yoga can help with.

Yoga is definitely recommended in like, every cancer-recovery booklet I've ever read, so I definitely want to give it a serious effort.

CANCER—DAY 119 FRIDAY, AUGUST 21, 2009

So get this headline: "Happiness may protect against breast cancer, study suggests" (Telegraph.co.uk). I wonder if anyone saw that on the sidebar of my website earlier this week? I swear, sometimes I go check my own reader-facing blog page just to see what the breast cancer headlines are, and this one really caught my eye.

The first sentence says "Positive thinking and happiness may protect against the [breast cancer] disease. . ." [Puh-leese, how in the heck can someone study that scientifically?? But it went on] ". . . traumatic events like divorce and bereavement may increase the chances of developing breast cancer, a research study has found."

So they weren't really studying happiness per se, that was just a catchy title to get me to read the article. Which worked, I read it.

One interesting thing is that they focused on younger women only, between 25 and 45 and still pre-menopausal. They also said that "the impact of adverse life on cancer risk appeared to be cumulative . . . a significant effect was only seen after two or more events had occurred in a person's life."

But here was the kicker: "Two or more negative life events increased the chances of the disease by 62 percent."

Now come on, there are so many things that go into suffering and facing severe adversity that it's hard to put any credence behind a scientific hypothesis that there is a clear and direct correlation between adverse life events and breast cancer. They didn't really test for all known breast cancer factors such as family history (well, BRCA 1 and 2 genes anyway) or body weight, or other elements already correlated with increased breast cancer risk. So, let's not get all upset about the findings of this one little study. Granted, I do fit their profile for being at higher risk of cancer since this is, by their definitions, my third hard-core adult "negative life event." If they go further with this research, it will be interesting to see if they start breast cancer screenings earlier in young women with these additional risk factors. Not that I would have been happy about starting mammograms before 30, but I probably wouldn't have declined them after being told I was at 60% higher risk for breast cancer because of previous traumas in my life.

What I am annoyed with at the moment is that an entire article about the potential relationship of severe life adversity and getting breast cancer starts with the word "Happiness!"

CANCER—DAY 121 SUNDAY, AUGUST 23, 2009

You know, when people tell me they feel bad that I'm going through this, I'm never quite sure what to say. If people are talking about the side effects, I usually say "Well, it is what it is, so I just have to get through it." I usually try to tell them that it's not so bad, and "It could be worse." That's really very true. I just found out yesterday that Tia Maria (Artie's aunt, so, like, an aunt-in-law to me) has breast cancer. She just found out two weeks ago, and it's big. It's so large and dense that she has to go through chemo *before* surgery in order to shrink the tumor so it can be excised. Right now the surgeon is telling her that removing the tumor now would leave a big indentation (I forget what she called it) because, it sounds like, the tumor is pressing against her chest wall. Big bad voodoo daddy stuff.

Tia Maria called me today because Artie's brother had lunch with her yesterday and gave her my cell number suggesting that she call me to talk about my experiences so far and let her talk about what she's being told and work through how she's going to deal with it all.

So here's me, five weeks into chemo, 121 days since diagnosis (how long is that, anyway?), telling a new diagnosee everything I can about what I've learned about breast cancer, and trying to be helpful to someone who's still at that "is this really happening?" stage. We talked for an hour and a half or so. I have to give her a lot of credit for even calling me. When I was first diagnosed, everyone was trying to find someone for me to talk to, but it's actually pretty hard to find someone my age with breast cancer. Now I'm of the mindset that anything anyone would have told me still wouldn't have prepared me for what it's actually been like. I just cannot begin to tell you how awful and sick and weak and debilitated you feel from chemo. It's like every element of my body has had some kind of reaction to this treatment and is fighting it tooth and nail, and all the while I'm trying to have a good attitude (which I'm apparently failing at on a daily basis now, if my caregiver's recent moods are any reflection), though people who see me "out" like at River Tango or Firehouse 9 seem to think I have a great attitude. But it's a constant struggle. It would be so much easier to just be severely cranky and mean all the time instead of still *trying* to be nice and good to people. Oy vey, it would be soooo much easier to just stop trying.

But wrong. I really believe we all influence the energy around us, and that it's important for me to stay the course of always trying to become a better person—more kind, more forgiving, more accepting. How I'm feeling physically is no excuse for making someone else feel bad by taking it out on them. It's sort of like being on stage for a performance. You go out there and do it even if you don't feel 100% up to par, because the audience is there to see the performance and they deserve a good one. I guess I've taken that mentality fairly deeply into my psyche and my attitude that if I'm feeling low, that does not need to be projected onto others. So I try not to do that. I try not to complain or whine about poor me. I don't claim to succeed, but I do try.

Who is this "poor me," anyway? By external comparison, my situation sounds so much easier than so many other cancer patients. I have a "caregiver." At least there's usually someone around if my heart fails or something awful happens that I can't take care of alone. I'm on disability and not working, focusing on my health and chemo recoveries. I'm almost never alone in the house, though I am expected to be in charge of my own care and well-being, according to my caregiver. I have evening plans with other people every week to give Marco a break from being the "caregiver," though having breaks from me doesn't seem to help much. We're going to have to talk about that at some point. Soon.

Other people dealing with cancer don't have all the luxuries I do, though. They have to go it alone, literally, maybe leaning on friends for the most difficult things but mostly just taking care of themselves, completely alone. Other people have to still try to work full time and struggle through a daily grind of being "on" for other people, whereas I can stop whatever I'm doing any time to rest (though I can't sleep to save my life right now, I've slept about twelve hours since Thursday of last week). My tumors were still small enough that they could do just a lumpectomy, instead of *having* to do a radical mastectomy (although, esthetically, I suspect a double mastectomy with implants would be better than how I've ended up visually).

Other people have other major life issues at the same time they're in chemo . . . divorces, kids getting sick, other people to care for like aging parents or children. My only "parental" concern is that I can't take care of my cats during chemo because of potential cat litter bacteria, and I can't wait to be done and get them out of the kennel (nice as that place is, it's still a kennel, and not a place Mizzou and Seoul should have to live for months on end). But that's my worst problem. Living on 36% of my income isn't easy, but that's why financial planners tell you to have at least six months savings in case of life disaster, and I have savings to get by and family that will help me with absolutely anything if the going gets too rough. I really have it very easy, for a cancer patient.

Aside from having every side effect known to chemo, that is.

Tia Maria teaches grade school. She can't take time off for chemo, and she can't suffer in front of the kids, they won't understand. She has to go through chemo twice, though she'll probably have a mastectomy and not have to do radiation. Her sons are adults now and don't live at home anymore, so she goes home after work and has to make her own dinner and take care of herself. Alone. And here's me, complaining because Marco doesn't vacuum or keep the kitchen reasonably clean. Sheesh, if that's my worst problem (aside from chemo side effects, again, can't forget about that), I sooo have nothing to complain about, and I am incredibly thankful I have had it so easy. But when Marco is stressed or crabby, I have to admit that in a way

I'm jealous that Tia Maria *doesn't* have a caregiver. What an awful thing to say. For shame, Cynthia!

The thing is, Marco's love and caring is, well, bipolar. It's hard to believe it's real or has any depth in a positive way toward me sometimes. But even when he's being a grouch, which is more often than not recently, even when he doesn't seem to want me around, I still think that somewhere underneath his stress and frustration he still loves me. Still, he's been in such bad moods of late. When he's stressed or frustrated, he says things that seem so hurtful, especially given how overly sensitive I seem to be now. But it's not an exaggeration, it really does hurt emotionally to have him tell me I'm self-centered and only think of myself, just a few days after telling me that his "not" taking care of me, leaving me to take care of myself, is part of his "caregiving strategy."

The one thing I need that I can't conjure out of my own determination is to feel cared about, to feel loved. I didn't realize how spoiled I was having two cats before all this, doting on me and loving me all the time no matter what. There's an irony for you—I get more emotional support from my cats than my caregiver.

Oy vey, I need to live with my cats again. It's so depressing without them, and Marco completely balked at my willingness to pay rent on the condition that I can keep my cats locked up in a spare room here instead of paying a kennel to keep them. If he's really that allergic, he's never going to tolerate the cats, and I can't stand being without them much longer. If for no other reason than that, I will have to leave him or get him to leave me, eventually.

But even though he's not taking care of me and he pretty much acts like he hates having me in the house all the time, when I ask him, when I *tell* him that he doesn't have to be my caregiver, he says that he committed to doing it and he's going to do it. But what if I don't want him to? What if I want to fire him from being my caregiver?

Then again, how do you fire someone from a job they're not performing to begin with? Take away their stapler? (Ha! If that doesn't make you laugh, you absolutely *must* see the movie *Office Space* so you understand the significance of a red Swingline stapler in the process of firing someone.)

CANCER—DAY 122 MONDAY, AUGUST 24, 2009

So, the story for today is offering up some Truth that I have been avoiding both in my blog and in my mind, even though I have written about some little episodes in my private journal. I found myself in an e-mail conversation with one of my tango friends today that, down the thread, got me venting about the living situation here. I don't even remember writing the first reply to Dietrich about his friend's cancer-diet thing, that one was late at night and I'd had either an Ambien or other sleeping pills, I don't remember which, but I know they didn't help me sleep because I was up at 3 a.m. Facebooking.

Anyway . . . Dietrich wrote "Whoa, you are cleaning up after the care-giver? I didn't think it was supposed to work that way. I believe my friend did the special diet first before any of the harsher treatment stuff. Nice to dance with you again. I must say you were looking quite well."

And man! I must REALLY have needed to get this stuff off my chest, because I wrote this long reply: "Uh oh, now you're going to get me venting. Yeah, I would definitely prefer not to clean up after other people, especially my supposed 'caregiver.' You'd think it would be enough to clean up after myself and that a lot of people wouldn't even expect a lot of that from someone in chemotherapy, but I just can't stand what the kitchen gets like, it grosses me out to re-use knives or cutting boards that haven't been washed since the previous use, or to have stinky dirty dishes piled up in the sink for days and days instead of simply putting them in the dishwasher. Not being able to walk in the closet or bedroom for the clothes on the floor bugs me (especially since there are two huge laundry baskets right there inside the closet), so I tend to clean up the kitchen and the bedroom as I pass through them. The only thing I can't do really is vacuum, it's just too tiring, but it's also painful to ask Marco to do it, since it seems to really annoy him to be asked to do any cleaning (he lived here over two months without ever vacuuming or dusting, and Randy lived here four months before that without ever cleaning at all. I finally went out and bought a vacuum cleaner for this house because neither of them even owns one. I never go barefoot, there are stains everywhere from Randy's dog that isn't toilet trained, which is disgusting). I've also done all the laundry since at least the beginning of chemo five weeks ago, but I decided this weekend that I'm not going to do that anymore. I have plenty of clothes so I'm just going to wait to see how long Marco waits before finally doing a load of laundry himself. The one concession I got from Marco in this whole thing is that he will pull the covers up on the bed in the morning now. He still doesn't "make" the bed, but at least it's not completely disheveled. I'm not big on the messy house look. I miss my house in the mountains; I haven't been home in six weeks because I get too carsick to make the drive across the divide to get there. That kind of exacerbates things, we thought I'd be able to go home during this third week of each chemo cycle to give everyone a break, Marco in particular, but I haven't been able to tolerate car motion. I appreciate your compliment; I keep trying to use the milongas to make myself "be" better, for what sense that makes. Makeup, a wig, and a smile do a lot for making me seem better in a way, at least to other people. I guess it makes me feel more like a regular person than a cancer patient too, as opposed to when I stay home because I just can't muster the energy to go. Thanks for the dancing too; yours was the best tanda I had all night."

Dietrich has become a good friend. I definitely felt better after my little rant to him, when I finally told someone some little bit of what it's really like here. I've been covering it up with my friends and family because I don't want to worry them. At the same time, while I know Dietrich won't breathe a word to anyone, it's worrisome to myself, admitting those things, openly (to myself) recognizing the fact that so many issues exist. And the issues I told Dietrich about were just the tip of the iceberg.

I have to figure out a way to get through this, though. I can't bottle it all up forever. Can I?

That's it. Nausea be damned, I need to go home to my own house, where I have space to think, even if it means giving up dance completely until I come back for the next treatment.

CANCER—DAY 123 TUESDAY, AUGUST 25, 2009

I drove home last night! It was far from comfortable and I pulled over several times to stop the motion and swallow down the carsickness, but at least I didn't throw up. I was nauseas all night after the drive even though I took all three of my nausea meds before I left Sac, but I did make it all the way home. I'm going to stay here by myself until Saturday night when I'll go back for the milonga and then my third chemo on Monday. At the moment I'm at home in Volcanoville resting, lying in my hammock, looking at the forest, listening to the wind in the trees. I spent the morning tidying up the house a little before my parents come out next month, but I wore out before noon so it's rest time.

You know, I'm writing this while trying incredibly hard not to sound totally upset when I pretty much am. Marco and I had a disturbingly unpleasant IM (instant messaging) conversation this morning, and it's still swirling around in my head. Might as well journal on it and see where that takes me, since some pretty amazing personal insights have come up that way in the past . . .

But, Ugh. That's about all I can say. Just trying to reread the thread to figure out how it became so awful is turning my stomach. Why do I care about this guy, again?

The killer line of the IM thread with Marco was a remark he made after I told him that it bums me out to feel too sick to go to most of the milongas because I really want to go to the dances. He wrote:

> **"You have to suck it up that you can't do that right now and take better care of your caregiver."**

Are you *kidding* me? *I'm* supposed to "suck it up" and take better care of *him?* I don't think I would believe he even said that to me, except it was right there on the screen in front of me, in writing. He threw my "selfishness" in my face again, in the same conversation. He tells me I'm selfish because I only think about cancer and chemo and treatments and managing side effects and trying alternative medicines and alternative treatments . . .

Am I really supposed to be responsible for my caregiver as well as myself? That's a new one. How am I going to do that?

CANCER—DAY 124 WEDNESDAY, AUGUST 26, 2009

All right, so the gauntlet has been thrown down. There is no mistaking the meaning of the statement: "you have to suck it up that you can't do that [dance] right now and take better care of your caregiver." Apparently I've been exceedingly selfish in taking care of myself during chemo, and someone thinks that needs to change. Marco wants *me* to take better care of *him*.

I can't imagine a greater challenge. Putting someone else first in life isn't that big a deal, it's actually one of my greatest failings in relationships. I have a tendency to morph into whatever the guy wants or needs, and it takes me a while to recover my sense of self when the relationship ends. But how am I supposed to put someone else first while I am in chemotherapy treatment? I'm already entirely taking care of myself in treatment now, managing the meds and side effects and trying to keep a positive outlook on it all knowing the treatment and pain is only going to get worse over the next three or four months. To do all that and somehow "take better care" of Marco at the same time just sounds like an impossible goal. I mean come on, I want to become a better person, but I'm no Gandhi!

I will not put my life in jeopardy for a personal development or spiritual growth goal. At least, I don't think I would put my life in jeopardy. Then again, look what I got myself into here. Like it hasn't been hard enough just taking care of myself, now I'm supposed to put someone else's needs ahead of my medical care when I'm in treatment for *cancer*? Sounds pretty stupid to me.

But hey, why not at least try to do what he wants and put him ahead of myself, if not always, than at least as much as possible? What could be a better thing to learn as a human being, what could be a better way to learn to be a truly giving soul, than to put someone else first when you're navigating one of the most difficult medical treatment regimen a person can undergo? Maybe focusing on someone else will actually make it easier to *not* dwell on how awful I feel. Well, ok, let's be real, even focusing 100% of my thoughts and energy on making Marco happy and content would not stop me from getting or feeling or having to deal with chemo side effects. I don't have that kind of subjective reality control over objective physical existence.

Let's not forget though: I made a choice early on, maybe 100 days or so ago. My options then were to go stay with my parents in Nebraska during chemo, or stay in Sacramento with Marco during chemotherapy (and radiation) treatment. Flip back 100 days, it's right there on the page. I did NOT choose to stay in California because it would be easier. I chose to stay in California because it would be more challenging and I would grow more as a person if I had that more challenging experience. I knew I would try harder to be (or at least act) well and reasonably healthy, because I would have to in order to make it through chemo here, trying to be around people and going to milongas to dance or at least see my friends.

I think I've kept up The Act decently for other people when I'm out socially, but recovering from that takes time and concerted effort. Back at the house afterward is where I recover from the forced happy demeanor of doing "OK" that I put in front of everyone else. I knew it would be difficult emotionally to stay with someone I hadn't known very well for very long and to trust that person with potentially everything if I were completely debilitated by chemo. I knew it would be easier to go live with my parents where I could keep my cats with me and I would feel cared for and loved all the time no matter what.

Admittedly, in choosing to stay here instead of going to stay with my parents in Nebraska, I didn't think any of it would be as difficult as it has actually been. All of the side effects and the severity of them and the emotional challenges—everything has been more challenging than I expected or was prepared for, more than my doctors expected or prepared me for. But, it is what it is, and now is the new starting point to take my life development to a completely new level: discovering what it means to be a truly giving soul.

Chapter 17.
Finding Inspiration

Cancer—Day 125 Thursday, August 27, 2009

I texted with my VP today and I found out that my company, the ENTIRE COMPANY, is going to walk against breast cancer as "Team Cynthia Swan" in Atlanta in October. I was speechless, but found plenty of tears at the ready as I tried to comprehend it . . . to think, an entire group of people, everyone at my entire company, would care so much and give me such a wonderful gift. I find that utterly humbling.

I also got a call from my oncology nurse . . . this is pretty neat. The Marshall Oncology Center called and asked me if I would be a mentor to a new breast cancer diagnosee, Alice. I don't know if Alice and I are close in age or not, but I told them that of course I'd do it. They confirmed my phone numbers and said they hope she'll call me, but possibly not. If she's like me, she's not going to call, but maybe I'm the only one who's so weirdly stubbornly independent as to prefer to research everything on my own on the Internet instead of asking one-on-one questions of someone whose experience may or may not be similar to my own. I probably should have talked to more people at the beginning, but I just didn't. I thought it was neat that they called to ask me to do this, though. I know they have dozens of women in treatment right now, so they easily could have asked someone else, but they asked me. It felt good to think that Dr. Lombard and Heddi think highly enough of me to make that kind of recommendation of me.

I'm still trying to get my head around Marco's blowup and telling me to take better care of my caregiver. Unbelievable. What a thing to say to a cancer patient. I just can't imagine speaking to someone that way, I would hate myself for how badly that could make the other person feel, and gosh darn it, it's important to me to NOT make other people feel bad about themselves or anything else, least of all me. There's enough negativity in the world without me adding to it.

And yet, here are all these other people, my entire company, planning to do a breast cancer walk as "Team Cynthia Swan." That seems like such an enormous showing of caring and support that it gives me inspiration to keep trying.

Cancer—Day 126 Friday, August 28, 2009

Randy is moving out this weekend. Actually, he pretty much already has. Before I get back to Sacramento tomorrow, Marco is rearranging his things to fill up more of the house, but all I was renting from Randy was my office, so none of my stuff is getting moved around that I'm aware of. I bought all our bedroom furniture, but I did that as a thank you gift to Marco, so he can move it wherever he wants and I won't fuss. Apparently the current line of thought is that we're going to get at least 60 days eviction notice when the house forecloses, which is plenty of time to find another rental and this one is so cheap now without a housemate, we're not going to do anything about looking for a new rental place to live until the time comes (when an eviction notice is received), and in the meantime Marco is really excited about having this entire house to himself for the rental amount he agreed to back when he moved in here three months ago; his rent isn't changing with Randy moving out. I say "to himself" because he made a point recently of informing me, during the "take care of your caregiver" conversation, that I am merely a guest in "his" house so I should behave like one and be more appreciative of the fact that Marco "lets" me stay here. Oh boy, you can imagine how that made me feel, given that I've been paying Randy rent all summer and doing all kinds of things to help with the house and furnishing it and being as generous with money as possible. What I don't do is specifically pay a fixed portion of Marco's rent to Randy, and that seems to bother him. But I paid more than two months' rent buying him furniture, I spend several hundred dollars a month to keep my cats at the kennel because of Marco's allergies, and I pay rent to Randy for my office room (which I pretty much do just to be nice). It seems to me that staying here costs me plenty on a monthly basis. Between spending plenty of money on all that, and, you know, living with him as his girlfriend, especially since that day he said "You have two homes now" (here, and my house in the mountains), I have generally considered myself a roommate in the house, not a guest. But apparently I was way out of line on that, according to Marco. I need to more fully appreciate that he lets me live here. That's how he sees the living arrangement now.

Oh well, one good thing about people having different perspectives than my own, it's a great way to learn. It's a hard way to suddenly live in the same house with someone though, with this committed thing of being with him at least through chemo treatment (so we're talking into October at least, and through December if we include radiation treatment as well, which was the original plan).

CANCER—DAY 127 SATURDAY, AUGUST 29, 2009

The verbal I-love-you phase is over almost as suddenly as it began. It lasted about a month in human days, which is equivalent to about one-fourth of the entire existence of Cancer Girl. (I cannot get my head around how time has become both insanely drawn out and unfathomably compressed at the same time, since I was diagnosed.)

When I came back tonight for the milonga, Marco was OK, not warm, not cold, but OK. I did say "I love you" as usual before he went to sleep, testing the waters a little after being away for several nights, but his reply was "Thank you, honey." So much for that. And here I am again, awake at 3 a.m., journaling it out.

I mentioned to Marco that I am still interested in the U Street house. We had been about to make an offer on it. Since we're expecting to get a foreclosure eviction notice any day now, we had been considering buying a house together, fixing it up, and then reselling the remodeled house. That plan was concocted back when our relationship seemed very solid. I was going to put up the money, he was going to put in the labor, and then we'd split the net gain 50/50. But when I mentioned it today, Marco said "Good luck with that." So much for that, too. And what else is gone from the relationship?

Well, it seems that he has, in a matter of a few days, written me off completely in his mind, and I'm now someone he will NOT have in his future. But why is he keeping up the charade then? Tonight we went to the milonga just like always and everyone still sees us as this fabulous couple, affectionate, still saying good things about each other in our conversations with other people. Still acting like we're in love even, or at least that's how it must still look to everyone on the outside seeing us acting affectionate in public. For me, it was all an act because I didn't want to make people feel sorry for me or make them think poorly of Marco. But why is Marco doing it?

The devilish side of me thinks I should just 'out' him to the world in my blog, move out, and let him deal with the fallout that would create in the tango community here, if everyone who thought Marco was so wonderful were to know the truth. But, alas, that's just my shadow side, and I don't really let that side dictate a darn thing I do anymore. Basically, if a thought comes from my shadow side, I know it's something I have to deal with within myself, to *not* act upon my injured ego reaction.

When I can't figure things out for myself and I feel like I need a way to find a way to approach a problem, I often turn to the Nordic Runes. I wrote about this once before, way back when I was trying to decide where to do chemo. Drawing a Rune often gives me a starting point for my thought process. On this subject, the Runes keep giving me *Teiwaz*, which, in response to relationship issues, means the relationship is both timely and providential. "There is work for you to do together." I can't count how many times I've gotten this Rune in response to worries about Marco in the past year. At first I figured it was all about our professional dance partnership, and partnering on that without ensnarling our lives romantically, but then all this other stuff happened. Now it seems obvious to me that the work involves me NOT being in love with him, because he's withholding love from me, he now says he can't love me. Therefore, in my thinking, I can't love him. It is a two-way street after all, and loving someone who doesn't love you back is an agony I try to avoid. So, I need to convince myself to stop loving him. I can do that, but I hate the process; it depresses me. And it takes time.

It is sooooo hard to be what he wants, to be someone who puts him first and herself second even when she's fighting cancer. I get depressed when I think about how much of my Self I'm giving up to play this role with him. It's exactly the role I thought I was attempting to NOT take, actually, adapting myself completely to be whatever he wants. I thought the relationship side of this would be a chance to possibly learn how to be in a relationship without losing my identity in it. I keep reminding myself to accept him for what he is since that's been such a big goal of mine in the last couple years, but it always comes back to remembering that it's what he *is* that may be very, very wrong for me. And the one thing I absolutely do NOT want is to become like him. I have to figure out a way to not become like him but still give him what he wants so I can get through treatment in Sacramento.

HA! I just brought myself full circle again. Basically, by trying not to let him rub off on me and not let his moods and negativity and meanness rub off on me, I *am* essentially saying that I have to keep my identity even while I'm taking care of my caregiver like he wants and being what he wants regardless of how I feel health-wise or emotionally.

You know, it sure would have been easier to just stay on that Buddha all-is-connected-in-me mountaintop place when my heart failed five years ago. The ER doctors shock my heart back to life from that so I can live through *this*?

Again, Cynthia, remember: Life has a lot to teach you, and this is not just the greatest spiritual growth opportunity you've had so far in your life, this is above and beyond anything you could possibly come up with to challenge yourself. This is the single greatest opportunity for your spiritual growth that will *ever* happen in your lifetime. Surely there can't be another life trial in my future that is even *more* difficult than this to survive and learn from.

CANCER—DAY 128 SUNDAY, AUGUST 30, 2009

My mind has been whirling around this new challenge, and I know that what I need to do is conjure up my inner strength. I've never really let myself think of this as a fight against death, rather I've always told myself it's just another, very difficult, medical process I have to survive. And to survive, I need love and strength. I used to think Love came from my family, and it does, but I also am getting an enormous amount of love and support from all these people who just seem to believe in me, like my company, and the tango community, and the University, and the West Coast Swing community, and my ballroom friends, and even people whom I've never met except through my cancer blog. I have an insane abundance of love in my life, regardless of the emotional situation with Marco. And inner strength? Well, for some reason I've always had quite a lot more of that than I ever think I have. I don't know how to conjure it up on demand though.

In terms of getting through cancer treatment, I often seem to have a Scarlet O'Hara *Gone with the Wind* kind of mentality. There's a scene in the movie when their daughter dies in an accident, and Scarlet and Rhett are both completely distraught and suffering in their own ways, Scarlet alone in her room, Rhett locked up in the den with the body of their daughter, whom he refuses to let be put in a dark coffin in the cold dark earth. When a friend arrives to try to help them, she asks Scarlet's Mammy how the two are doing. Mammy tells her something like, "I know Miss Scarlet will get through, she has a way of conjurin' up more strength than she even know she has when she need it. It's Mr. Rhett I'm worried about." And several times in the movie when things seem beyond her, Scarlet basically tells herself to get through the current disaster and worry about what happens next when the time comes. The last three lines of the movie really sum me up some days. The movie ends with Scarlet saying,, "I just can't think about that right now. I'll think about that tomorrow. After all, tomorrow is another day."

You can get through a lot, one day at a time. Thinking like that is often a kind of inspiration for me to get through the current day. Don't worry yourself about tomorrow until it comes. One of my common phrases for it is "I'll cross that bridge when I come to it."

Lately I've been reading and thinking about how people get through cancer treatment, whatever their cancer or situation. All I've been able to figure out is that the *how* of survival is both complex and mysterious. Medical treatment is a process, but survival is more of a journey. And for me, much of survival comes from determination that is based on inspiration rather than desperation.

I have this book my mom bought for me when I was a little kid, it's called "Michelle," and the story of it has stayed with me my entire life. When I was home in Volcanoville this week, I dug through my boxes of books in the storage shed and found it. I brought it back to Sac with me to read again. I remember it being so very inspiring to me even the first time I read it as a girl that I thought it would be a good thing to read again now, with my new personal context of understanding.

Michelle was an eight-year-old girl with bone cancer in her leg. Her leg was amputated, and even though they were planning tons of chemo, she had only a 4% chance of survival going in. But she survived it all. Not just a survivor, the spirit this little girl maintained throughout treatment was amazing and inspirational. So I'm re-reading the book.

It's a young adult book, so it's a quick unchallenging read but a compelling story good for the spirit no matter how old or young you are. To me, two things really stand out in the book: her bravery in undergoing all the horrible treatments required for bone cancer, and her ability to always be thoughtful and considerate of others, and giving. At eight! There's a line in the book that sums it up really, it's her mom reflecting on some comments made about Michelle's spirit and loving nature: "Michelle seems to give without being concerned whether you can give anything in return, even in her pain she still cares for others."

See? So there's nothing unusual in this desire I have to use this experience to be a kind and giving person even in the throes of adversity. Well, maybe it's still a bit unusual in that maybe not everyone takes that approach to it, but it's not like I'm the only person to ever try, and this little girl Michelle, she lived her young life that way, always giving even when she herself was in pain. It inspired me in grade school and it still inspires me now. I wonder what happened to her longer term, after the time period of the book? I think she was in her mid-teens when the book was published, but that was when I was a kid. When our Internet is back online, maybe I can do some research and find out if there is anything more out there about her long term survival.

There are a couple of great metaphors and other quotes that stood out enough to me to put Post-It notes on the pages, and these are the things I want to do or be in my cancer journey, so to save them for posterity in my chronicle of cancer survival, here they are:

"She watched the gray sky grow darker until rain wept onto the roses outside the window."

"Michelle realized she'd learned much about herself and her world. She learned a lot about conquering fear . . . She learned that, as she had suspected, we are truly handicapped most cruelly by our own choices. 'If you're going to be brave,' she quipped, 'you've got to do something that scares you.'"

"You can't let fear overcome you. You have to live each day and make the most out of it every minute by living on a day-to-day basis."

"So many of the children she's seen just seemed to lose their spark. The days and weeks of illness and limitations place on them so often beat them down, robbing them of their color and personality."

That is the one that's been on my mind lately. Losing my spark. It's so hard to find it for phone calls, or to write with any upbeat momentum for the blog or even to dance, and the spark isn't there in my eyes in photos anymore. I used to always have a genuine spark of happiness in my eyes that would always be captured in photos because I was always genuinely enjoying the moment I was in. Now, with almost every moment a challenge, I feel like that spark is gone from my eyes and my smiles are forced and tired. No one seems to have seen it yet, not even my parents or Brian, who are about the only people I fear will notice the difference. I seem to be covering up my lost spark very convincingly, but I know it's gone, at least for now. May all the good intentions and prayers and faith of so many wonderful people save me from that as a permanent fate. I can't be like this forever . . .

I thought that was going to be the end of my rambling on finding my internal strength and inspiration, making this an entry I can come back to again and again to remind myself of what I am trying to be when things get especially difficult with Marco and the new expectation that I am to take better care of my caregiver.

But towards the very end of the book, there's a good final quote that I just read and this just says it all so I have to quote it . . .

"She's smiling but it's painful,
Courage demands a toll.
Her strength is somewhere deeper
In the unseen living soul."

I read this book when I was like, 12 years old, and I never forgot about it and I never lost track of the book. It was inspirational then, and it's still inspirational now. Strength is in the unseen living soul.

I can do this.

Chapter 18.
Third Chemo

CANCER—DAY 129 MONDAY, AUGUST 31, 2009

The day I've been dreading for the past five days is here. Third round of chemo, here we go.

CANCER—DAY 130 TUESDAY, SEPTEMBER 1, 2009

I think all I did was sleep today. No, wait, I went for a very short walk also, to get a croissant at Tupelo's around the corner. Ha! I didn't sleep ALL day.

CANCER—DAY 131 WEDNESDAY, SEPTEMBER 2, 2009

Nothing much to report, I was too wiped out to go to yoga, so we had a little road trip to Fry's Electronics tonight to get a new power unit for Marco's computer, which is apparently on the fritz. I slept almost the entire day though, waking up only to take meds and then dozing back off.

CANCER—DAY 132 THURSDAY, SEPTEMBER 3, 2009

All the side effect meds are still kicking my ass, I was only awake maybe two hours today, and I wouldn't even have made it that long except we had to go back to Fry's and get a motherboard and pretty much everything else for Marco to build a new computer. We got back, and I didn't even make it to the bedroom to change into comfy napping clothes or take off my wig. I fell asleep right away in my office for three hours, at which point the work day was gone and Marco was well along in his happy little project of building his new computer. I tell ya, nothing makes this guy happier than to build things.

The do-not-bend-forward side effect is back. Whenever I bend forward, say, slouching at my desk, or not sitting up completely straight at the dinner table, or . . . here's a really annoying one . . . trying to curl up for a nap, I get this scrunching pain in my chest that I can get rid of by overextending my back for a few moments, then staying exceedingly straight instead of curling up again. It makes it hard to get comfortable to rest.

CANCER—DAY 133 FRIDAY, SEPTEMBER 4, 2009

Ugh, new unpleasant development, not sure what kind of side effect to call this, but I'm developing a gag reflex to swallowing. Exacerbated by swallowing anything non-liquid, i.e., pills. More fun on the Cynthia Swan Medical Merry-Go-Round.

On the up side, with sooooo many pills to take (they've added a couple *more* to try to reduce the side effects of the medicines they're giving me for the chemo side effects), about all I have time to do and think about is managing and staying on my schedule regarding which pills to take when, which pills require food and so forth and so on. I sleep a lot, and I am having less of the esophagus and intestinal warfare I was having in earlier rounds of chemo, which means the additional meds are helping somehow. Sometimes I think I would prefer to tolerate a little of that pain to get some tiny percentage of my brain power and energy back. But what drug should be reduced to achieve that? I see a phone call to the oncologist in my near future . . .

CANCER—DAY 134 SATURDAY, SEPTEMBER 5, 2009

Wow, sleep is eluding me tonight. I finally went to bed around 2:30 a.m. I think. We did go to the Firehouse 9 milonga for an hour, until about midnight, so realistically getting to bed around 1 a.m. and then taking some time to actually fall asleep isn't that odd for me at night. Except during these days right after chemo of sleeping all day and all night, that is.

Anyway, I now firmly believe Trazadone is evil. Better not to sleep than to have nightmares like this.

I just had the worst nightmare of my life. It's freaky that I remember it in such detail and it feels like I lived it. Sometimes I really hate how my brain can't tell dreams from reality. When I'm dreaming, it's the same to my brain as waking reality, and I get really confused about what is "real" and what is not.

Anyway, here's the nightmare:

I'm some kind of researcher or investigator and I'm working on the history of this ancient Chinese temple/fortress, including specific undocumented horrific supernatural events rumored to have occurred there. I'm on Day Three of my trip to the place, no telling when I'll be leaving because this could be turning into an enormous project. The first day I just explored and felt what I could of the energy of the place, got my impressions of what little portion of it I was able to see (because it's so huge, like a small city in size and complexity, rather than just a palace). The second and third days I started recording the sounds around me and taking notes on where I was and what the rooms were for, sleeping rooms, tea rooms, etc.. . .

Night Three, I'm back at my little room of the fortress (little meaning like the size of a house in Beverly Hills) and I lie down to listen to three recordings I'd made where something a little more interesting than silence seemed to have been happening. Well, I don't remember anything from the first two recordings, except that they both started too soon. I started making comments or verbal notes too soon in the recordings, and it affected the quality of what was recorded around my voice, in the silence.

The third recording scared the hell out of me. It has a long, silent, open air sound beginning. As I listened to that whispery silence in the recording, I could feel the room getting colder, and I'm all tucked in with the blankets [this was true of the room I was sleeping in in the dream, the room I was listening to on the audio in the dream, AND the room I was actually sleeping in last night, next to Marco]. It feels like there's something big and heavy on my legs [back in the dream now], like when Mizzou and Kingsford used to both want to sleep between my feet or knees, and Mizzou would always end up half over one my legs, and I tell ya, a 16 pound cat can immobilize my leg with little difficulty! Then I start to hear the breathing of an incredibly large, solid, hefty dog, or maybe it's a wolf. It's breathing heavily—low, not agitated, but aggressive breathing. This ghost dog-wolf-beast comes across the room (eases off the lower part of my bed?) and comes right up to my throat. I can feel its hot breath from my esophagus to my lower left ear, that's how huge this dog's jowl was, because it's mouth was barely open. I want to say it was a Rottweiler-based beast, but that's a vague guess because it was pitch black. Anyway, I'm scared stiff and tucked in my blankets from the cold, so my arms (and legs) are pretty useless, trapped. And then it happens. The ghost dog-wolf beast takes my throat between its jaws.

I tell it to "let go." I tell it to "Let Go!" Instead, the massive jaw clamped down preparing to rip away my throat. Then, feeling hot blood gushing from my throat as it starts to tear open in the jaws of this massive cur, I yell through its jowls "LE' . . . GO . . . 'OW!!" I yelled with as much strength as I could muster while trying to push it away with my arms from under the covers. But the words I tried to yell at the top of my lungs were just a raspy whisper, and my throat tore away in the beast's jaw. I couldn't even gasp out a scream, trapped in the bedcovers with dark blood gushing from my torn throat out into the blackness.

That thrashing effort, though, did finally let me escape the dream and wake up. You know, when I have dying dreams, I always wake up before I actually die in the dream. I read a psychology thesis once that purported that if you die in your dream, you die for real. Well, I can't refute the hypothesis. Before I actually die in a dream, I always wake up. Anyway, back to the current nightmare and waking up from it.

Apparently I said all three of those "Let go" sentences out loud during my nightmare, and the third one was loud enough and scary enough that Marco understood it and woke me up. He asked if I was OK. He kept shaking me by the shoulders and asked me twice more before I could hoarsely whisper "yeah . . . nightmare." He asked what happened and I told him "A dog tore my throat out." He thought he misunderstood and I had to tell him again. At that point he must have realized what a horrific nightmare it had been, and he became comforting, patting my arm and saying it was OK now, I'm OK now, it's over, I'm OK.

Wheeewwwww, doggy! It took a while to calm down from that one. Actually, I can't really say I've calmed down yet, given that two hours later after thrashing awake from that dream I'm still more than a bit hesitant to get back in the bed. No more sleep for me tonight.

One thing's for sure. Ambien may not be working to help me sleep at night anymore, but Trazadone is definitely NOT the solution. Trazadone is evil!

CANCER—DAY 136 MONDAY, SEPTEMBER 7, 2009

Aarrrggggrrrrrrrrrrhhhhhhh! It is soooo frustrating to try to type when your numb burning clumsy fingertips don't function and you can't see the computer screen because of your failing eyesight! Going from 32 years old to something like 82 years old in physical capabilities practically overnight is definitely a challenge to adjust your mind to.

I actually came across some good, brief definitions of what are now the most annoying of the side effects I've been having, and I thought the brevity may be useful to other women trying to get their arms around this whole wide mess. It's continually shocking to me that any of these side effects can manifest themselves as debilitatingly as they do. But, they do.

Chemo Brain. Difficulty Thinking Clearly. It is believed that chemotherapy can temporarily affect the nerve cells in the brain, causing confusion commonly referred to as "chemo brain." Chemo brain is described as a feeling of "fogginess" that sometimes is mistaken for depression or aging. A lack of focus, general confusion, and decreased ability to think clearly are all signs of chemo brain.

Fatigue. Fatigue is when a person feels weak or tired sooner than usual after physical, mental, or emotional activity (or possibly lack thereof). Fatigue is a major side effect of chemotherapy. It can last for months after treatment.

Neuropathy. Certain chemo drugs can affect the nerves and can sometimes makes the muscles weak, tired or sore. These nerve and muscle effects are called "peripheral neuropathy." You may feel tingling, burning, weakness or numbness in the hands or feet. Some people experience a loss of balance and difficulty walking.

Depression. Cancer may disrupt the lifestyle and threaten the purposes and goals that give meaning to people's lives. The physical and emotional stress that cancer and it's treatment places on the body can often lead to depression.

Anemia. Anemia is a side effected experienced by over 70% of patients undergoing chemotherapy. Chemo reduces the bone marrow's ability to make red blood cells that carry oxygen to all parts of your body. When there are few red blood cells, your body tissues don't get enough oxygen to do their work. This condition, known as anemia, may be characterized by feelings of extreme fatigue, weakness, tiredness, dizziness, shortness of breath and confusion.

Also, this isn't one of the core common side effects, but I have to note again that my eyesight has degenerated further to non-seeing levels even with the new super-strong contacts prescription, so I'm taking another trip to the eye doctor. I wonder what they'll say? Could my vision have changed enough again and so badly that I need another new prescription? And am I going to have to go through this again three weeks from now in the next chemo cycle? It's cumulatively degenerative, and cumulatively depressing, in all honesty.

CANCER—DAY 137 TUESDAY, SEPTEMBER 8, 2009

What a singularly strange experience, while in your thirties, to live in a body of limitations double and triple your actual age. And to go through the aging process quickly, in a matter of weeks, not decades, is definitely a shocker. Hard to handle. Depressing.

Nothing works. Can't see. Can't type. Can't write. Can't think. Bowels don't work, either flush everything upon ingestion or hold for eternity and a blockage. Shaky. No balance. Afraid to ride my bike, or even go for a walk, too tippy, too clumsy, bumping into stuff all the time, bruises everywhere. Worrying about dehydration, trying to get calories to stay inside the body but not gain any weight.

Trying to keep a good attitude. This is definitely a trial of staying stubborn about survival, instead of giving in to the accumulation of challenges and letting cancer win.

I may not have specifically done enough to "take care of my caregiver" in the week I had my third chemo treatment, except that I insisted that he go to yoga two nights to get him out of the house and doing something for himself besides the night he's out teaching. I do know that I did not ask a single thing of him all week, I set alarms on my phone to remind me when it was time to take each medicine, and I managed all my meds by myself. I always got food for myself, and I forced down lots of liquids to stay hydrated without a word from him. My presence in the house was simply in case some insanely awful thing went wrong. Which it didn't, at least nothing severe enough that I had to ask for Marco's help, anyway.

Third round of chemo, and I'm taking complete and absolute care of myself, exactly as my caregiver intended my care to be.

Chapter 19.
Staying Strong for Just One More

CANCER—DAY 138 WEDNESDAY, SEPTEMBER 9, 2009

Now that Randy has moved out, there is no living room furniture, no dining room furniture, and an empty spare bedroom. The only furniture Marco owned before I moved in was a futon bed, a desk, and the LoveSac bean-bag thing. We set up the futon in what used to be Randy's bedroom, and that's become a new escape for me, a place to take naps completely out of Marco's sight, a place to be out-of-sight, out-of-mind so my presence doesn't annoy Marco. He said one of the reasons he gets frustrated and mean is because we're together all the time, every minute of every day. I honestly don't feel that way. When I'm working, when he's working, we are not together. I actually feel like I'm completely alone in the house when I'm focused on what I'm writing or reading or whatever. I can segment away from any sense of "togetherness" when I'm in my little office room, sans door or not. But Marco says that because I'm in the house, even though we're not talking to each other and he's working, he still feels like we're together all day and that frustrates him, which is stressful for him and makes him surly and even mean. It's really hard for me to put myself in his position, because I just can't make myself think like he does on this one.

I've always had great focus working in a home office, so when I'm in my little office room here occupying my attention with something, I don't even realize Marco is in the house. I don't hear the phone ring, I don't hear music playing . . . I'm just . . . focused. And when I'm working, that's how I am: focused beyond realization of my surroundings. I seem to have maintained that little trait during cancer treatment. So when I'm in my little office room at the house doing something alone, it is definitely *not* like spending time with Marco to me.

But he says he doesn't like spending all day every day with me the way he does. I just don't get how being at work in his office all day is spending time with me, but Marco has a lot of issues and perspectives that I can't seem to grasp no matter how hard I try to understand where he's coming from. My way of understanding different perspectives is to put myself in the other person's position. I completely understand that a caregiver cannot be with the patient every minute of every day, but my mistake in trying to put myself in Marco's position to try to understand what he may be feeling, is that when I'm working, I'm working, and that's not how Marco thinks. I've been misunderstanding him all this time because I didn't know he can't focus on his work the way I can. That was a bad assumption on my part, thinking that as a rule, people who work from home are able to focus on what they're working on without feeling like they're "spending time" with someone else just because someone else is in the house.

Anyway, in the interest of trying to get more out of Marco's sight to give him more space while I'm taking care of myself in recovery, the spare bedroom has become my sanctuary. It's also kind of a music room for me. I keep my flute in here, and when my hands can handle covering the holes and pressing the keys, I like to play. If I can't dance, at least I can still make music. Marco said he can't hear me playing when the door is closed, it's like I'm not even here. What's good for Marco's mood is good for me, but in this case, it's much more than that. I've been a musician since I was four, it's part of who I am and another source of inner strength and calm when I'm struggling emotionally. I'm really struggling to stay strong for just one more round of chemo. But playing my flute helps. Music is good for the soul.

CANCER—DAY 139 THURSDAY, SEPTEMBER 10, 2009

Here are the tears. Again.

I had absolutely no motivation for going to yoga tonight. It was all I could do to encourage Marco to go to his yoga class and "take care of my caregiver." By the time all that emotional energy was spent on Marco, there wasn't anything left to encourage myself to go to my own yoga class. Now here I am in tears twenty minutes before class just agonizing over the fact that I used to be very frequently accused of being the most motivated person people knew, and here I am, so down with the mumps I can't even compose a coherent sentence that explains why I'm so run through that I can't even muster the energy to stand up and walk to the car to drive to yoga just six blocks away.

Getting Marco to go to yoga was completely draining emotionally. For as much as Marco complains about spending too much time with me, he's strangely reluctant to leave to go do anything by himself. I managed to convince him I'll be fine without him here and that he should go to his yoga, and he finally left. But rather than happily leaving the house to go to my own yoga class, which I really like, I'm sitting here crying and wondering what the hell has me feeling so anxious and worried. There has got to be something going on with all these meds. One week I'm a zombie with sleep, the next I'm sleepless and anxious for no apparent reason. That's where I am right now in the chemo cycle. Sleepless and fearsomely anxious for no reason. Weak.

So I tell myself, if I used to be so damn motivated, there is no reason not to be that way again now. I went all Tenacious C on myself, essentially, telling myself that I absolutely *must* make every effort to go to yoga today because I am, in truth, actually physically capable of getting through it tonight. Tenacious C has more willpower than Chemo Girl, so after that emotional battle with myself, I went.

But then there were more tears. I managed to get there a couple of minutes early to talk to the studio owner to ask her how I should pay for the sessions because I'm in this three-month beginner series yoga class but I have only been able to attend every other practice with chemo, and it's sporadic at best when I can go to any other drop-in practices to make up the sessions I miss. I completely expected to pay her the full amount for the beginner series, but I was hoping she might be willing to allow me couple little extra passes to use later for weeks I can't make it at all because of chemo. When I brought this up with the studio owner, she told me not to worry about any of it, we'll just let it go. I didn't understand. "What?" I asked, confused. She said, "You're not working, right?" I replied, "That's right, I'm on medical disability." So she told me "Then don't worry about it, we'll work something out later when you're working again and things are more steady for you. You don't need to be paying for this right now." I was dumbstruck, speechless. I've only met this woman twice, and here she is telling me to come to biweekly yoga practices at her studio for free, just to be kind to me during my treatment. I gave her a huge hug and said I didn't know how to thank her for such generosity and that I really appreciated it. And so, tears, flowing, I went and set up my yoga mat for the practice.

She doesn't even KNOW me! She's just a good soul being a good soul at a time and place when I desperately needed another one to enter my life. And now it will always be so much easier to motivate myself to go to yoga, to not let her down for putting herself out to let me come to her yoga practice for free. I owe it to her as well as to myself now to go every day that I am physically able. I don't have to get all my strength from within myself, there are all these wonderful people around me providing support too. That should be motivation enough to keep going.

CANCER—DAY 140 FRIDAY, SEPTEMBER 11, 2009

All right, let's face it—things have gotten cumulatively more degenerative for me physically. They said this would happen, but it's still hard to believe until it actually happens. You just can't believe it really can get worse until it actually *does* get worse.

My eyesight's still degenerating and now (after already having gone to the eye doctor and gotten a new prescription three weeks ago) it is again to the point that I can't see well enough to risk driving a car, and I'm wearing magnifying spectacles in addition to my new super-strength contacts in order to see the laptop screen right this moment, while my fingertips are alternately numb, thorny or burning, and always clumsy for typing. Not being able to be at the computer messing around much of the day has been more annoying than I expected. I didn't realize how much I research and read news and communicate online on a daily basis. But I'm reading a couple of good books now (inches from my nose, it seems) and resting almost all the time now. I don't have a lot of options but to rest and heal because there just isn't any energy left for anything else! My balance is off, so I'm not even taking little bike rides for exercise now, and my little walks are limited to just the six or so blocks between the house and the hospital because I seem to trip over my own feet and on every little twig and seam in the sidewalk. It's slow going, anything that I do.

I tell ya, I have a new appreciation for the very elderly now, an appreciation that I probably never would have developed without my body aging like this, in a matter of weeks instead of over decades like a normal person. My body feels about triple my actual age right now, with the exception being that I still have all my teeth (I don't really expect to have all my teeth at ninety, does anyone?). It's been absolutely surreal. Thank goodness I don't have kids to take care of and I can focus on recovery and managing the cancer treatments and meds. My oncologist says the side effects have been especially severe for me because of my age (early to mid-30s cancers are apparently especially brutal in comparison to over age 40 cancers) and so, being young, my body is fighting hard against the chemo. Which is good in a way, it means there's a strong healthy body in there battling for survival, but wow, does that battle take a lot of energy!!!

After chemo finishes I will go into radiation (in late October), and my understanding there is that radiation fatigue is even more debilitating than chemo fatigue. I can't imagine being more fatigued than I currently am, but just because I can't imagine it doesn't mean it can't happen. There may be some chance I'll be able to work 1/3 to 1/2 time during radiation because all of the other chemo side effects should go away except the fatigue and maybe the neuropathy, or I may not be able to work at all until sometime in January. It's impossible to tell right now, but I keep trying to get a sense of it so we can plan what help I can be at work or not. It's really important to me that the performance of my team at work does not suffer because of my health and limitations. I really want to come back strong as soon as possible, and stay healthy from that point forward, of course.

Whenever I think about how hard other people must have it in chemo, and being in chemo longer than me, gosh, I feel like such a baby for all the complaining I do about the side effects and how difficult it is. Almost anyone else going through this has a more difficult situation than mine in terms of support or insurance or something, and though the side effects may not be as bad for some other people, that doesn't mean the overall situation isn't actually much more challenging for someone else than for me. It could always be worse.

CANCER—DAY 141 SATURDAY, SEPTEMBER 12, 2009

So here my parents were supposed to leave Nebraska today, Saturday, to start their drive out here to visit, but they called yesterday and were already in western Wyoming somewhere, and today they drove all the way to Nevada (Winnemucca, I think) so they're sure to be at my house in Volcanoville on Sunday. I guess that's not sooo much earlier than what it would have been if they hadn't left home early, but it threw me off, because I suddenly thought I had to get things here in Sacramento ready more quickly!

Of course, there's nothing to get ready, not really. I can tidy up my office just a bit, but there are only so many places to stash so much stuff, so the space can feel cluttered with books and computer equipment even when the room is about as tidy as it can be. I also made the bedroom as tidy as possible. I threw all of Marco's dirty clothes from the bedroom floor into the closet, where there is now zero walking space, but better for his piles of dirty clothes to be in there than carving a little path through the bedroom. Sheesh, my mom can't see that! The bedroom, and the whole house could (as usual) easily bear multiple passes with a vacuum cleaner, but short of me getting an infection from stepping on something on the floor to motivate Marco to vacuum the house, I've given up on asking for it to be done. It seems to be a weird sort of sore spot with him, vacuuming, and the thing's too heavy for me to maneuver without exhausting Chemo Girl's pathetic weak body, so, dingy the carpets will remain even though my parents are coming to visit.

I do need to talk with Marco about what time we'll be spending with my parents and how it fits in with his work week and yoga and all that . . . since Mom & Dad have my house in Volcanoville to stay at, they can be relaxed and enjoying themselves out there when there's other stuff going on down here that they wouldn't participate in, like going to tango at Cell Block Wednesday night, or my yoga classes that I don't really want to skip if I can help it. I still get carsick, so we don't really expect me to be driving back and forth between home and Sacramento, and everyone seems to be in general agreement that I should continue to do my regular activities of yoga and dance as much as possible even while my parents are visiting.

Today I went over to the cat spa/kennel to pick up the cats and moved them to Brian's house. It's one of those ironically convenient timing things . . . Brian is traveling in Japan, his housemate is out of town for the week, and Brian's house is just empty this entire week. It's perfect timing for my cats to take over a whole house and have a pseudo-normal cat life for a few days, and for me to have a place with living room and dining room furniture (also sans grimy floors) to meet my parents at for a relaxing wine time, without being underfoot and possibly annoying Marco. Other than the fact that my parents won't get to visit with Brian, it's ridiculously good timing. Sometimes the timing of how things work out is just, well, too perfect to be random, you know?

CANCER—DAY 142 SUNDAY, SEPTEMBER 13, 2009

"Cancer, Day XYZ." It's like Star Date Something Something from some Sci-Fi show that I'm too young to have seen. (I don't really get Trekkies, no offense.) But other than numbering, I can't imagine actually titling each daily entry. Oh and tagging, don't get me going on tagging, I just can't seem to get in the habit of adding tags to make later blog searching easier. Besides, overall I'm lucky if I can keep the numbering straight most days! One of my long-time dance students, Mice, has corrected the numbering of days in my online cancer journal twice! How can I screw up the count when I make an entry every single day? One plus one plus one equals . . . four? No wait, let me guess again, I'll try counting on my fingers this time . . .

This is my last recovery week before going into another infusion. Ach, each one just gets worse than the last. Each recovery is harder to make, and I never get back to the strength of what "normal" was when this all started. Every time I find myself settling for a new "lower" definition of normal, just to call it normal, rather than dwelling on how much health and energy I had six months ago before all this cancer stuff.

CANCER—DAY 143 MONDAY, SEPTEMBER 14, 2009

Now this is cool. One of my old friends in San Jose whom I haven't seen in at least a couple years was in an all-weekend event run/walk for the cure last weekend, it was a three-day Susan G. Komen thing. They do these intense run/walk events, some 10 kilometers or more, some even multi-day (60 miles?), to raise funds and awareness to fight breast cancer. And, this is so cool, my friend even put my name as one of the four people she was walking for on her t-shirt.

What a neat thing to do! It's amazing to me that so many people always have me in their thoughts and do things like this, because they're just good people. She's getting me even more excited about the American Cancer Society breast cancer walk that my company is doing in October!

CANCER—DAY 144 TUESDAY, SEPTEMBER 15, 2009

We had a bit of a scare last week. Well, not really a scare exactly, but on Friday I finally called my doctor's office because this anxiety thing is so excessive I think it must be related to the combination of meds they have me on now. There just had to be something they can tweak with the meds to make the anxiety more tolerable and less freaky for me. After I talked with the oncology nurse for twenty minutes on Friday, Marco ended up taking me in for a blood draw (I still can't really see well enough to drive). My oncology nurse wanted to be sure the anxiety was associated with my meds, and rule out other problems like my electrolytes being low which could indicate other problems. So Marco takes me in for a ten-minute blood draw that of course turns into two hours. If it were simple and straightforward, the name on the chart couldn't be Cynthia Swan, right?

I do have one funny story about while we were there, though. So, it's Friday afternoon, right? For the most part, the staff is doing end-of-week work, finishing up file notes, that sort of thing, and there are practically no patients around. Well, the last time I had chemo was on the Labor Day holiday, so we had it at the other, older, chemo infusion center a couple blocks away. Apparently my physical file was still over there since they would have transferred it between the two facilities this weekend or something but here I am at my regular infusion center for this unexpected extra blood draw Friday afternoon. When the techs went into Dr. Lombard's office across the hall from the infusion center to see if they possibly had my file in there, Heddi (my oncology nurse) heard them mention my name, and she and Dr. Lombard came over to see how I was feeling and ask about my symptoms. I reiterated basically everything I'd told Heddi on the phone and filling in some gaps as more things occurred to me, talking about what may be going on and that it's probably fine, of course. The funny part of the story is the effect Dr. Lombard's presence had on the infusion center. All of a sudden they got very quick and professional about getting me set up, and working on my port (which they ended up having to TPA because the blood inside had clotted too solidly in the reservoir, no big deal, just a little hassle from being thin and not having much spare body fat covering the port, they said). Anyway, you should have seen the professional hustle and bustle of that infusion center when Dr. Lombard was there! I get the impression they don't see the actual medical oncologists all that often, at least not on a Friday afternoon.

Anyway, that's the funny story from the afternoon of the extra blood draw. There wasn't anything wrong in the lab tests they ran, so they gave me another medication that's for anxiety as well as nausea to maybe help with the carsickness more.

The unfunny story from that afternoon is how annoyed Marco was by the length of time we were there. After 30 minutes I asked him to just leave and I could call him to pick me up later, but he seemed to think it was his duty as my "caregiver" to be present. But having him there was more stressful than being alone, I swear. He was constantly annoyed and working on his blackberry, asking me every ten minutes when I would be done. Hmmm, you think this could have anything to do with my anxiety?

I really wish I didn't have a "caregiver" right now. Sigh. I wonder if he'll behave appropriately in front of my parents?

CANCER—DAY 145 WEDNESDAY, SEPTEMBER 16, 2009

I finally spent some time with my parents last night. They arrived at my house in Volcanoville on Sunday, and since I had yoga Monday afternoon, they stayed at my house Monday and came in to Sacramento Tuesday to see me. Conveniently, Marco teaches on Tuesday nights, so early Tuesday afternoon I drove over to Brian's house to spend the afternoon and evening with my parents. They haven't even seen Marco yet.

Ach, have I mentioned what wonderful people my parents are? I felt so much better talking with them. (We did not talk about Marco or the living situation in the house. I avoided that subject entirely.) I told them all about all the wonderful things, like my yoga teacher telling me not to pay for classes until I'm out of chemo, and my friend that put my name on her cancer walk t-shirt and e-mailed a photo of it to me, and all the people in the tango community that I see every time I go to a milonga and who are all so very concerned about how I'm doing, telling me to hang in there.

I also told them that, even though it's been really, really hard emotionally to go through treatment here in Sacramento, it was a good thing to do because I try really hard to stay upbeat and positive when I see my tango friends or go to yoga or anything. I'm definitely trying harder here than I would have to do if I were staying with them in Sidney during all of this, letting Mom take care of me but away from my friends and everyone I know. Seeing people frequently has been a big part of how I've managed to make it this far. I keep trying to act like I'm fine, or at least getting by OK, and in putting on a wig and a smile for The Act, I can even convince myself that I'll be OK. If I were home with Mom & Dad, I don't think I would try as hard. I mean, I would try to act well so I didn't upset them if I were staying with them during chemo, but I'm pretty sure I wouldn't be putting all the effort that I am into taking care of myself and putting on the good attitude for everyone else. If I had the luxury of being in my bedroom at their house with my mom to take care of me, I wouldn't have to try at all. And where's the lesson in that? If you're going to be brave, you have to do something that scares you. If you want to learn to be more giving, you have to be in a situation where it's challenging to do so, otherwise you won't learn anything.

Anyway, it was beyond wonderful to see my parents and have our familiar five o'clock wine time (I drank juice) with the usual kind of chatting. Even though I was keeping up The Act so my parents wouldn't worry, it was still the least stressed I've been in months.

And like Mom and everyone else says, it's just one more chemo. I just have to stay strong for just one more.

CANCER—DAY 146 THURSDAY, SEPTEMBER 17, 2009

So, good news on the genetic testing front! They tested for BRCA 1 sequencing and a "5-site rearrangement panel" and for BRCA 2 sequencing, and no mutations were detected anywhere. This basically means that I have a normal risk level of a new breast cancer or of ovarian cancer for someone with the rest of my profile. My profile, meaning, for someone who already has cancer and is getting chemotherapy, radiation, and then Tamoxifen.

It's funny, but that was exactly what I was expecting to hear. I even told my parents that before I went in for the appointment. I just had such a strong gut feeling there wasn't anything genetically wrong that I was completely expecting to hear that I didn't have any gene mutations, and I didn't know what the heck I was going to have an appointment with the genetic counselor about. It turns out the appointment was less than ten minutes because there was nothing to talk about. Did I call it or what?

CANCER—DAY 147 FRIDAY, SEPTEMBER 18, 2009

You know, I had meant to do all this writing today and get "caught up" on my blog this week since it's my "recovery" week, but I just feel crummy, besides having a pretty busy week. Today is a busy day too, relatively speaking. I'm waiting on the Sac pharmacy place to deliver my Emend, which is always stressful because they've missed almost every delivery they've committed to, and the Emend is apparently ridiculously important for chemo infusion day so it's really important that they deliver today, and they were supposedly delivering before noon but of course they haven't shown up yet. After my one o'clock blood draw, I'm off to Brian's to clean up everything from the cats (thankfully he has all hardwood floors so it's just sweeping, no vacuum cleaner to push) and pack up the cats to take them back to the kennel, then it's an early dinner at Logan's with my parents and Marco so there's not a lot of quiet time. I wonder if Marco will keep up the affectionate act that he does at milongas in front of my parents? Probably. Hopefully, actually. If my parents get the sense that he's mistreating me, it's going to get very ugly very quickly. I don't want my parents to worry about me any more than they already do.

And, of course, I have the usual looming dread of Monday's infusion and how awful I know I'm going to feel next week, and the week after, and the week after that. Just one more infusion, I know. We all keep saying that, "Just one more," and I agree it's good that there is only one more chemo infusion, but that still doesn't make me want to go through it. No offense to anyone who's tried to use that in a "stay positive" note to me this week. I do appreciate all the little notes; all my friends and family have been wonderfully supportive.

At the blood draws on the Friday before my Monday chemo infusions, they always ask how I'm feeling, and we always get into this lengthy discussion about what symptoms I'm having and the severity and all that. Today I really didn't want to have that conversation because talking about it all makes it seem worse, but it turned out to be important that I did give an honest report to the tech, because the severity was such that the tech then reported it all to Heddi, who then reported it to Dr. Lombard, and then both of them came over to the infusion center (again!) to see me and ask me more questions. The neuropathy has gotten quite a bit worse. Dr. Lombard had me walk down the hallway because I told them I've been bumping into stuff, and it turns out I can't actually walk straight down a hallway! At least I didn't bump into anything during Dr. Lombard's walking test though (it was a wide hallway). Dr. Lombard also had me hold my hands a certain way and he could really see the tremor in my right hand, and I told them about the burning sensation on both my hands (and my left foot, oddly) that seemed to be like an advanced stage of the fingertip prickling thing that started back with the first chemo.

Anyway, summary diagnosis is that I currently have a moderate level of neuropathy (a little more than level two of four). The bad news is that it's been continually degenerative with each round of chemo, and continuing chemo makes the neuropathy more severe more quickly with each subsequent round of chemo. Given this, Dr. Lombard is thinking about canceling or delaying my final chemo infusion that's scheduled for Monday, because this neuropathy is a side effect of the Taxol chemo drug and, get this, neuropathy can be *permanent*. The burning in my hands could get worse and be seriously for-the-rest-of-my-life permanent? Uff da. Just when I think I have my brain around the side effects and can get through them for the last round of chemo, I find out things could get worse *and* last forever. I just can't imagine that, not really. Is this a whopper of a life trial, or what?

We're going to go ahead with the pre-chemo appointment with Dr. Lombard on Monday, but they're not going to mix my chemo drugs until they get a go-ahead from Dr. Lombard after he sees me on Monday. And he may decide that we should delay my final dose a week or even two, to see if the neuropathy improves or continues to get worse during this time. The concern is that he doesn't know with certainty that the neuropathy will reverse itself completely over time. He had one other patient where it was about the level I have and it took about four months but she did have a complete recovery, but he just can't be sure, and he's being very careful about evaluating me and considering the long term effects of the neuropathy versus the benefits of completing the chemo (which apparently are pretty high, because he would rather delay a week and get in the full dose than give me just a partial dose on Monday).

He's a good guy. Gosh, I can't even imagine what would be happening right now if I were with that first medical oncologist I met with. You know, the one who made the chemo recommendation for six months of standard chemo including Adriamyacin without running any additional blood tests to confirm chemo would even be beneficial or possibly harmful in my case. Thank goodness I trusted my instincts more than that doctor and I went through the effort I did to find Dr. Lombard back then, instead of blindly agreeing to do whatever the first oncologist ordered just because he was a doctor. Hey, just because someone is a doctor, doesn't mean they're a *good* doctor! Dr. Lombard is definitely one of the good ones though. Actually, he's one of the great ones I think, and I'm definitely lucky to have him as my medical oncologist.

As for potentially canceling the last chemo because of the potential of permanent neuropathy, we'll know more on Monday.

CANCER—DAY 148 SATURDAY, SEPTEMBER 19, 2009

I take it back, we know more today. You will not *believe* what the new information is, though, so hold onto your hat, this roller coaster is about to do a nauseating loop-the-loop.

I just had a phone call from some administrative person at Marshall. The woman told me that Dr. Lombard is leaving the Marshall practice, and they've assigned me to a new doctor for Monday. This has to be a joke, right? Some doctor who only knows what's written about me in a chart (if the new doc has time to even read my chart before I get there Monday morning), this new unknown-to-me doctor is now going to be making a decision that will forever affect either my risk of cancer recurrence or possibly cause permanent nerve damage that could mean I'm in pain for the rest of my life? How's *that* for drama? Someone I have never met and have no reason to trust is suddenly in charge of my cancer treatment, at a *crucial* moment in my treatment. That's just great. This whole cancer thing just keeps getting easier and easier.

Not.

CANCER—DAY 149 SUNDAY, SEPTEMBER 20, 2009

I hit my head yesterday morning. Hard. Under my desk, turning the aquarium back on after changing the fish water. And as I was standing up after hitting my head, I blacked out. I wobbled and sunk to the floor with a groan. It was a weird darkening sinking sensation, slowly losing my consciousness instead of suddenly blacking out and being gone like when my heart failed. Marco bolted over from his office (good thing he was back inside from mowing the yard). He helped me sit on the floor and WOW did I suddenly get nauseous. And besides the pain in my head where I bonked it, I got this searing pain in my right arm, all the way down and especially in my hand. My whole arm was burning the way my hands have been burning with the neuropathy.

At that moment, for the first time in what seemed like forever, it was good to have a caregiver.

Marco got some ice for my head, and I sat there on the floor with it for ten minutes, then he slowly got me up and walked me over to sit in his office a while so he could "keep a close eye on me." It was awful, my right hand was shaking and useless; I couldn't grip a thing.

This was before I received the call about Dr. Lombard leaving, and the last thing he said to me on Friday afternoon was, "I'm on call this weekend so feel free to call and let me know how you're doing." After the bonk on the head fainting thing and how my right arm was burning, I told Marco I thought we should call in. He seemed resistant to that, and wanted me to rest longer, so I did, but after another fifteen minutes my right arm was still really bad so I called in, but it was a different on-call doctor (this was about 30 minutes before Marshall called to tell me Dr. Lombard was "leaving" the practice). The on-call doctor listened to my description and saw in the chart that I had just seen Dr. Lombard about the neuropathy on Friday afternoon and that I have an appointment with Dr. Lombard (or so we thought) on Monday morning, and he told me we probably didn't need to worry about it this weekend. He asked if I needed pain medicine and I told him I've been taking Ibuprofen and that's probably enough for the headache, and I've just been putting up with the neuropathy pain. Meds don't seem to help with the neuropathy pain. So, yesterday was a pretty tough day.

Wow, my head still hurts and my right hand is still totally weak, though not as shaky. Only my hand is burning again, not my whole arm like yesterday. I wonder if they'll do chemo tomorrow, or wait a week, or cut down the meds, or cancel my last chemo altogether or what? My vote at this point is to wait a week, given how this neuropathy thing is going and that I suddenly have a new doctor I've never heard of, can't find any good information about in my research, and don't trust. It's not like I can find a new medical oncologist in a week, but at least I won't feel like this substitute oncologist guy essentially committed me to permanent nerve damage by just automatically giving me the last round of chemo despite how bad the neuropathy is. But if the neuropathy doesn't get any worse next week, then maybe we can feel more secure in the notion that it won't get any worse and I can finish chemo. I certainly don't want to cancel the last round of chemo and risk wasting all the hell I've been through already. I know people do have to stop their chemo for a multitude of reasons, but I've been told more than once by more than one doctor that you pretty much lose the value of doing chemo at all if you cancel out partway through. With chemo you basically either run the whole course or don't enter the race. As it is I generally feel like I've wasted three months of my life so far, and it may be longer with radiation if I keep being so darn sensitive to all the treatments and not able to work. The time seems just lost, gone. Not that three months is really a long time in the greater scheme of a lifetime, but if you knew my personality before cancer, you know how much I hate wasted or lost time. Every moment is precious and there's no reason to waste it when you can be enjoying the moment for whatever it is. But, well, let's face it, there hasn't been a lot enjoyable about the last three months, and the time is just, well, gone.

But I've made it this far. I can make it through one more night. I have to. No matter what the outcome is, tomorrow is going to be an important day.

Chapter 20.
Last Chemo

Cancer—Day 150 Monday, September 21, 2009

I had to decide myself whether to do the last chemo or not today. The new doctor (Amagwal, a lung cancer specialist rather than a breast cancer specialist) refused to make a recommendation. He was leaving it entirely up to me to decide what I felt was right and what I can handle. Heddi, my oncology nurse, was there too, which helped a lot because she knows my case history and she was there on Friday when Dr. Lombard was testing the level of my neuropathy, so she knew exactly where we were at with that just a few days ago. We talked about what is known regarding the 4-series chemo regimen and how it was started and why it has continued in medical practice (basically because it works and they have all the stats on how much it reduces the 5-year risk of recurrence to do the 4-infusion series on a strict schedule). We also talked about my neuropathy, which is about a 2 on a 0 to 4 scale, so I'm halfway to the worst possible neuropathy and doing another chemo will very likely aggravate the neuropathy further. We did not talk about *how much* worse my neuropathy can get, which in hindsight was dumb on my part, because it was the consideration of potentially permanent neuropathy that was making us all hesitant to do the last chemo. They have no way of knowing who is going to have permanent neuropathy or who is going to recover from it completely. The fact that I've had neuropathy since the first chemo infusion is not a good sign, but the fact that I've had scattered intermittent good days gives me hope that with time it will be fully recoverable. It'll make my work really difficult when I start trying to work for my company again if my fingertips burn with every keystroke. But here I am, typing away to keep my journal up to date and keep everyone informed of where we're at. At least on a big day like today, I have to make the effort even if it burns.

So the two big considerations were: 1) the known value of completing all four chemo infusions on schedule, and 2) the unknown about the potential severity and permanence of the neuropathy. I'm told plenty of people quit their chemo before completion because the side effects become too unbearable but no one does less than four rounds as a standard course of treatment because clinical trials have shown at least four infusions are necessary for chemo to have a beneficial impact and reduce recurrence risk. As for the neuropathy, there doesn't seem to be much information about how much more severe it may get if I do more chemo. They know each round of chemo makes neuropathy cumulatively worse, but they don't know how much worse the neuropathy will get from one more infusion. As we all talked, I mulled it over in my mind. The neuropathy hasn't been as bad today as it was on the weekend, and Saturday was the worst I've had, where my whole right arm was useless and burning and my right hand couldn't even close, let alone pick anything up. I did have that knock on the head, which could have had a lot to do with the effect in my right arm that started right after that massive whack under my desk. My whole arm didn't hurt until that little head-bump incident, whereas the neuropathy presented immediately after my first chemo (I didn't even know the side effect was called neuropathy back then). The neuropathy has indeed been progressively worse with each round of chemo, so it would be naïve of me to think it will simply stay the same and not get any worse if I do the fourth round of chemo.

The question in my mind, regarding the neuropathy, was pretty simple, but also completely incalculable. How much pain can I live with?

Marco was leaning towards NOT doing the final chemo, at all, because of the potential neuropathy damage. His position seemed similar to how he resisted chemo altogether until we got the Oncotype DX score indicating how much chemo (and Tamoxifen, darn it, I don't want to deal with the known side effects of Tamoxifen) would reduce my recurrence rate. I think Marco's current resistance is partly because he's so close to it all now, he does know better than anyone how much pain and trauma I've had with all these side effects, and it has to just kill him to see me suffering and not really have anything he can do to help me feel better. If I were a caregiver in this situation, I would feel helpless like that, but there's still the element of emotional support that can make all the difference in the world to a cancer patient. That is the key element that has been the hardest thing of all for Marco and the greatest thing seriously lacking in my "care" that I think I would have felt so much better having.

He actually told me (via instant messaging while I was home last week) that he is not capable of providing the love or emotional support I said a cancer patient needs, and that it frustrates him that I would expect such things from him as a caregiver. Ugh. He should have known that of himself before saying he wanted to be my caregiver. But I've toughed it out so far, and this is the last time. We're two-thirds through all of my chemo, only three or four weeks of bad stuff and then hopefully a small window of goodly health time before radiation. I hope I can get home to my own place in Volcanoville for some of that break time between chemo and radiation. There's an extra recovery week, maybe my carsickness won't be so bad as to ruin my time at home if I can get there again. And then I can get my cats out of the kennel! Whoohoo! I'm allowed to take care of them during radiation, no more worries about the bacteria and my immune system. I miss them so much, I can't wait to have them here with me (even if they are locked up in just the spare bedroom like Marco said he'd allow . . . it's unlikely that arrangement will last long with Mizzou, and if you have to put money on a battle of will, well, Mizzou is a better bet than Marco since Mizzou is tenacious like me and doesn't give up what he's after if his first attempt fails).

Which reminds me that I need to tell everyone: I mustered my tenacity and decided to go forward with the last chemo. No one else (at least, not anyone with medical training) was making a decision, and the conversation was going in circles.

I was externally participating in the conversation, but I was engaged internally, sensing out my feelings in two extreme scenarios:

1) I ***don't*** have the fourth chemo, my neuropathy gets better, but I have a cancer recurrence in say, two years. What if that recurrence would have been delayed or eliminated by doing this last chemo?
2) I ***do*** have the fourth chemo today knowing that the neuropathy can worsen and/or become permanent, but also knowing that I have done everything that can be done to prevent a recurrence.

Those are the extremes. Two years out—alive with constant burning pain or, worst case, dead. Well, if you've read this far you know that I am not one to shirk away from what must be done just because I'm afraid it will be hard or painful. So I decided to tough it out, take the last chemo infusion, and deal with the side effects. If the neuropathy gets worse, so be it. It is what it is. If it gets worse *and* turns out to be permanent, well, I'll just have to deal with it.

What I cannot do is quit on my family and everyone who has been wishing and praying so hard for my recovery. I am determined to suffer, as gracefully as possible, the very worst cancer treatment has to impose if that is what I must do to stay alive and not abandon the people I love.

You know, it may very well never come to that. I may never have a recurrence, ever, and we may never know if doing the fourth chemo mattered or not. But if I ever have a recurrence, at least I won't blame myself for chickening out on the fourth chemo.

To be brave, you have to do the things that scare you. Likewise, is there any other way to learn compassion, than to suffer what others must suffer? If I do this and I survive this and I learn from it, maybe I can be a compassionate giving soul that helps others deal with trials and tribulations like breast cancer.

CANCER—DAY 151 TUESDAY, SEPTEMBER 22, 2009

The appointment with Dr. Amagwal (the substitute medical oncologist) was at 11:30 a.m. yesterday, and they started my chemo around 12:30 p.m., and I wasn't out of there until 5 p.m. or so.

Bless Marco, he missed the whole afternoon from work to be there for me, he stayed off the blackberry, and he never left my side for an instant. He was kind and caring throughout the infusion and the entire evening. He was a completely different person from the annoyed guy harassing me to hurry up my blood draw last Friday. I think the whole thing was pretty overwhelming for him with the enormity of the decision I had to make, and then realizing that I consciously chose to take the more difficult path. Anyway, though I became groggy during the chemo infusion, he let me win a game of Scrabble (I scored over 350, my highest score ever!), and then he read to me from *The Celestine Prophecy*, which is this thoroughly entertaining adventure book that actually really gets you thinking a lot about spirituality and similar matters. I've read it several times so I was still following along though my head was a fog. It would be neat if he continues to read this book, because it would instigate a lot of fun conversations about spirituality and faith and beliefs that would be really interesting to have with Marco, who is a die-hard there-is-nothing-after-death atheist.

Side effects have already kicked in hard. Before even getting back from chemo, I started having esophagus pain, the swollen burning feeling in my esophagus that spreads down into my guts where it expands to what I think of as the intestinal Battle of Cynthia Island. I have this new med now called Reglan that I'm supposed to take before eating, and it seems to take the edge off the submarine warfare though my esophagus still hurts. I've started drinking my juice from a hospital mug that measures quantity consumed and has an enclosed lid with a straw. That seems to help, having a straw can prevent me from smelling or having to taste water all over my mouth to drink it, if we run out of juice.

CANCER—DAY 152 WEDNESDAY, SEPTEMBER 23, 2009

Well today I'm apparently ready to go back in time because I initially wrote the date as 2004. Weird, chemo brain, weird. Actually, I kept trying to get to my journal all day, but I just couldn't stay awake, like, at all. Wake up to take pills, nap. Wake up again (with an alarm) to take more scheduled pills, nap. Wake up to the alarm again to take the next round of pills, nap. Be careful not to disturb or distract Marco from his work. Such is my world during infusion week.

CANCER—DAY 154 FRIDAY, SEPTEMBER 25, 2009

I've been wearing my granny magnifying specs to see the computer screen. It bums me out to realize how very severely limited I may still be after the "official" timeframe for chemo is supposedly over. I want to just jump back into my normal of way being and my normal way of doing lots of different things, yet here I sit unable to see the computer screen to type a sentence with less than 50% typographical errors in it and burning my fingertips on the computer keys in the process. I wanted to dance at Boogie by the Bay out in SF, and I wanted to fly back to Atlanta for the "Team Cynthia Swan" walk against breast cancer in October, and I am doing everything in my power to make it to L.A. for the six-year-mark of Artie's death coming up on October 19th. If anything, that's the one thing that will happen because it's such an important time to me and to Artie's family. Someone will have to drive me if my eyes don't get better or the nausea doesn't go down, but it's still a few weeks away, there's lots of recovery time between now and then. Just a quick, quiet little drive to L.A., no dancing, no excessive socializing. I can do that, can't I? Just spend the time I need to at the cemetery and come back.

CANCER—DAY 155 SATURDAY, SEPTEMBER 26, 2009

I sent Marco off to the milonga without me tonight. There's just no way I'm up to the socializing and physical activity of tango tonight. Besides, Marco needs more than one night off from me in a week. The weight of this thing, and how never-ending it seems is hard to bear even when we know the upturn has to be just around the corner, somewhere, some gradual improvement, infinitesimal even, but please oh please let me improve. It's depressing for me, and I'm surely not easy to be around right now. Marco bears it reasonably well during chemo week though, except when he has his little bursts of wanting more free time to himself.

You know, we actually had a nice couple of hours this afternoon talking about the plants outside and how to take care of them and stuff which Marco is really interested in and I know little about, so it was nice to get his mind off of me and onto something he enjoys. Besides having to put up with me, apparently there are layoffs coming up at Marco's company and he's genuinely concerned about possibly losing his job. Uff da, more stuff for Marco to stress on, getting all frustrated and negative. The more I can get him talking about things he likes, regardless of whether or not I'm actually interested, is a good thing, methinks. Take care of your caregiver.

CANCER—DAY 156 SUNDAY, SEPTEMBER 27, 2009

Wow, almost seven days into it this time and I can't seem to stay awake long enough to accomplish much or be coordinated enough to think and type at the same time. It's driving me batty. I made dinner tonight (it wasn't particularly good in my opinion though Marco complimented it), but the whole process completely exhausted me. Bad idea. On the upside, at least the additional anti-nausea meds seem to be helping. The odor of food cooking doesn't drive me out of the house now. That is definitely an improvement!

My brain seems addled though, and it's driving me nuts because there are all these things I want to think about and start planning, like how much or when I can work or teach dance again. I wonder how long it's going to be before I can think through this fog of chemo brain, or be less fatigued, or when the neuropathy pain will lessen to a tolerable level.

I have to hold onto things to sit down, like a very frail *very* old woman. It's not looking good. The substitute oncologist said he hopes I'll have some recovery by week 4 (he doesn't expect to have much improvement in weeks 2 and 3, given my past history of slow chemo recovery). Week 4 is three weeks out; that's not so long, right?

Frail, ancient old woman, that's Cynthia today. Not forever though, it can't be forever. I just have to get through this a little while longer.

CANCER—DAY 157 MONDAY, SEPTEMBER 28, 2009

I'm trying to go through the motions, but I can see why people just have to retire at some point, when continuing to work is just no longer feasible given declining physical limitations. I just can't function, the simplest tasks exhaust me. It takes me three tries to get off my office chair and that's while holding onto both the desktop on one side and the bookcase on the other. It's so debilitating that I can't really believe it's happening. Besides the eyesight thing being so annoying and all the other stuff (submarine wars in my GI, non-functional fingers, inability to walk straight and keep my balance without holding onto something, the mouth sores, increasing neuropathy pain), besides all *that* garbage, the bone pain is back. It stabs into the center of my spine and just radiates this spike of constant deep pain from there. It can't be reached with any kind of deep tissue massage or anything. The heating pad does give me some relief for the bone pain though, which is definitely better than no relief at all.

Marco should be back from yoga soon, and I hope to go to mine on Thursday. Though, if I can't ride my bike I don't know how I'll get there (I *definitely* cannot drive a car!). My bicycle is off-limits with this balance problem. I'll have to walk. Darn it, that really exacerbates the neuropathy burning on the bottom of my feet. Sigh. It's not very far, maybe I'll take the car and just be really, really careful. I hate to miss yoga now.

I do have something funny to note today though, instead of just complaining incessantly. One of my friends sent me a piece of flair on

Facebook today (flair as in those round buttons people working in certain chain restaurants wear on their suspenders or something. You know what I mean, the yellow smiley face, a shamrock with "Kiss me I'm Irish," or "Life is too short to wear ugly shoes . . . " that kind of thing. On Facebook it's digital but they look like buttons, and the buttons are called "flair." Anyway, it took me three tries to read this one with the font and all (and I didn't understand it the first time I could actually read the words), but when I finally got it I laughed out loud.

This flair button had the pink breast cancer ribbon in the middle of it, and in dark pink script it said "Help Save Second Base!"

CANCER—DAY 158 TUESDAY, SEPTEMBER 29, 2009

So you must be wondering . . . whatever happened with Dr. Lombard, and why was he suddenly dismissed without notice from Marshall Cancer Center on an unexpected Friday evening? (There is no way he knew it was coming, because at 4 p.m. Friday afternoon he told me he was on call that weekend.)

I had a private conversation with my oncology nurse, Heddi, and it sounds like it was administrative politics, and not the kind that increases the quality of patient care. Dr. Lombard was spending *too much* time with patients, His mother, his grandmother, and his sister all had breast cancer, and he's incredibly sensitive to the patients as a result. Heddi said he was working long hours every day to see to it that all of his patients got the quality of care he felt they deserve and he would usually stay late to finish up his paperwork in the evening. The administrative powers-that-be didn't mind him working long hours, but they still didn't like his approach. Essentially, spending more time per patient means less patients seen overall, and sometimes he would be with a patient and be late for or miss staff meetings as well, which didn't help his standing with administration. Meanwhile, they have a business to run. I get that. My dad is a hospital administrator, and this is one of the fundamental clashes that frequently pop up because it's hard to balance time in patient care with keeping the business afloat. It's basic economics, but it's emotional economics.

So, anyway, Dr. Lombard was deemed unfit to the mold of what the Marshall Cancer Center wanted in its medical oncologists, so he was summarily released, basically without notice. Heddi said he did get a "warning" a month or two ago that he had to adjust his methods to see more patients per day and not be late for meetings, but neither he nor the medical staff had any idea he was being dismissed until it actually happened at 5 p.m. that Friday. Dr. Lombard wasn't allowed to contact any of his patients to say goodbye or reassure us somehow that we were going to be OK even through the change. I think it's a travesty. It must have been difficult for Dr. Lombard, at least on a personal level, to be leaving patients like myself at a crucial point in their treatment. It was definitely devastating for those of us entrusted to and depending on his care. I didn't go to Marshall for Marshall, I went to Marshall because I wanted Dr. Lombard as my medical oncologist. I think the way Marshall handled the patient communications was atrocious. Of course, I was particularly sensitive to that because it was the most critical moment in my entire treatment, so I'm biased.

I had printed a bunch of business cards with my website on them so that Heddi could hand them out to other new breast cancer patients that may be interested in reading about my experience but not really up to a phone call (I remember those days extremely well), and Heddi said she would give one to Dr. Lombard too, so maybe he's gotten to see in my blog that he was deeply respected and appreciated both for his expertise as well as his bedside manner and empathy. Heddi said she is going to bring my cards up at their staff meeting too, so that everyone working the desks will know my blog is out there as another resource, because people are always asking them how to get real information from actual patients without disturbing them.

So, that's what I understand of Marshall v. Lombard. It's very abridged, but still enough information to piss you off that it couldn't at least be handled more professionally and less like patient abandonment.

Aren't there laws against that? Call it mistreatment of patients or something? Can a medical facility really fire your doctor without allowing the doctor to tell patients he's leaving and force you to switch to another doctor without notice? Overnight? I don't know how the legal side of medical service works, but the only way I can describe this as a personal experience is that it's patient abandonment. And I know Dr. Lombard would never willingly abandon a patient.

CANCER—DAY 159 WEDNESDAY, SEPTEMBER 30, 2009

I'm down to focusing entirely on one thing at a time now. I don't think about the next thing until the current thing is complete, because I can't multi-task my brain at all anymore.

One thing at a time. That basically means one thing in a day for me, give or take.

I had to fill out DMV forms to make my Rubicon a non-operating vehicle today because when I stopped being able to go home I stopped the insurance on the Jeep since it's just parked in the garage and is therefore covered by my homeowners insurance, and I need to do everything possible to cut costs while on disability (which is paying, at the end of the day, about a third of what I used to make in total in a year because I had other jobs without health or disability insurance, like teaching dance classes and grad school courses). Now that the Jeep renewal is due, I decided to file it as non-operating. This should be a relatively simple task, right? Research online, find the right DMV form online, get it filled out, mail it in (after buying stamps). That simple process, ladies and gentlemen, took me ALL afternoon. Unbelievable. On the other hand, I stayed awake all afternoon to get it done, no nap. I'm starting to wake up.

CANCER—DAY 160 THURSDAY, OCTOBER 1, 2009

Carsickness be damned, I wanted to visit the cats today after lunch. I'm also getting things ready for them to "come home" to Marco's house, to live in the guest bedroom at the end of the month. Marco finally said that if they were kept in the spare room, never let out, and the $300 a month I was paying the kennel would now go to Marco, then the cats could be here. I've been rearranging the empty storage boxes and the gi-normous dog bed Randy left behind. It made a nice window perch for the cats to be lazy on and hopefully not meow all day from being locked up in one room. That room is also my "music room" where I play my flute when I'm well enough. I haven't played since the last chemo though. No energy. But when I feel up to playing I can, and that feels good to be able do. Even when I can't play and just go in there to nap, I like seeing my flute and music stand, reminding me of the old me, a part of the old me that I don't want to lose. I've already said this but it's worth repeating: music is good for the soul.

Disregarding carsickness, I still don't think I can drive the distance to the cat spa kennel. My hands burn and shake with the neuropathy. It's gotten worse, and everything I touch hurts my hands. I keep trying to put on hand lotion to sooth them, but even the coolness of that feels like little slivers. One thing I am definitely doing tonight though is yoga. It's less than six blocks away, and I'm going even if I have to do my drunken-sailor neuropathy-feet double-limp walk to get there.

With separate yoga studios and times, there are now three more nights every week that Marco has off from being a caregiver (in addition to Tuesday nights when I usually hang out with Brian—Tuesday has been his scheduled night "off" from me from the beginning). Whenever possible, I encourage him to engage in his own activities without me. I excuse myself from most of the wine club parties now so Marco can go by himself. One night I took myself out to a movie alone to give him space on a night he was particularly frustrated. He has other stresses on his mind besides me and cancer though, and he says his frustration isn't only because of me—he's also worried about the upcoming layoffs at his company, and finding a place to live when the foreclosure happens, and how he's going to work out his finances to afford an apartment again, because his rent here is dirt cheap. Any decent apartment in Sacramento would easily cost double what Marco pays in rent now, and it's worrying him.

I really have been taking care of myself completely, though, just as he intended. He doesn't have to worry about being a caregiver in the traditional sense of what you would expect given the job title "caregiver." I take care of my meds and food/diet and fluids as well as managing all the doctor stuff. So, just like it could always be worse for me as a cancer patient, Marco could have it worse as a caregiver. If I were a demanding, dependent patient, it would drive Marco mad. That would definitely *not* be the right way to take care of my caregiver.

CANCER—DAY 161 FRIDAY, OCTOBER 2, 2009

Today I'm going to Jolynne Miyao's (*great* last name, pronounced 'meow') for another Reiki session, which is this kind of energy massage that Jolynne and Bitsy do. So this morning I wanted to do make up and make myself presentable to be with other people, which is quite a process these days, I tell ya! So I'm sitting here doing my two-hour makeup process and trying to just be in the moment of just doing what I'm doing and not think about pain or side effects or radiation or worry about my relationship with Marco . . . but it's not really happening for me.

My eyes keep watering, and tears slip down my cheeks. Marco happened to walk in at completely the wrong time, because I had just finally lost enough tears that I had to grab a tissue to catch them from all falling all down my cheeks and ruining the makeup I'd done so far. He asks, "What's wrong?" Well, I can't explain it very well of course because I don't really know, at least not that I can explain to him without upsetting him. I think I told him I had torn a contact lens or something. I definitely did not get into a heart-to-heart chat with him about why there are tears on my cheeks.

I've been feeling so very much alone, with Marco. I can't blame him, not really, not since he openly and honestly told me that he cannot give me emotional support and part of his frustration is that the cancer patient (me) needs emotional support more than anything else when that's the one thing he cannot give. So I try not to bother him with this sort of thing.

The tears come because I've suffered through all this, all this pain and doing this the hard way by staying here with him and having to take so much more responsibility for myself instead of trusting that it will be OK without a huge debilitating drain of effort from me . . . I've suffered through this here instead of being somewhere that I'm loved and safe and can totally trust my caregivers because they love me unfailingly. I've suffered through all the pain and side effects and trying to be a good patient during chemo weeks so it's as easy as possible for Marco and I've tried to be encouraging of him going out and doing things without me so that he doesn't feel so pressured as a "caregiver." And I put a *lot* of effort into keeping all the pain and emotional strain deep inside me so that I don't take it out on other people. So when I'm by myself, that anguish has to get out of me somehow, and I think that's what these tears are. I let them fall now so that I get some of it out of me before I swallow it all down again to go be with other people.

But you know, those other people are my emotional support. My family, all the faraway people that e-mail me all the time, and my tango friends, countless people like Jolynne Miyao and Bitsy, or Kym, my yoga instructor. All these people genuinely care so much that even though I don't get any emotional support from my caregiver, I don't really need it because I actually receive so much emotional support from everyone else around me, and from people all over the country and other parts of the world, even.

CANCER—DAY 162 SATURDAY, OCTOBER 3, 2009

Everyone sends these nice little thinking-of-you notes, and of course everyone always asks how I'm doing when they see me, and I never know what to say. My standard response is "I'm doing OK, how are you?" I put on the brightest smile I can muster so they don't see that I'm in pain, and I force the old brightness into my voice from the days before cancer when I could honestly always say "I'm great! How are you?" I don't talk about treatment or any of the physical side effects unless someone asks specifically about it. And I never say anything about emotional strain. That's just a burden I do not want to force on anyone. I know people are genuinely concerned and sincerely want to know how I'm feeling, but it seems so wrong to just spout off a bunch of true but awful stuff when the person was quite possibly just trying to be polite in asking how I'm doing because they heard I had cancer.

Physically I'm not great of course, here in week 2 of the chemo cycle, but I'm finally "waking up" from the chemo into that state of knowing I can't do anything or even think straight but remembering that I used to be able to, six months ago. This is also the point (week 2) at which I stop sleeping at night or being able to take naps even though I'm too fatigued to dress myself or do anything in any reasonable amount of time. After the physical pain part, the week 2 chemo recovery segment is a kind of mental torture for me.

Emotionally tortured is probably a good summary statement for where I am right now. But every day is different, slightly. The physical limitations aggravate the emotional issues because I don't have any way to kill the time until some of the physical things improve enough to be able to do anything useful or the fatigue clears enough that I can think. I can't remember the last time I felt like that, actually. When did I last have a truly clear-headed thinking mind?

Physically, as I said, things are not great. My balance is gone. I can't walk straight or ride my bike. I'm shaky and unreliable from neuropathy in my hands and feet so the doctor told me not to drive a car. With my feet suffering from neuropathy, with the bottoms all numb but somehow also with spiky pains, I can't balance or be on my feet long enough to dance at a milonga even if I had the energy to go to one. The fatigue keeps me from even bothering to get dressed and certainly blocks the energy I need to muster for makeup and preparation to go out in public. My hands are damaged worse than my feet by the neuropathy. I sometimes can't feel my fingertips to type properly or grip anything, but usually, much worse than being numb, they burn. My hands are altogether clumsy and claw-like in use, and the pain in the whole underside of my hands feels like everything I touch, including the flat surface of my glass desk, burns my hands. Opening a pill bottle is just agony to my hands, with those little cap ridges slicing like razor blades into my fingers and palm. It's an exquisite form of torture only a medical person could conceive of, I'm sure . . . the child-safe pill bottle cap has become my nemesis. My eyesight fails within an hour or two of any concentrated focus, so reading is of limited duration, watching anything on the computer, writing . . .everything is limited. It's honestly a pretty miserable existence, temporary as it may be.

I've learned that eyebrows are a pain to create when you have no eyebrows, and my lower eyelashes are mostly gone too. Not having eyelashes is kind of hard to disguise, though thankfully I still have my upper eyelashes, which feels somewhat normal to make-up and eyeliner does wonders for hiding the fact that someone may not have eyelashes, so that's a positive side note.

That's enough complaining. Tomorrow will be different. Right now I just have to get through today. I'll deal with tomorrow when it gets here.

Marco is going to be gone all day tomorrow. It's the Big Crush, and the wine club gets a bus and goes wine tasting all day.

Marco thinks the nausea will be too much for me. I just begged off on the excuse of still being in chemo recovery (though the more important element of the equation is that Marco is in constant need of breaks from me). So, I'm not going even though I was originally excited about it. I genuinely like the wine club people and the day trip sounds like tons of fun.

They're going to have a long day of wine tasting though, and when Marco gets back, well, he's not exactly going to be sober, you know? As for having a day alone to myself, well, aside from the fact that I'm obviously going to disobey doctor's orders and drive my car to visit the cats and run errands, well, it will be nice to have a day of quiet where it doesn't matter what I do or when as long as I keep on my meds, which I've been doing just fine all along. Besides, we're going into week 3 of the chemo recovery cycle, which is usually just my flu-ish week when I'll have a mild temperature and feel like I have the flu all week, while the other side effects of the chemo poisoning should decrease in severity.

Ach, darn it, now there's a stabbing neuropathy burning in the toes on my right foot. Why does this stuff have to keep getting worse??? Just as I was writing that things are going to get better!

CANCER—DAY 163 SUNDAY, OCTOBER 4, 2009

Tonight Marco and I did something we should have been trying to do once a week or at least every 2nd and 3rd week during chemo . . . we went to a friend's house for dinner.

Food and nausea have been a problem throughout chemo, of course. The physical act of eating hasn't been such a terrible problem, but the smells of food cooking generally drive me out of the house. I ended up doing a lot of cold meals or things that heated very simply and very quickly, or that could be cooked outside on the grill, without lingering odors in the kitchen and throughout the house. Still there were plenty of nights where I was driven outside to the back yard by nausea, just eating a slice of bread or some crackers . . . something without a smell or even much taste, because once I'd had a nausea episode, my stomach was in turmoil for the night, it seemed. But I could still usually eat when necessary. Throughout all of this, even if it was just soup, I've pretty much been able to eat and my weight has stayed completely stable (surprisingly so, to me). No weight change makes for happier doctors. No weight loss, no weight gain, that's what they wanted. I'm more in the just-don't-gain-weight camp, myself.

Early on I'd read cancer things saying to let people make/bring you food, but we'd kind of written it off as unnecessary for us. I mean, I live with my caregiver, so why do other people need to bring me food, too? That was our thinking at the time, anyway. But last night we went to Bitsy's house and had a "John Wayne" Cheese Casserole that takes an hour to bake (baking smells are the worst for me) and there's no way we could have prepared it here at Marco's house, but arriving at Bitsy's house with the dinner already prepared (and the windows open thanks to the always thoughtful Bitsy), the smells didn't send my nausea through the roof. She also made some yummy broccoli (my favorite veggie), and cornbread. I haven't had cornbread in forEVER, and that was a treat, too. So, we went "out" for dinner last night and had a nice home-cooked meal that didn't make me nauseas in the preparation because we didn't prepare it. What a novel idea. I can't believe we're in the last throes of chemo treatment before making this little discovery. This approach to cooked meals is something that should have occurred to us as soon as the smell of food cooking started making me nauseas months ago.

It was nice to have a real dinner with normal-people conversation too, since I generally eat alone in silence so that I don't disturb my caregiver. Bitsy has become a wonderful friend through this. Six months ago, I didn't really know any of the other tangueras very well, because when I went to a milonga I would dance, literally, all night. Now I can't dance the entire evening (well, much at all really), but I've become great friends with some wonderful women in the tango community. Bitsy, for example, always comes over to me immediately to give me a hug when I arrive, and she always keeps me company through at least one entire tanda, always genuinely concerned about each element of my treatment, but also very sensitive to my concerted effort to *not* focus on it and instead make conversation about other, more enjoyable topics.

CANCER—DAY 164 MONDAY, OCTOBER 5, 2009

I went to my first "regular" (beginner, as opposed to introductory level) yoga class tonight, and I was wiped out about halfway through, my body would just shake with the impossibility of holding a position long enough to really benefit from it. And it's not like any of it is actually hard. I mean, come on, I graduated from introductory level to *beginner* level, not into some high level yoga. And even the beginner level stuff is a strain for my body. I noticed how weak I am yesterday too, when I was running errands after visiting with the cats. I needed an ink cartridge at the office store, and they were on the bottom shelf. Normally getting up from a squatted position like that, I try to go slow to make sure I don't get light-headed while I'm still off my heart meds, but yesterday my legs actually *shook* with the effort of trying to raise myself from a squat without using my arms to assist and it was an agonizingly slow ascension. It's not just fatigue now. I seem to have some serious weakness to recover from, too. This poor body.

CANCER—DAY 165 TUESDAY, OCTOBER 6, 2009

Each day does seem marginally better now in terms of my feeling slightly less lost and fogged out of my own brain as time passes, though all the side effects continue to shift: some lessening, some worsening, some things reappearing that I keep hoping I am done with. Like night sweats.

I haven't had too much trouble with hot flashes, at least not severe ones in the traditional sense. Tonight I'm constantly much too warm or much too cold, and I guess it's coming in waves that could be considered hot flashes by my oncologist. Not hot like *unbearably* hot, though, like I'm going to sweat into a puddle on the floor in the next thirty seconds, which is what I understand a bad hot flash to be like.

My most severe heat extremes occur in bed at night. I'm generally much too warm when I go to bed and I try to keep the ceiling fan on as long as possible to cool the room as much as possible before actually going into the room to sleep. More often than not though, by 3 a.m. I often wake up so completely boiling that I've sweat completely through my pajamas and soaked my pillow and sheets so that my whole side of the bed is just a wet muck that can't be slept in. So I get up for a while, and this is where my long sleepless nights come in, because once I'm awake, it's incredibly difficult for me to fall asleep again. I'm one of those ridiculously light sleepers; I've just always been that way, my entire life. Being a light sleeper didn't matter when I lived alone in the woods just a little over six months ago, but it's a real problem trying to sleep here in a city where there's traffic and garbage trucks and people who snore, and, well, just a lot of noise that I am not accustomed to, as well as a complete lack of the white noise I used to fall asleep to every night with the quiet constant forest sounds. Wind in the trees, now there's a sound to sleep all night to. Why do people want to live in these crowded noisy places anyway? I'm here because I have to be. Will I stay when it's no longer necessary for my cancer treatment? Ha. With my home out in El Dorado National Forest begging to house the cats again? It's nice to be near the dance stuff because it takes less effort when the milonga is just ten minutes away instead of two hours away, but other than that, I don't have much reason to drive down to Sacramento from my home. I see my friends at the milongas and when I'm teaching. That's enough for me, but the truth is I wouldn't be doing any of that at all now if I weren't staying here in Sac, very close to everything I may want to go to.

I'm rambling. This entry started out about night sweats. So anyway, after I wake up at 3 a.m. soaking wet, then I have to get out of bed and change into something dry. I've gotten in the habit of keeping everything I need right there on the floor next to the bed so I can either try to change just my top and hope to go back to sleep, or, more typically, get completely dressed in sweats with socks and a hood or hat and everything to come back to the office (because it's always cold back here at night since my office doesn't have a heat vent). Then I mess around on the computer or read. At 6 a.m., my first meds alarm goes off so I take that medicine and keep doing whatever. Usually I'm doing my daily Rune around then, writing in my private journal about the messages the Rune for that day contains and trying to relate those messages to my life or the kind of person I am trying to be.

When my meds alarms go off, I pull out my cancer treatment calendar chart so I take and then check off the correct medications by time of day. We certainly don't need me overdosing or mixing together the wrong meds at the wrong time. The 6 a.m. meds ingestion includes Reglan, which is the drug that helps reduce the esophagus pain I refer to as the Battle of Cynthia Island. Ironically, Reglan makes me sick to my stomach if I don't eat something within half an hour, so the early morning meds are usually followed by a touch of breakfast, like half an English muffin with peanut butter, then ninety minutes later my regular alarm goes off for me to go wake Marco (the first week I was here Marco's barking bleeping alarm scared me to death, and then he would keep hitting snooze so it went off again and again . . . finally I convinced him that we could use my alarm because it's a quiet slow song that doesn't scare me, and then I have to wake Marco because he can't hear it; but that is vastly preferable to having my wits scared out of me every morning when his alarm goes off). I wake Marco and sit with him a few minutes so he doesn't fall back asleep and he does actually get up for work, then I brew some tea for him and we're pretty much into the day with me having had about three hours of sleep thanks to waking up with night sweats (well, and being a light sleeper in general). I zombie through the day, and try to nap whenever there's the slightest chance I may be able to fall asleep. Problem being, I can be falling asleep sitting at my desk reading on the computer screen, but by the time I get off the chair and onto the LoveSac to snooze, I'm wide awake again because I had to move around (even though my chair and the LoveSac are actually so close together that they're touching, how ridiculous is that?). I tell ya, being wired as a light sleeper has some serious drawbacks sometimes.

Anyway, that's my rant for today. Night sweats. I'm already expecting it'll happen when I go to bed tonight, because I'm constantly hot and cold just sitting here now. But tomorrow I have a long morning appointment with the new radiation oncologist. Marco can't go with me to help take notes because he (conveniently, for both our sakes) has a conference call, so I need to get my game on for that, to be alert and be able to ask all the questions I asked six months ago the last time I had a radiation oncologist consult. Yeah right, like I'm one-tenth as alert now as I was back then. A twentieth even? Nope, not even close. The good thing is that I still have my notes from the radiation oncologist appointment I had back in April with a different oncologist. My gosh, April? That was a lifetime ago! I'm not even sure I quite remember what life was like pre-chemo.

But praise be, no more chemo for me!!!

Chapter 21.
The Cortina

CANCER—DAY 167 THURSDAY, OCTOBER 8, 2009

In Argentine Tango, you always dance a tanda (a set of tango songs) with each dance partner, and the sets are separated by these 30-second blasts of completely non-Argentine music so people know the tanda is over. At the milongas I've been to in Buenos Aires, that 30-second blast is when they play American music, which always confuses the non-tango Americans present. I sometimes wonder if the Argentines don't do that as a little inside joke on the Americans, testing their knowledge of the traditions of authentic Argentine Tango and bemused (or maybe annoyed?) when the Americans do not understand the brief break in the style of music or why the American song is always cut off after about thirty seconds. This little break between tandas is called the cortina. And that's what I feel like I'm in now, between chemo treatment and radiation treatment. This is my Cancer Treatment Cortina.

Once a tanguera, always a tanguera, eh? Even with chemo brain, I still have tango brain.

Yesterday I met with the new radiation oncologist. (Argh, the painful shaky hands neuropathy thing is going to be a severe bother today, I can tell already.) Besides all the important information we discussed (and which I will note in detail when radiation starts and hopefully my hands don't hurt as much), this appointment was probably even more important to me as a milestone. Chemo is over, and this appointment was like the big change in music for the cortina. Staying with the tango metaphor, the next tanda of my tango with cancer will begin with radiation.

The decision to go to a new radiation oncologist was actually just for the convenience of keeping everything local to Sacramento now. When I met with the first radiation oncologist, six months ago, I still thought I was going back to Nebraska for chemo and then returning home (to my house in Volcanoville) for radiation, which would have meant a daily drive 45 minutes each way from home to the radiation treatment and weekly appointment with the radiation oncologist at his office in Cameron Park. Then when we decided I was going to stay in Sacramento for everything and live here with Marco for all the cancer treatment, I called the first radiation oncologist and he referred me to a Sacramento-based radiation oncologist in his medical group, a woman this time, who is also a breast cancer specialist. I was pleased with the idea of having a female radiation oncologist, I just like the feel of it. The more female doctors in the world, the better, I think. So when the confirmation forms came in the mail saying my appointment was with some guy named Dr. Andrew Lewis, I had to call them up again and ask that they make my appointment with the female doctor that Dr. Goldstone had specifically referred me to, Dr. Janeen Rue.

As you can see, Tenacious C is still alive and kicking. In a way, I was glad for the opportunity to see the tenacious me again. Chemo didn't knock the tenacity out of me, though in all other respects it wouldn't be lying to say chemo kicked my ass. But chemo didn't win; I'm still here and chemo is over! Take *that* ya darn breast cancer!

CANCER—DAY 168 FRIDAY, OCTOBER 9, 2009

I had a good yoga practice last night. Afterward, I sat quietly as usual and reached for my water and my hoodie behind me without turning around. the woman next to me, Susie, was trying to remember if I was the breast cancer girl from yoga the week before. We talked a little bit, and it turns out that last Friday (the morning after our last yoga practice) she had a lump examined, and it wasn't good. She then had a mammogram on Monday, which also didn't look good, and she just had her biopsy today, so she's waiting now on the official pathology to tell her formally that it's cancer. Unbelievable, yet serendipitous for her to end up right next to me for yoga tonight so we could talk quietly together for a little while afterward. Actually, our yoga instructor saw us talking closely together sitting on the floor and she knew what we must be talking about, so she let everyone leave but didn't start shutting off lights or closing down the studio until she knew we finished our talk. My yoga instructor is an awesome person.

Susie said she thought I was inspirational with I how seem to be handling cancer treatment. (So many people use that word about me now, "inspirational," but I have a hard time accepting such a compliment; all I think I'm doing is simply surviving, doing what has to be done to get through it, and trying not to drag anyone else down with my problems. None of that seems inspirational to me, but maybe that's just because I'm on the inside looking out and really have no idea what other people see, looking in.) To reply to Susie, I said a few things to encourage her like: "Just keep moving forward one thing at a time," and "It's all going to happen really fast so don't be afraid of that," and "I'll be thinking lots of positive thoughts for you all week, just hang in there, you can get through this."

Wow. Right there right next to me in yoga, someone that I could help face breast cancer even in just a small way. Beautiful serendipity. That's what I want to do when this is over. Encourage and inspire other people facing breast cancer. Being an on-call "survivor" for Marshall is a step in the right direction, but I want to do more. Somehow. I'll have to think about it more when my head is less foggy.

It's getting on 6:30 a.m., I've been up since 3:30 a.m., couldn't sleep. You know this well by now, I just can't stay asleep. Usually if I wake up at 2:30 a.m. or so there's some hope I'll be able to sleep again, but usually if I'm still lying awake and it's getting on 5 a.m. I'll just get up. That's how I was until the last week or so, but now if I'm wide awake at 3:30 a.m. I don't bother trying to sleep again; I go ahead and get up.

So what do I do with the time in the wee hours of the morning? Pretty much the same stuff I do when I'm awake during the day. I try to read, though my comprehension is about a tenth of what it used to be, if that. I often start writing in my journal (later in the day I use my journal to start my blog post for the day, though I often write something on a completely different subject for the blog, if the journal writings are just too personal that day). My writing and typing are getting more and more limited by neuropathy, so if I can't type, I switch gears to reading. I do a lot of research online to find things I can do to help with my side effects, or what other people have experienced in chemo/radiation/breast cancer treatment. I also study up on each of the multitude of meds they've given me. The research on radiation is very simple because it is much more standard both in process and side effects. I did a lot of reading as to what hormone treatments are available—at least, I did until I found out there actually is only one hormone treatment for me, Tamoxifen, since I'm only 32. I read up on why we have to do it (Tamoxifen) and the side effects of that and other risks caused by it. Heck, I just do a lot of research on breast cancer in general. What can I say? I'm a data pack rat. The more information I have, the less afraid I am. Keep your friends close but your enemies closer, right?

It's amazing how I can feel like time is crawling by in treatment and yet each day somehow fills with rest, reading, rest, writing, rest, research, rest, and more rest, keeping me occupied day after day. There's the regular life stuff too though, like doing laundry or making something to eat. In all honesty, I spend a good deal of time just managing my meds, making sure I have everything and I am taking it all on the right schedule along with the times I am supposed to eat certain amounts of certain types of foods relative to what med is taken when. Putting everything about my treatment regimen into a calendar schedule made it easier to keep track of it all.

The med calendar also helps me in another way, though. It shows me, day after day, that I have survived another day, time is passing, and, some day, treatment would be over. My treatment/meds calendar has become an interesting manifestation of mind-body healing. There are all kinds of studies that show that a person's mental health (reduced stress, belief in survival, etc.) is every bit as important to the person's physical health, and that you can't really treat one without treating the other. I forget the name of the doctor who published that study, but it was very interesting and I agree with his position that in treating the body we cannot overlook the mind, and vice versa. He says we need to treat the mind-body, not just the body, in order to aid the patient to a complete recovery. I started my cancer calendar to keep track of meds and appointments—the physical stuff—but there's a strong psychological benefit now as well. As each day on the calendar fills with tiny print, each week draws closer to an end, meaning the beginning of a new week is closer and closer. And since my calendar is by week, I set aside the thoroughly scribbled calendar of the previous week to move on to the fresh, clean calendar of the next week (which has only my scheduled meds and doctor's appointments on it).Even though the time may pass achingly slow—hour by hour, day by day—I'm getting through it, and I see it right there on the paper. And now, I'm also seeing fewer insertions of "as needed" medications. I can hold up this week's calendar to last week's calendar or the chemo week calendar, and I can see that fewer drugs are needed and that means I'm feeling better.

But it's slow. I'm slow. Each thing I do just seems to take a lot of time because I'm so slow. I walk slowly, both because I don't have the energy to move quickly and to be sure I don't trip on a rug or bang into the wall corners or smash my hands on things because of the neuropathy. Everything is in slow motion because of the fatigue.

Now there's something that just continues to blow my mind. That the fatigue can keep getting worse. It really worries me for radiation, when fatigue is one of the primary complaints/side effects besides getting burned. I had no idea fatigue could be like this. Last night after yoga I went in the bedroom for something easily forgotten, I don't know what . . . to take off my shoes and put on my fuzzy night socks, I think. You would expect that to take just a few seconds but such a trivial action takes me several minutes to accomplish because by the time I get there I don't remember what I went in for. Last night after yoga, when I walked into the bedroom, I saw again that my headscarves on the bottom shelf of my wig cabinet were messy and I really should fold them. So I sat on the floor for what should have been two minutes to fold these scarves but of course it took me ten minutes to do and then I was so tired I could not for the life of me get up off the floor. Fatigue is a strange beast. I can't count how many times I've given up on trying to get up off the floor from something and instead let myself nap there for ten or twenty minutes because I don't even have enough energy to get off the floor.

Which is why it annoys me so much that Marco has issues with vacuuming, because this carpet is just plain nasty dirty and here I am sleeping on this filthy carpet because I'm too fatigued to stand up. You'd think that would bother Marco as a caregiver, me sleeping on this dirty floor. It's happened sitting on the floor to change socks, that's how bad the fatigue is. Fatigue is a normal state for me now. How am I going to deal with that getting worse during radiation?

CANCER—DAY 169 SATURDAY, OCTOBER 10, 2009

Cue tears from my company, AGAIN! They called my parents because they want to pay all of Mom & Dad's travel expenses to go to the Team Cynthia Swan Breast Cancer Walk!!! That seems so over-the-top generous—I couldn't help but cry again at how wonderful these people are and how good they are to me. I can always count on them for a good healthy cry, it seems.

Then there's Marco's company, which is completely different. I am insanely lucky that all this happened now, while I'm with this company, rather than at some other point in my life when I worked for companies with no heart. Marco's company has been "supportive" of Marco taking care of me in that they allow him flexible time so he can go with me to chemo and appointments when he needs to. One of my chemo sessions was on a holiday, so we're talking about just three afternoons off in three months for him, and an hour or so in total each week for other chemo-related appointments and such. But really, aside from the constant of keeping an eye on me from across the hall during chemo week, we're not talking about a huge impact on the work of someone who works from home and can make up lost time in the evening if necessary. Marco's work is just like mine that way, it's the way things are when you work from home, I think. You get used to having extra time over lunch or in the early evening or whatever to finish up when something really needs to get done. Working from home means flexible time almost by definition, I think, because you don't lose time to a daily commute. That's how I look at it anyway, and so from a work perspective, I don't feel like this has had much impact on Marco's work.

But his company made a big deal with him about the fact that they've been so "supportive" of his taking care of me, and they used that to try to pressure him into making another trip to Phoenix while I was still in chemo, after Marco had already talked with them about not traveling again until after chemo was done. It was one thing for him to go out there and run that move they had . . . he was "vital" to that happening and he absolutely had to be there, which is why he went and I had all those other people checking on me and helping take care of me that weekend, way back in the first round of chemo. But this second trip his company was pressuring him to take recently didn't have that kind of importance as far as Marco could tell, they just wanted him out there for a meeting and Marco pushed back a little because he didn't agree that he needed to fly out there for a meeting that he could just call in for, and he didn't want to leave me alone again during chemo. That's what he said he told them, anyway. (Never mind that it's been nearly three weeks since my final chemo infusion and he really doesn't need to be here for me. So things became tense and Marco was venting a lot about it, and that just continues to highlight how very special my company is and how wonderful the people at my company are. The supportiveness I've received has been amazing. The fact that the entire company is walking against breast cancer this month just because of me is still utterly amazing to me, and they keep doing things that I would never expect of a company. I've always thought of my company as a "best of the best" in terms of people, because we have so many of the best people I've ever worked with. Most intelligent, most dedicated, and well, just downright "good" people. And I keep getting reminded of it now. Best company I've ever worked for, no comparison.

CANCER—DAY 170 SUNDAY, OCTOBER 11, 2009

The neuropathy pain is an eight, or worse. All the time. Touching anything feels like my hand is pressed on a sizzling frying pan. The touch of sheets burn my toes like frostbite. Neuropathy sucks.

The carsickness test yesterday was a success, though, so that's good news. I can get home to Volcanoville and back without throwing up, with just average nausea really. I'm so relieved that I'll be able to go home sometimes now. Not driving because of neuropathy is not an option. Going home is important for my sanity, so my body will just have to tolerate the neuropathy burning as the price that must be paid for going home once in a while.

More another day when my hands aren't in so much pain, the hand and finger-burning is just too unbearable right now; it's making me cry.

CANCER—DAY 171 MONDAY, OCTOBER 12, 2009

Back when we were trying to get cancer medical information on my birth family, I had to choose to either fill out the forms to get just medical history—but that meant they would delete all contact information so I could only have the medical information and would never be able to find out who my birth parents were. Alternatively, I could fill out the forms to request both medical history and contact information. I've never had an urge to find my birth parents. I don't know why I have never felt a need to find out who gave birth to me. It's just a simple fact of me I guess. Finding the birth mother or father or other family just never mattered.

I filled out the forms for medical info only but then at the last minute I check-marked the box to get the contact information too, because I didn't want the contact info to be deleted forever. Just because I've never gone looking for them in the first 30 years of my life doesn't mean I know with absolute certainty that I will *never* want to know who they were, you know?

When the medical forms came back with the immediate family tree (which didn't have too much history of cancer, just the birth father and his sister and one grandmother), it was interesting to find out I have a couple of real sisters and several half-siblings, the birth father has already died, and the birth mother lives in Wisconsin. Apparently the birth mother was about sixteen when I was born and put me with the adoption agency. But a few years later, she actually married the birth father and had two more daughters before he died and she remarried, so I have two real sisters out in the world! How wild is that?

Even after receiving this information, I still didn't feel any need to contact them, though. The birth mother told the adoption agency that she never told her children that she had birthed a baby when she was younger, and she asked the adoption search counselor to ask me if I would please not identify myself as a daughter if I called her. I didn't feel the need to call her, so no worries there. But when the adoption search agency counselor made such a fuss about how my birth mother was so very helpful and prompt with the medical information, I did want to send a thank you note. I also thought it might be nice to let her know the gene testing showed I do not have any gene mutations, which means it's not genetic so she and her other daughters do not have to worry that they are genetically at higher risk of breast cancer. So I sent her a brief letter in a thank you card.

September 2009

Dear Anne,

Thank you for your time to complete the Family History Questionnaire Medical & Genetic forms for the Department of Health and Family services. With an additional genetic test and the information you provided, we were able to determine with certainty that I needed to undergo chemotherapy, but also that the chemotherapy treatment required only four infusions instead of six or eight, so that my total chemotherapy treatment is only four months long, truly a blessing.

Even more importantly, the gene testing showed that I have no genetic mutations for breast cancer, which means neither you nor your daughters are at higher risk for breast cancer.

I also want to thank you for your willingness to reveal your own identifying information so that I could thank you. I never felt the need to seek out any blood relations, quite probably because of the wonderful childhood and family I do have in my adoptive family. My parents are amazing people, and it was another blessing for me that they were bumped up in the adoption list over hundreds of other couples to save me from my sixth foster home in five weeks . . . miraculous really, and it was all of fundamental importance to the person I became.

I don't mean to dwell on my life here, I simply wish to express my sincere appreciation that you responded so quickly to the request for medical information and to tell you that it was helpful for my oncologist to have that information to decide the best course of treatment for my breast cancer. Should you have any personal interest in getting to know a bit more about me and what is going on in my cancer recovery, I do maintain a public Web log; you can access it online at www.cielemel.com.

Warmest regards,
Cynthia

CANCER—DAY 172 TUESDAY, OCTOBER 13, 2009

I am sooooo glad chemo is over. All the side effects lasted longer this time, and I can't imagine how bad it must get when you have to do six months of chemo instead of three or four. It's week 4 after my last chemo session now, and I'm still in week 3 flu-symptoms mode, along with still getting nauseas from food cooking smells or much riding in the car, and I still have a hefty dose of fatigue. The neuropathy is the toughest to bear—it has gotten much, much worse since the fourth round of chemotherapy.

My hands drive me nuts, burning all the time, especially the more that I use them. After yoga last night I was in tears again, the pain was so bad in my hands. Same thing with eating using utensils, especially forks for some reason. Last night my hand was shaking uncontrollably while I was trying to eat with a fork and the edges of it felt like I was holding a double-sided knife blade in my hand. My feet are bothersome but don't hurt as constantly as my hands (probably because I don't use my feet much, in comparison to how much I use my hands in any given day), but when my feet do hurt the pain is worse. There's something exquisitely painful about putting your body weight on your foot when it feels like you're walking on fire. With my hands it's the palm side that hurts, not the back of my hand (not the top of my feet either, just the underside). I find myself sitting with my palms turned up a lot so that my palms and fingers don't touch anything. It looks a bit odd, but it's less painful than having my palms and fingers touching anything. My heels are less painful than the balls of my feet, so I walk slowly and when possible I walk with the heel of my foot more than the ball of the foot, which looks funny. Standing in place for any length of time is unbearable. Even walking is better than just standing there with the burn increasing from the constant pressure. I still go to milongas, but I don't dance much, just a tanda or two in a night. I do a lot more sitting than dancing at milongas now, but I still go. I don't want to give in to the pain and give up the last thing I love and the reason I'm even here in Sac instead of with my parents in Nebraska—tango is like breathing to me. I can't imagine my life without it, but the neuropathy makes it really painful. Ach, the neuropathy has to get better, it just *has* to!

I went to see the substitute medical oncologist today to follow up on the neuropathy and other remaining side effects. Going in, I wasn't expecting to get a lot of value out of this appointment. Everything I've read on neuropathy says that you pretty much have to tolerate it and wait it out . . . there aren't any medicines that specifically target neuropathy to make it feel better or to heal it. We've tried a few different pain medications, but regular painkillers don't help with the neuropathy, and they make me nauseous besides. In terms of the neuropathy side effect wearing off, well, it can take two months to recover, or six months, or two years, ten years, a lifetime . . . some people have neuropathy for the rest of their lives after chemo. The doctors don't know who is going to be most affected or how, or for how long. Similarly, there's nothing the doctor can do about the fatigue. So what was the point of this appointment today?

Mostly I went to meet the new medical oncologist and see what kind of rapport we have. That was OK. He did give me a prescription for a medicine for diabetic neuropathy that sometimes helps some people with chemo-induced neuropathy, so that was a huge point in his favor. I'm willing to try anything at this point. He said it takes a few weeks before the medicine has a noticeable effect, so he wants me to use it for a month before deciding whether I think it's helping or not. We'll see. They have already tried a couple other medicines that can help with neuropathy, but so far nothing has helped with mine. Neuropathy seems to be a mystery to medical science, at least in terms of treatment.

CANCER—DAY 173 WEDNESDAY, OCTOBER 14, 2009

Last year, just about a year ago now, I was in Albuquerque to dance for a West Coast Swing movie called *Love 'N Dancing*. While I was in Albuquerque dancing for the movie, my dad's cousin passed away in Phoenix. Since I had driven to Albuquerque for the three weeks of filming the dance scenes of the movie, I decided to drive back via Phoenix so that I could go to the funeral. The timing was too serendipitous to disregard.

I got in late the night before. Thanks to a time zone change that I hadn't realized I'd crossed, I was an hour early for the funeral the next morning . . . there was no one there and I thought I'd missed it! I found the rectory office where they told me the funeral wasn't for an hour, and I realized I'd missed the time zone change, thank goodness!

So here I am fresh off the movie set, right? My hair was long and super-blonde and had fresh dark stripes in it since that was my competitive show dancer hairstyle at the time (I wonder what color my hair will grow back?). I haven't seen anyone from this side of my family in more than fifteen years I think, so I was kind of a stranger to them. I didn't go to anything night before and no one knew I was coming to the funeral because I'd only figured it out myself a day or so beforehand. And with how I was looking for the movie, it's no surprise really that my cousins (my second cousins, actually, I think, since our dads are first cousins) didn't recognize me until I introduced myself at their mom's house after the funeral.

Well, last week there was another death in the same side of my family, so here they are already going through the difficult emotions and memories of a year ago, and they have fresh grief to deal with too. The funeral is this Friday. I was e-mailing with one of my cousins today letting her know I was sending them all my love and asking if they're getting by OK, and she told me this great story from last year.

So I'm at the funeral last year, sitting kind of in the middle back because I didn't really know anyone except the immediate family in the front rows, whom I haven't seen in years and years, since we were kids really. They had a full funeral Mass, so I went up for Communion. This is when my cousins first saw me, and wondered who the heck I was because no one recognized me. As I walked past the first row where they sat, going back to my seat, my cousin Tommy was sitting at the end of the pew watching people file by in silence, and he briefly made eye contact with me and I lowered my head in sympathy. Without thinking, as I went past Tommy I gently touched his shoulder for just a moment.

Krystal told me today that she thought I must be "Tommy's new chick," and when I walked by she whispered some off-color remark to him about how cute I was compared to "how ugly his mug is," and they got the giggles. Krystal said it was that kind of "I should stop now, I'm in church!" giggle, like being kids again, and I can tell you that is one of the best laughs you can have. Anyone who has ever caught the giggles in any church where you're supposed to be quiet knows exactly what I mean by that, I'm sure. But the really neat thing Krystal said today was about how good it felt to have that giggle right then, during such a somber and difficult time, and she thanked me for giving them that moment of levity just when they needed it most.

It was really moving when she told me that today—to think that, just by being there (literally!) I'd helped them feel just a moment's relief from the depths of grief during their father's funeral last year. I just love the idea of that.

After the funeral I went to their house and re-met a bunch of people and cleared the mystery of my identity, which was kind of fun. I didn't get to talk to everyone, but I was still so glad that I'd gone since I was the only Swan that could make it to Phoenix for the funeral last year. They really appreciated having me there.

Have I mentioned before that I have a wonderful family?

CANCER—DAY 174 THURSDAY, OCTOBER 15, 2009

I've been gradually catching back on my e-mail all this time, and I finally worked my way back to all the e-mails I got from people when they first heard about my diagnosis, back in May and June. I hadn't realized how very many people had written to me back then; there were pages of names in my Inbox from that first week. PAGES! It took the better part of two hours today just to read them all. I know I'm overly emotional now, but to be reminded now that so many people care and were concerned, well, you can't expect me to read all those well-wishing e-mails and *not* cry (in a good way)!

CANCER—DAY 175 FRIDAY, OCTOBER 16, 2009

I think too much. I try to distract myself from myself by thinking about anything other than myself, but some nights I just cannot sleep. I'm scared. I'm afraid of losing my identity like my Dad's friend said happened with his wife . . . she was never the same after cancer treatment, her personality was forever altered. And I worry. Worse yet, I scare myself because I seem to have forgotten myself.

Who was the pre-cancer Cynthia Swan? What did she do with her life? What did she contribute in the world? How did she live her life? I know I miss my home and my cats. That's about it. It's all just messed up in my head, making no sense. And then I feel like I haven't grown or changed at all, that the last six months are just gone from my life, like the time that didn't exist after Artie died.

Which isn't true, of course. The last six months of my life have not been an absolute waste of time. Every time I talk with anyone, they can't believe what I'm going through and how well I'm handling it, with so much inner strength that they find inspiring. When people tell me things like that, all I can tell them, all I can think, is that "I'm not doing anything special, I'm just surviving the best I can." I am learning from it, but uff da, if I get an A in this course it's going to be with a LOT of effort and late night studying. But hey, if it were easy to get an A, then everyone would always do it right?

Without darkness we cannot comprehend or appreciate light. Without sorrow we cannot know joy. Right?

I asked Marco: "So as an atheist, are you a single-lifetime atheist, or a multi-lifetime atheist?" He said single. I didn't really understand that, so I asked "So the whole karma thing is, like, what you get in this lifetime is what you deserve in this lifetime kind of thing?" He said he kind of plays around with karma but doesn't really define it like that, it's more that he just believes there's more left to chance when it comes to karma. Can't say I agree with that. Much of any of it, actually. Except his questioning of whether or not there is "A God." The existence of "A God" as worshipped by religions is very debatable in my book. But there is *something*, so if you want to call it God, well, that's what faith is, right? I guess I just think of it all in terms of spirituality now. Marco is not a spiritual person. When you die, you die and that's it, in Marco's opinion. We've never talked about my "experience" with death during my heart failure, except for me to tell him I am not afraid of death because of that experience.

I'm not sure what to think about Marco's level of atheism except that it's probably another "we're not so compatible" point on the list for I-wonder-how-long-he'll-take-to-dump-me-when-radiation-is-over? Or maybe even before radiation is over? Likely not, because everyone would want to know why. I think we'll pretend to be in a relationship until after the tango workshops we're teaching together in January. After that, there won't be any need for us to "stay" together, and we can both move on with our lives on our own paths, if that's the way it goes.

With everything else going on in my head, my relationship with Marco is far from the most urgent concern in my life (which seems to be a problem for him, but there's not much I can do about the fact that cancer treatment comes before all else—including family—while I'm in treatment.

CANCER—DAY 176 SATURDAY, OCTOBER 17, 2009

You are going to love this; it's I think it's the funniest story in my journal. My entire company roared with laughter, and it was great to hear about it from my mom tonight.

First of all, my company's cancer walk was a *huge* success! Team Cynthia apparently even included seven kids in strollers because everyone brought their families, and Mom said it was just a wonderful gathering. Overall the walk had more than 12,000 participants and Mom said "It was just "awesome!" (If you know my mom, you know 'awesome' is not a word in her usual vocabulary!) My "team" had more than 40 participants all in matching t-shirts, and they had a wonderful presence in the walk. I was completely bummed not to be able to fly out there for the weekend and do the walk too, but I'm just glowing as I think about my company doing such a wonderful thing.

After the walk, everyone in the company—with their families and all the kids and my parents—went out for a celebration party/dinner. During the pre-dinner social part, my CEO quieted everyone down and thanked them for participating in such a special event and he said what a pleasure it was to meet my parents and that he knew he spoke for every person in the company when he told my parents that they all wish me the very best towards a speedy recovery, and then something about unfortunate it was that treatment has been so trying and they all felt for me and my parents in how difficult it must be for them, knowing what I'm going through.

There was a little pause, and everyone was looking at my parents, giving them a chance to comment, probably hoping to hear things are getting better, but my mom said, "Well, like Cynthia always says, 'It is what it is.' "

The restaurant BOOMED with laughter. Everyone that I work with just roared themselves to tears, they were laughing so hard. My parents didn't know why that was such a hilarious thing for my mom to say, until my CEO explained: "That's what we *all* say here!"

CANCER—DAY 177 SUNDAY, OCTOBER 18, 2009

Radiation is about to begin. The 30-second cortina between my tango with chemo and my tango with radiation has ended.

I considered not writing today, but this story is actually of fundamental importance in explaining my determination to survive breast cancer.

Six years ago, I received the phone call that changed my life forever. I had dated my boyfriend, Artie, about five years, and the phone call was to tell me that he had just been killed in a horrific motorcycle wreck.

The loss destroyed me. We'd lived together and he'd been a part of my life for so long, and I completely believed we would have the happily-ever-after, kids, the whole partners-in-life deal. And then he was suddenly gone, in this horrific wreck that just made it even more difficult to deal with the loss. The San Francisco Chronicle said: "On Saturday, October 19, at about 10 p.m., a San Mateo man, identified by the County Coroner's Office as 30 year-old Arthur Grant, died when his motorcycle collided with another vehicle on Highway 101 south of San Francisco International airport. According to the California highway patrol, a driver of a 1985 Lincoln lost control of her car while entering southbound highway 101 near San Bruno Avenue. The car spun around across the southbound lanes directly in Grant's path. Grant was throw off the cycle and was struck and dragged by two other cars whose drivers did not see him. He was pronounced dead at the scene."

It was brutal. My depression was, well, suicidal. But I survived. Getting through that was an emotional survival like no other. But when I sunk lower than low, when I hit rock bottom and sank lower, somehow I pulled out of it. There is more inner strength in me than I could even fathom, if I had not gone through that survival experience.

My parents knew I was depressed, but they expected me to "snap out of it." Maybe 'snap' isn't the perfect word, but, like, they knew I had the inner strength to get through it. Writing this now in my private journal, I've decided that I'm going to tell them the truth about it when I go home at Christmas and be honest about how bad it got, how deeply mired I had been in depression after his death, not wanting to exist anymore, botching a suicide attempt, and how they, my parents, brought me out of that without even knowing it. It's a gruesome story so I'm not going into any details whatsoever. The story does have a wonderful ending though: I survived Artie's death for the love of my parents.

I'm close to Artie's parents. We don't talk all the time, but often enough. I go down to L.A. to visit them a couple times a year. They are like in-laws to me, another set of loving parents caring deeply for me and appreciative of the very deep love I had for Artie. The unspoken truth is that I knew Artie better than his family did when he died. Artie and I were together for many years, and he hadn't lived at home since he was in sixth grade when he went off to military school and later boarding school, then college . . . you get the idea. He had left home as a child, and I spent years with him day in and day out as an adult. There were many facets to his personality and his life, and it seems I was the only person that knew all of them. He was one person for his family and another for his friends, and something in-between for work. His brothers and sister were just starting to get to know him as a person when he died. I mention all this because it's important in explaining my current close relationship with his parents, many years after he died. When we talk, I often give them a perspective of Artie that they never knew, and a lot of his personality rubbed off on me and vice versa. And, like my parents, they're good people, and I prefer to spend my time with good people.

Right after Artie died, I spent a lot of time with his mom, helping her sort through his belongings and decide what to keep and what to leave with me and some specific items for his friends, then the rest went to Goodwill. Having to even think about dispersing his things was such an emotional strain for Artie's mom that I helped as much as possible, understanding what she wanted and then taking care of it for her, like taking things to his friends to remember him by, and packing up everything for Goodwill and arranging the pickup and all of that so she didn't have to deal with it. I had always gotten along great with Artie's mom, but this was a pretty unique experience to have with her when we were both so vulnerable and, in a way, lost.

Now I have roses placed at his grave every week, and every time I go anywhere near Los Angeles, I make time to go out of my way to go to the cemetery where he's buried in Rancho Palos Verdes, and to see his family. Every year on the anniversary of his death I go there to put more roses on his grave and have a morning or afternoon or day to spend there to just let myself grieve, alone. It's actually a beautiful place with a rose garden and a little path through the roses to a large pond with a fountain, and there is a gazebo to sit in while you listen to the waterfall. It's a peaceful place, and if you have to mourn a loved one, well, I don't think I've ever seen a more serene place for mourning than the Garden of Reflection where Artie is buried.

Last year was probably the worst October 19th for me, emotionally. For some reason the fact that it was five years—that he had then been gone as long as we had been together—was especially painful. It's still going to be many more years before he will have been gone as long as I knew him, but that five-year mark was definitely a hurdle.

It's not painful on a daily basis now like it was the first couple of years, and obviously over time my life has gone on because I'm still around and working and teaching and dancing in competitions and shows. I have a very full life (although I do avoid dating, with a multitude of excuses), or at least I did right before cancer. Moreover, other than neuropathy, there's no reason to think I won't get back to being that kind of person again.

Back when they were scheduling my chemo, I kept counting out the weeks on my calendar to make sure October 19th was in the third week of a chemo round when I was supposed to have the least difficulty with side effects so that I could make the trip to L.A. again this year. It's amazing that I ended up getting only four months of chemo so that October 19th ended up being at the end of week 4 of the last chemo. But then my first radiation treatment was scheduled for October 19th, so I'm here a day early this year.

I've spent my morning near Artie's grave and with the fountain and roses and serenity of the Garden of Reflection, reflecting.

It all comes back together—everything about Artie's death, my relationship to my parents, my relationship to his parents, and how I survived his death and the ensuing depression—each are of fundamental importance in the evolution to Cynthia Swan, the survivor.

Artie's death was by far the most difficult emotional experience I have ever endured. On the emotional side, surviving cancer *pales* in comparison to what I survived emotionally then. As a result, I knew I had the internal fortitude to survive cancer and cancer treatment no matter how awful it became.

Being with Artie's parents through their suffering (which continues to this day, as you would expect) showed me with absolute clarity that the only emotional pain worse than losing your significant other is losing your child. My very close proximity to their pain made me realize something else, too. I would never, ever, put my parents through the emotional anguish Artie's parents had to survive. I will do anything and everything in my power to prevent that. I have to survive cancer and cancer treatment because if I gave in and died, I would be putting my parents through what Artie's parents have suffered. No matter how terrible any of it gets for me, there are other people in this world who will be emotionally damaged, possibly for the rest of their lives, if I died.

I often remind myself of a decision I made at the beginning of all this cancer stuff, in the week between the "It ***looks*** like cancer" phone call and the "It ***is*** cancer" phone call. I made a conscious decision then, and a promise to myself, which I will absolutely pursue with every fiber of tenacity in my being.

With Artie as my inspiration, I am determined to survive cancer for my parents.

Chapter 22.
Radiation

CANCER—DAY 178 MONDAY, OCTOBER 19, 2009

The first appointment with my new radiation oncologist was much longer than I expected. Even though I have the gist of the mechanics from my long conversation with the other radiation oncologist in April, there's apparently still a lot to talk about regarding what's happening next.

We're doing radiation to close off (as much as possible) any potential that the cancer will recur in the same breast. We need to do this because I had a lumpectomy. The only way we could have guaranteed not having a breast cancer recurrence in the right breast (where I had the two tumors removed in surgery) *or* the left breast (which we didn't operate on after the four biopsies there were benign) would have been to have a double-mastectomy. Dr. Thatcher, my surgeon, hadn't recommend that, and it didn't have a lot of appeal to me at the time, so I did the single right-side lumpectomy knowing that I would have to undergo radiation treatment to that side after chemo. The radiation kills off any lingering cancer cells in the treated area that may have slipped beyond the margin they cleared during surgery. In my case this is especially important because Dr. Rue (my radiation oncologist) feels the one-millimeter margin Dr. Thatcher left is too slight given that the tumor was deep, right on my chest wall. This tight margin means that she is going to do 36 radiation treatments instead of the standard 33 treatments. So instead of 6-1/2 weeks of radiation, it's 7 weeks and a day, just a few extra radiation treatments to make sure she gets in some extra slices where the margin was so close to my chest wall. This means though that I will be getting a little radiation to my chest wall and probably a hair of my right lung, which has implications I'll get to in the side effects in a minute.

We also talked a little bit about the hormone therapy I'm going to have to do later, Tamoxifen. I've been resistant to the Tamoxifen hormone therapy, partly because it's known to cause secondary cancers and also because I don't want to have my body chemically forced into menopause or the other known side effects of Tamoxifen. Dr. Rue was insistent that the majority of risk reduction in my cancer treatment is coming from Tamoxifen, much more so than from the chemotherapy or radiation treatments. There aren't any other hormone therapy options for me because of my age and the fact that I'm nowhere near menopause yet. For post-menopausal women, there are some other drugs they can try like Arimidex and Raloxifene, but those haven't shown any benefit at all for women my age, premenopausal. So, Tamoxifen it is, for five years or possibly more. I'm going to be doing a lot of reading on that, once we're well under way in radiation and getting closer to the start of hormone therapy.

They tattooed me with these blue freckle-sized marks and ran a simulation to determine exactly what my 3-D body image will be for radiation. They ran mathematical models with the body scan to simulate where the radiation beams are going to intersect in me for the radiation. On my skin it will end up being a square field from below the middle of my collarbones to just below the breast bone on my right side and then around to my mid-side on my right side. They make these little blue tattoo marks so they line up exactly where they're radiating every time and it's consistently precise. We certainly don't want to radiate the wrong place, not by a millimeter.

Given all the other scars I have now, having a little blue tattoo freckle in the middle of my chest, on my side, or just below my collar bones doesn't bother me much. Dr. Rue said a lot of women get upset about the blue tattoos, and I guess it's going to be hard to cover up a blue freckle with make-up, but hell, I'm still wearing wigs and drawing on eyebrows and coloring in eyelashes, so what's one more little effort of trying to cover up a blue freckle?

Dr. Rue explained the rest of the process and then started telling me the side effects I am likely to have. There are "acute" side effects that everyone gets with radiation, and then there are other non-acute side effects that occur later. In terms of acute effects, I'll get a square sunburn over the entire radiation field. Because I'm fair-skinned, they're expecting the skin reaction to be fairly severe with heat rash, itchy soreness, and very dry skin that I have to put rash cream on. Radiation burn is pretty miserably uncomfortable, from the sounds of it. Once I had a sunburn so bad it rashed, and yeah, miserable is about the only word to describe how it felt—this constant burning pinged by more intense burning with the rash bumps. Hmmm. That's basically a toned-down version of neuropathy. What fun! Not.

The radiation burn kicks in fully by the second week of radiation, and will turn to tan a few weeks after all radiation is done. This is also about the time I should start growing my hair back after chemo, btw.)

The last acute side effect is fatigue, which is worsened by the fact that I did chemotherapy and am already at a fatigued level from which the only direction I'll be traveling is further south to more severe fatigue cumulatively through the radiation process. I'm trying not to be too grim here, but at the same time, I want to be realistic about all this, especially since it has such huge implications for whether or not I should work during radiation or instead stay focused on the treatment and recovery and just stay on medical disability through the rest of treatment to give my body the very best chance to heal as completely as possible, without work stress and busy-ness.

There are going to be more blood draws, so I'm keeping my port rather than have the port-removal surgery now and getting my arm poked over and over for the blood draws (which was really why I got the port in the first place—the feeling of blood being sucked from my veins makes me faint and nauseas).

There are also non-acute side effects that don't happen to everyone. When Dr. Rue she told me that I have about a one in one hundred chance of having these side effects I was *not* reassured, because one in a hundred is a much, much higher probability than the statistical probability that I would ever have gotten breast cancer at my age in the first place. But, whatever, OK, one in a hundred odds for having these other side effects. It is what it is. Let's move on.

There could be a few other side effects as well. At six weeks, I could develop a severe pneumonia or bronchitis or just a bad flu, which is an allergic reaction to the radiation. My right lung could also be specifically affected, especially with the margin thing and my radiation needing to go so close with the chest wall. At six months there can be another allergic reaction that's more like a bad achy-ness that lasts a month or longer but can generally be addressed with Motrin.

In terms of physical changes . . . the breast skin thickens, which makes the breast smaller and pulls the skin up so it's higher than the other breast. I hadn't thought about radiation making me more deformed that I already am from the lumpectomy. In hindsight, I do believe a skin-saving mastectomy with full reconstruction would probably have been the better way to go, rather than the lumpectomy. Oh well, it is what it is. The radiation also increases the encapsulation of the reconstructed breast, which makes it more firm and not as pliable, and also raises the breast further. If it's significant enough, all that means a second trip to the plastic surgeon. Oh well, I'll cross that bridge when I come to it.

The big downside of radiation is that they know it causes cancer. So to prevent a breast cancer recurrence in the same breast in the short term (the next 5 years), they do radiation, knowing this fact. They know that at some point, maybe not for 20-30 years, I'm going to have a cancer recurrence somewhere else in my body anyway, even with everything we're doing to try to prevent a recurrence. They say it matter-of-fact like that. Like being professional while skimming over that kind of statement makes it easier to hear. Yeah, right. Dr. Rue says that's the risk everyone faces with cancer in the long term though, it's just not always as big a deal because most people with cancer have it much later in life, so worrying about developing a second cancer 20 or 30 years later if you live to be 90 or 100 years old, well, that doesn't have quite the impact versus having your recurrence countdown start in your early thirties.

There's a cold fact here that I've been told by multiple doctors and read about, and it's a simple one. Actually, it was about the only thing I knew about cancer prior to my own diagnosis. Once you have cancer, you have cancer. Cancer has learned how to grow in your body. And if your first cancer is at a young age, then it's more likely that your cancer is going to come out of remission at some point in your lifetime, and chances are that recurrence will be a more aggressive recurrence, which is why we do everything possible as aggressively as possible and as early as possible. We do everything we can to detect the recurrence as early as possible, and that is how to look at it. I have cancer, and it's in remission, possibly forever, but not necessarily. So we stay on the lookout and keep it in remission for as long as possible, but they expect it to come back. Maybe not for 20 years, but it's in there. So, well, it is what it is I guess. Remission is good.

For the cancer patient, every single day of remission is another day of grace. I was already living a life of daily appreciation before diagnosis, so this notion is not new to me. For all of us, each day we wake up is another day of grace.

CANCER—DAY 179 TUESDAY, OCTOBER 20, 2009

The cats are here!!!!! Granted, they're locked up in the guest bedroom (hereafter referred to as the "cat room"), but they're here in the house, and I go in the cat room to see them all the time. It is soooooo nice to hear them purr again. They never did that when I went to visit them in cat jail.

News on the neuropathy front isn't great . . . now besides the burning in my hands and feet they will also often have this piercing thing too that feels like little thorns or needles stabbing through my hands and feet, especially my fingers, the ball area of both feet, and, most painfully, my fingertips. I've developed this weird habit now of not only sitting with my palms turned up not touching anything but also frequently pressing my fingertips together trying to rub out or spread out the needling feeling. I don't even realize I'm doing it, not that it helps. I'm going to grow my nails out so they're long enough that I can type with the nail tips to save my fingertips from tapping the keyboard.

The first radiation treatment was this morning. It was over lickety-split; I think I was in the building a total of fifteen minutes. It takes longer to drive there than to get the radiation. Thank goodness I'm not driving 45 minutes each way like I would have to do from home to go to that other radiation facility. Of course, if I'd done a double mastectomy, I wouldn't have to have radiation at all, but that didn't seem like big deal when it was decided I would just have the tumors removed in a lumpectomy. At least, it didn't seem like a big deal to the doctors.

I've read that some women refuse radiation because it's every day for many weeks and they would have to drive so far to get to the radiation center and they just don't want to (or can't for some reason) deal with all the driving. That seems kind of short-sighted, given the potential lifetime effect, but then again, Marco's still letting me stay at his house for the duration and I don't have the long drive I would from my house for radiation, so who am I to talk?

When I got back from my first radiation treatment, I was ridiculously tired. I had a two-hour nap—in the cat room—nice!

CANCER—DAY 180 WEDNESDAY, OCTOBER 21, 2009

They told me today that Dr. Rue also ordered that a bolus (a "tissue equivalent substance") be placed at a particular spot to trick the radiation machine and draw the radiation closer to the skin over the lumpectomy scar. They put on this round sticker that I'm supposed to not wash off for as long as possible; that's their marker for where to place this bolus every other day in radiation. They said it does probably mean the burn will be worse in that spot, because the skin is getting more radiation there, so I have that to look forward to. I'm already getting itchy, and they said to start skin therapy (pure aloe) right away and not to wait until I look burned. And man, pure aloe is seriously cold straight from the bottle!

On a different note—when Dr. Rue (the radiation oncologist) heard how bad my side effects were the first time she met me, she said "Maybe you're just unlucky." How's that for a medical opinion?

CANCER—DAY 181 THURSDAY, OCTOBER 22, 2009

I saw Dr. Rue after my radiation session today. She's doing weekly breast exams with me, which will change to monthly checks after radiation is over, for the first year or something like that. Besides the radiation treatments, they do blood draws every three weeks, so I'll probably have my port-a-cath taken out right after radiation. I want to have the surgery to have it removed during this calendar year, before my deductible starts over again with my insurance January 1st. No matter how fatigued I get from radiation, I want that surgery done in December.

The good news from Dr. Rue today was that the MRI they did on Monday was completely clean, no indication of any new tumors. It would have been pretty freaky to have heard any other kind of result on the first post-surgery MRI, so I guess I was expecting it to be completely clean. I'll probably always have that general expectation, since they got the entirety of the two tumors out, the lymph nodes they removed were node negative, and I'm doing everything I can (chemo, radiation, hormone therapy, alternative medicine, etc.) to prevent a recurrence. I continually tell myself not to expect a recurrence, trying to stay in a "Think Positive" mindset as much as possible.

CANCER—DAY 182 FRIDAY, OCTOBER 28, 2009

Uff da, with so many reminders all the time that I'm in cancer treatment, who could forget and effectively be normal? Neuropathy and fatigue taint anything normal that I try to do. I tried to go to a tango workshop Wednesday night (meaning, I was physically present at a tango workshop Wednesday night), but I was really frustrated by "chemo brain" forgetfulness. Trying to stay focused after the first fifteen minutes or so was nigh impossible. That was also about the time I started feeling excessively fatigued, and my feet were screaming "Fire!" Trying to stay "on" and give the energy I used to in workshops was just impossible, though I tried my best. After a while even keeping a smile on my face felt impossible, though I kept trying because that's the Cynthia Swan everyone knows. I stopped and sat out for a bit, but other than that I did make it through the whole workshop. Then I had something of an emotional breakdown in the car on the drive home. It was basically like tears were the only way to let out everything I'd been holding in to get through the workshop. Even with the strain and difficulty, there's another side of me that's glad I went and did as much as I could. It reminded me how determined I can be, and that even if I'm not able to be as "on" as I would like or can't take in as much content as I used to in workshops, I should still keep trying to do the things I loved to do before the cancer diagnosis. If I keep trying, eventually it will either get easier or—at the very least—I will get more used to it, this dealing with how I feel physically and with the neuropathy while trying to do at least some of my pre-cancer activities.

My head is still foggy and "chemo-brained," making me forget things or not be able to remember well, and I still go blank a lot more than I think I should. I probably need to get used to another "new" normal, instead of expecting myself to be just like I was before.

I "attended" an online seminar a few days ago. It was a group of doctors talking about and answering questions about chemo brain. Many of the questions had to do with how long chemo brain can last, and what people can do to reduce the effects, especially with feeling less efficient at work. The general theme coming back from the doctors was that it can last the rest of your life, and that most people make adjustments in how they do things in order to continue to do their jobs . . . taking down more notes, spending additional time on a task that they used to do more quickly. They had just one example of someone who lost their job as a result of the lingering side effects . . . a trial lawyer who needed to think very quickly on her feet to respond in court. But I guess she moved into a related line of work after that, and found another good job. The doctors also talked about examples of how people dealt with the effects of chemo brain to still do their jobs but realizing that it was at a greater level of effort and cost to them than before. It will be interesting to see how I do working full time again, when the time comes.

Teaching, now that will be a trip if I still have trouble with this in a few months, needing to think quickly on my feet to answer students' questions. Or in phone calls with clients. Lucky for me most of my clients tend to use e-mail rather than call with questions about their modeling results. It's helpful to have a written-out answer they can refer back to or forward to others as necessary, so we use a lot of e-mail. Going back to work, the e-mail approach will allow me some time to think before I respond, if my chemo brain is slow.

CANCER—DAY 183 SATURDAY, OCTOBER 24, 2009

Now here's an interesting addition to the complexities of the Cynthia Swan cancer soap opera . . . Marco's car was stolen from the Safeway parking lot last night! We were in the store about six minutes getting just two items for the birthday party, limes and straws, and when we came out to the empty space where we had parked we were just speechless. We parked right in front of the store, walked in, walked out, and poof! The car was gone. Marco called the police and they filed a report and then he had to call his insurance company and deal with all that. Unbelievable. Marco's car was stolen from right in front of the store in a matter of minutes! Good thing I have my Camry here. I figure we can share my car through the end of radiation if necessary, and I could lend it to him while I'm gone for Christmas if it takes a long time for his car to be found or if he has to get a new car or something. Now, having me here (or, more importantly, my car) is a convenience for him. Does that count as a point for taking care of my caregiver?

CANCER—DAY 184 SUNDAY, OCTOBER 25, 2009

Oy vey, what a busy weekend. Friday night we had a birthday party to go to (after Marco's car was stolen). Saturday night there was a Halloween costume party. Marco was a brain surgeon in surgery scrubs and I was his patient wearing a hospital gown I "borrowed" from the radiation center. (I'm sneaking it back in tomorrow and throwing it in the gown hamper. Maybe they won't even know one went missing!) I also wore my surgery socks, and my elbow was still wrapped in purple gauze from the blood draw I had on Friday. We glued a gory open wound thing on my still-bald scalp . . . the wound had safety pins holding it together . . . and Marco drew a dashed line around my head indicating "Cut Here" for my rather inept surgeon. There was a couple at the party both dressed in surgery scrubs, so in the photos it looks like I have a whole team of inept doctors waiting to cut open my brain! That was fun.

Tonight Marco is DJ-ing the milonga at The Grind so we'll be dancing. Parties are easier to get through than the milongas, and I had a good time the last two nights with the birthday party and then the Halloween party. I'm getting better at keeping up a normal conversation with people again, though I still forget words and names all the time. Everyone seems to know about why I've gotten like that though, and they're very tolerant and understanding.

People are getting a kick out of how I wear a different wig every time they see me. People basically see Marco and if they see a woman with him they assume it's me no matter what color/length the hair is, I think, or maybe they just look carefully to make sure it IS me with another different color and length of wig . . . I think some day I may actually miss the wigs and changing my entire look in an instant.

CANCER—DAY 185 MONDAY, OCTOBER 26, 2009

This was a really tough Monday. I pushed myself to do wwaaaayyyyyy too much this weekend, and my body basically shut down yesterday and I slept a ton. But today I'm still paying for it . . . my hands and feet are terrible with neuropathy, my hands won't stop trembling, and my eyesight is so bad I can't see my own handwriting or the words on the screen. I put on my 3x magnifying glasses, and they help a lot with seeing the computer screen, but my hands are such mess of burning needling pains and shaking that I continually miss the intended key and end up typo-ing sooooo many words. I actually skipped the milonga last night, and right now I'm missing a surprise birthday party for one of my tango friends so I can stay home and rest more. I slept most of this day away. I am shocked by how tired I am. I really didn't think it would be this bad. But wow, just two particularly busy days and I'm shot.

CANCER—DAY 186 TUESDAY, OCTOBER 27, 2009

I'm starting to be burned from the radiation already. The whole big rectangle of skin that's getting radiated is feeling itchy and stings. My, aren't the next seven weeks going to be fun!

The shakes and vision blurriness are worse today. The neuropathy is particularly bad as well. I seem to have better days and worse days, today being one of those days I just can't seem to handle the burning and it puts me to tears. I toasted a tortilla with cheese in it and even after it cooled to room temperature I couldn't eat it because the toasted edges were sharp to my fingers and I couldn't use a fork and knife because pressing on the utensils to cut the tortilla just stabbed through my hands, more than I could bear. I ended up drinking a fruit smoothie for lunch.

I'm getting down and a little depressed from being in pain all the time, and from not being able to do things because of neuropathy or how worn out I get.

CANCER—DAY 187 WEDNESDAY, OCTOBER 28, 2009

I've been pondering where life goes after this. Am I going back to teaching dance? I really doubt it with the neuropathy in my feet. Forget training for performances, or even social dancing, probably, at least until the neuropathy gets better. I'm supposed to teach a graduate class at the University spring term, and I have to go back to my consulting job right after New Year's. But after this experience, do I really just jump back into my old life?

I pondered this a while, then I asked the Runes if I am supposed to go back to the same life I had before treatment. The Rune I drew was *Uruz* upright (which means Yes). *Uruz* is for Strength and it is the Rune of terminations and new beginnings. "Drawing Uruz indicates that the life you have been living has outgrown its form. Events occurring now may well prompt you to undergo a death within yourself."

Which life? My old life, or this new Sacramento life? Both? Guess I'll keep pondering. Whatever life is after this, it won't be the same as before cancer or the same as it is now, in treatment. It will be a new life.

CANCER—DAY 188 THURSDAY, OCTOBER 29, 2009

Well here's a neat little story. My mom wore her pink Team Cynthia Swan t-shirt to her exercise class on Monday morning. It seems everyone in the entire town of Sidney, Nebraska knows and loves my parents, and so everybody is always asking Mom about me and how I'm doing.

So today, when her exercise group got together again, everyone was wearing pink t-shirts. And they apparently even brought cookies with pink frosting. OK, it doesn't sound healthy for an exercise group, but still, what a creative way to show Mom that they care!

CANCER—DAY 189 FRIDAY, OCTOBER 30, 2009

I wore my neon pink wig for Halloween today, and it was a happy thing because so many people get a smile on their face when they see my super-bright wig, on Halloween at least (other days too, but not as much as today when wearing a neon pink wig is less outrageous). It's not like I was in costume, but it was neat because it made me smile to make them smile at my crazy-bright pink wig, and that was a good thing, a very good thing, actually.

When you are in pain and the state of being in pain becomes your standard state of being, you don't realize that you don't smile much anymore. I suspect the look on my face most of the time is probably something like fear mixed with pain, but I try to hide that with a smile, however forced, whenever I'm around people.

I had something of an "episode" at lunch today . . . my feet have been especially bad this week, and we'd walked two blocks to the crepes place for lunch and the neuropathy burning just kept getting more and more intense with each step, to the point that I just could not bear it. I was struggling to hold back the tears because we were in a restaurant. I was trembling all over because of the burning pain. I was nauseous with it and couldn't eat, and we left as soon as Marco was done.

Sometimes you just have to cry it out and wait for it to calm back down to something more bearable, which it eventually does. But trying to control it, trying to swallow it down and put on a smile for other people, can be absolutely impossible at times.

Uff da, there are times every day now when it's like it was today at lunch, just unbearable. I don't always have to struggle to keep it in though, since I'm alone a lot most days. When I'm just reading or resting and the burning or stabbing flares to an unbearable intensity, I just wait it out, hands upturned, bare feet touching nothing, letting the tears fall when the pain just cannot be contained.

Marco put up some black lights and Halloween lights for handing out candy tonight. I wonder if we'll get a lot of kids or not? It's been raining, but it suddenly brightened up in the last hour or so while I was sleeping. Hope it stays nice for the trick-or-treaters.

Weird. It's ironic that normal life things like Halloween and Trick-or-Treating seem foreign to me. Must be because I have cancer brain.

CANCER—DAY 190 SATURDAY, OCTOBER 31, 2009

Uff da, this stuff can really wear you down. Hurting a lot just plain wears you out. I can't really explain it. Like they said, it's cumulative . . . and it seems like there's never a break. If it's not my hands it's my feet. If it not my feet it's the shakes.

Last night we went to a cross-dressing Halloween party and then a milonga. We went as an old couple, Marco was the frumpy woman and I was dressed like Mr. Rogers; we went shopping at Salvation Army and a second-hand store on Saturday to find the clothes. The problem of course (and what made the shopping amusing) was that Marco is like a size 18 in women's (hard to find) and I'm smaller than small for a man. But we found khaki's and a shirt and tie as well as a frumpy old man cardigan sweater for me, and of course I went without a wig, just as bald as can be. I was really pale too, which in hindsight I regret because I look just ghostly in the photos. I should have worn base make-up on my head and found some way to draw on wrinkles or something. Oh well. We rounded out the cross-dressing affair with an umbrella cane for me and a frumpy handbag for Marco. For once it was appropriate that I had the shakes in my left hand—it made me look even more like a feeble old man needing a cane.

I only danced with four people at the milonga, sitting down for long breaks between tandas, but my feet were screaming bloody murder when I gave up for the night. Just walking aggravates the burning so, as you can imagine, attempting balanced, controlled movements entirely on the ball of the foot in three-inch heels really puts my neuropathy over the edge quickly. But it was fun to see everyone dressed up and in face makeup for the Day of the Dead milonga. And Marco was a hit in his matronly female attire, since we had just come from the cross-dressing party.

I'm really trying to stay upbeat and positive, but it's definitely a struggle sometimes. Sometimes I just want to curl up in a ball and disappear until it's over.

CANCER—DAY 191 SUNDAY, NOVEMBER 1, 2009

My dad sent me a graphics show file yesterday that contained photos of beautiful sceneries with a story about a man who had four sons. He sent each son on a quest to see a pear tree, each in a different season of the year. The first son went in winter and thought the tree was withered and ugly, the second son went in spring and thought the tree was full of promise, the third son went in summer and thought the blossoms were the most beautiful thing he'd ever seen, and the fourth son went in fall and thought it was full of life and fulfillment. The moral of the story is that you can't judge a person by only one season of their life. That really got to me, because this whole cancer thing has really been a "season" in my life and I have to remind myself that it won't last forever and that it's not who I am. I hope Marco realizes that, and that he doesn't hold Cancer Girl against me after this is all over. I'm still living with him during radiation, so I only have to drive about fifteen minutes from here to radiation every day, instead of the 2-ish hours each way it would be from my house. When radiation is done I'm going to go visit my parents in Sidney for a couple of weeks (it will be Christmas then). That will give us a break in our relationship. We've had some conversations about it, and we both think it's possible we could have a normal relationship when this is over and the stress is gone. I'll come back the weekend after New Year's, and then I'm planning to go back at work full time and live at home in Volcanoville again. Who knows where our relationship will be then, or even how I will be feeling health-wise after treatment, really. I can't imagine this neuropathy thing going on for months and still being a problem in January, though I guess it's possible. They'll also start me on Tamoxifen in January, which will be the third phase of cancer treatment that, if I tolerate it well enough, will continue for five years or more. I'm glad the tough stuff will end in this calendar year, though. It will be good to look at the new year as a beginning of a new life with all of this behind me.

CANCER—DAY 192 MONDAY, NOVEMBER 2, 2009

There is a woman who is often coming out of the radiation center when I am going in. My first time there she was coming out and her face was a little spotty and she had a scarf on her head like a chemo patient, and I wondered if she was getting radiation on her face. I've seen her a few times since then, and when I saw her again this morning, I felt so bad. Her radiation burn is a rectangle across her nose and cheeks now, and it's purple-red and looks really painful. I remember cringing inside wondering if it's going to get that bad with my radiation, and I had an awful moment of thinking that she's lucky it's on her face, so she doesn't have clothing rubbing against the burn all the time. It could be worse.

I'm not burned bad at all yet, it's just starting to get pink-ish with tiny little red blotches. Last week it was just itchy, which is annoying like any sunburn. After today's session it started to feel more like a burn, primarily where they put the bolus. I'm glad they're not using the bolus every day, just every other day, to radiate that area more but try to conserve on how much they zap my skin. Overall the radiation burn pain isn't bad at all though, compared to my hands and feet.

It's been dark and cloudy/rainy all day today and I can't get warm for some reason. It's crazy how short the days are all of a sudden. The gloomy weather doesn't help my mood. Summer sure disappeared quickly. I've been having trouble with my eyesight again today. It seemed good for quite a few days and I thought I was past this side effect, but today I'm struggling to see the computer screen again, and letters are all blurry. Darn it all, I'm ready to be done with all of this. How do people do chemo for six months or longer? How do people who have had sight all their life deal with suddenly going blind? I can't even imagine. Even though my neuropathy is now classified as stage 4, the worst it can be, even though that can cause incredible pain, losing my eyesight is something I fear beyond reason. I know people learn Braille and all that, and Brian gave me a book on CD to listen to (*Eat, Pray, Love*) so I can listen to the book without touching anything and not depending on my eyes to read. I know there are ways to cope and I know it's completely improbable that my eyesight will get so bad that it can't be corrected with lenses, but I tell ya, the idea of being blind scares me to death.

There are so many scary things other people have to deal with that I still constantly use my line of "It could always be worse" both when talking to other people and to bolster myself through whatever the current challenge is. There are a zillion things that could make life so much more difficult that I still have to feel blessed to only have to deal with what I have to deal with.

CANCER—DAY 193 TUESDAY, NOVEMBER 3, 2009

I had an appointment with the radiation oncologist today. She said my skin burn is not too bad for three weeks in, and that the burning that I feel is more on the inside. Yuck, I didn't think about that. Makes sense though. I do feel like I'm burning from the inside out. She also asked about the fatigue that I admitted is setting in, and she nodded like she completely expected it. With as many breast cancer radiation patients as she sees every day, I guess all this is old hat and nothing unusual to her. Same thing with the neuropathy, really.

She wasn't at all surprised that the neuropathy is still bothering me, severely, and she asked if it's getting better. I said I hoped so, though it seems to just vary day by day rather than actually improving. I told her what medication the oncologist gave me and said it didn't seem to help at all. She nodded again, same sort of thing, like there's nothing unusual about that either. Lots of people get stuck with this, I guess. Or else this is her way of being supportive and helpful, to assuage my fears by giving off the impression that what I'm going through is commonplace and expected. And heck, if lots of other people can get through it, some of them for a *very* long time, I can get through it, too.

~ Act III ~
Survival

Chapter 23.
Alternative/
New Age Medicine

CANCER—DAY 194 WEDNESDAY, NOVEMBER 4, 2009

I've tried quite a few New Age or Alternative Medicine kind of things along the way, especially more recently as the neuropathy continued to worsen all the way into the most advanced stage of the condition, the dreaded stage 4 of neuropathy (which is apparently quite rare, actually—lucky me). Western medicine has yet to provide any easement of the neuropathy side effect, and I have my doubts about the depth of knowledge my medical oncologist actually has in this area (it's superficial at best, no offense to the guy), so I'm pressing the oncologist to refer me to some kind of specialist, but he keeps belaying my request, "hoping" the neuropathy will get better soon. As the neuropathy continued to progress without relief from Western medicine, I have been more and more willing to try different Eastern or Chinese medicines as well as some alternative medicines and treatments that are, well, unusual.

Some alternative or new age treatments are a bit bizarre, but I try to be open-minded. I did *not*, however, try acupuncture. I already feel like needles are stabbing my hands and feet all the time, I hate needles to begin with, and the thought of intentionally allowing someone to put needles all over my body, well, that's currently more than I am willing to try just yet. Give it some time, maybe I'll be desperate and try acupuncture when all else has failed to ease the neuropathy.

In general though, especially with alternative medicine, you never know what may help, and my impression has always been that the downside is simply not having an improvement to what is being treated. Best case, it works. Worst case, it doesn't work, BUT, it doesn't generally leave you any worse off for trying. At least, I don't think it does, but I could be wrong. Alternative medicine is a slippery slope when you grew up with a hospital administrator father, registered nurse mother, and practically all siblings and cousins in medical occupations. Given that, actually, maybe it makes sense that I'm more into the New Age stuff than the rest of my family, because I don't work in the medical field.

The again, I'm the only Californian in my family too. Attitudes are different here versus the Midwest and the Great Plains. Some people may find some—or all—the New Age things I've tried to be a stretch. Some of this is decidedly *not* normal to the Western mindset.

For me, the New Age approach to medicine seems to be about energy and the connected nature of energy. In my own sense of it, there is a "oneness" of energy that connects us all, and the mind-body connection within ourselves is an even stronger energy that we must care for physically, mentally, and (this is a fairly new perspective for me) spiritually. At any rate, I think you have to be open-minded before even considering complementary new age treatments. Better yet, be open-minded without any pre-set expectations for the outcome, then no matter what happens, at least you're not mentally blocking the possibility of benefit.

BLESSED DIRT

I know I'm going to butcher the details on this one, because I had some serious chemo brain going on when I tried this and I didn't journal on it in any detail at the time. The neuropathy had already escalated to a burning sensation though, so this was around the third chemo, and the healing intent was to reduce, or better yet, remove the neuropathy pain.

I have a tango friend that is Jewish, and she traveled to a holy ground (holy land? I'm not sure) where there are healing springs and muds and clays and such, blessed because a saint was buried there. (My apologies, Rebecca, if I completely bumbled on why the springs and land there have restorative powers. I think I got the saint part right.)

Rebecca went to this healing place, and since she had recently sprained her wrist, she scooped up a little of the healing dirt. She rubbed some of it on her wrist and hand, and her sprain did indeed go away, immediately, not after some length of time like regular bodily healing. (I know, I know, some religious folks would say this sort of "miraculous healing" can happen just because you have faith in it, but whatever, this is the story of how I got and used the blessed healing dirt, not a discussion of religious faith in miracles.)

That all happened with Rebecca a couple of years ago, if I remember correctly. She brought a little box of healing dirt home with her, but she had not needed it again. When she heard about my neuropathy at a milonga, she wrote this nice note to me and included a tin with some of her healing dirt in it. She said she had no idea how I should use it for neuropathy, but she explained how she had used it on her sprained wrist. (As an aside, I have tried numerous lotions, ointments, and other topical applications . . . anything and everything anyone has suggested . . . but so far I haven't found a lotion or goo that helps with chemo-induced neuropathy, and I've tried a *lot* of them.)

Since my neuropathy is very specifically in the undersides of my hands and feet where the nerve endings are, I took some of Rebecca's blessed healing dirt and gently rubbed it between my hands and spread some on the bottoms of my feet.

But, no miracle for me. I left the dirt on for an afternoon, then I washed it off to make dinner. Maybe part of the medicinal powers of the healing dirt involves the person physically going to the holy site from whence it comes. At any rate, the neuropathy didn't change from the application of blessed dirt.

REIKE

The first Eastern medicine sort of thing I tried was Reike. It's a kind of energy massage that should be relaxing and ease stress and/or pain. Instead of relaxing me and easing my chemo side effects though, Reike seemed to have the opposite effect and I was so hyped up I didn't sleep for two nights. It was an insane Red Bull rodeo of alertness!

The Reike session in and of itself is very cool, though, if you are open-minded and have some kind of belief in the connected energy we have as beings, which I do.

Here's something you can try to see if you can feel the energy or something like it. With both hands flat, rub your palms together for a couple of seconds and then more your hands (palms still flat) slightly away from each other. At the very least you will feel a little heat that you created with the friction of rubbing your hands together. If you're more receptive though, you may feel like the "heat" is stronger between your joints, from the knuckles of one hand to the other. The really cool thing is to do this in the dark because you may even be able to see the energy as a kind of wispy white tornado-looking tendril spanning the gap between, say, the thumb knuckle of your right hand and the thumb knuckle of your left hand. Freaky cool.

In Reike, the masseuse (I guess that's what you call the person who does this) never actually touches you. They simply move their hands over your body until they sense an area that needs attention (the best I can describe it is that a trouble spot may feel too hot or too cold in the energy released from it for the masseuse to sense). So, much like a regular masseuse finds where you have knots and strains in your muscles, the Reike masseuse finds where you have bad energy, holds their hands over that area and, well, sends good energy into you through their hands.

Hey now, I didn't say this was going sound normal, did I? After all, it's not called alternative medicine because it's *normal.*

After a handful of sessions that always seemed to have the caffeine-hyping non-relaxing non-pain-relieving effect, I decided Reike is not for me, at least not to ease cancer side effects. But I haven't given up on alternative medicine. If you're not interested in and willing to try a variety of alternative medical treatments, I don't think you would fit in very well in California. We're kinda health nuts out here, for the most part. Blend that with Berkeley and you have a mental state like no other, that's for sure. (Haha, "mental" state, get it?)

TAPPING THERAPY

The same friend that does Reike also gave me a manual about tapping therapy, or EFT (Emotional Freedom Techniques). Similar to acupuncture, EFT focuses on acupressure points in one part of your body to address ailments in other parts of your body, but without needles, much to my relief.

Basically, the EFT manual tells you where to tap on your body to address different kinds of concerns, like, tap your forehead for this or tap your inside wrist for that. I don't remember exactly what any of them were, because even without needles this was an impossibility for me. Tapping my fingertips on anything is what causes the pain, so how am I going to tap on any body part? I did try a few of the recommended techniques for pain, stress, and anxiety, but I think I gave up on this one within a week when it became obvious that my fingertips were hurting worse from doing the tapping and nothing else was changing.

Hmmm. Maybe I should ask someone else to do the actual tapping so I'm not using my neuropathy fingers to tap. That's an idea, but it seems like a weird request to make of someone, and I'm certainly not going to ask Marco, since he is clearly mentally checked out on the caregiver thing. Anyway, I still have the manual, so maybe I'll read some more to see if they've done any trials where a second party is involved.

YOGA

OK, now this one isn't going to freak anyone out by sounding too "out there." Yoga can definitely help get clutter out of your head and ease your mind, just not when you're in poses that put pressure on the underside of your hands or feet if you have neuropathy. I started yoga before I had any neuropathy pain though. My first yoga session was around the time they put in the chemo port below my left collarbone. It had been many weeks since my lumpectomy, but I still had limited range of motion with my right arm, and the underarm, where they took out the lymph nodes, seriously hurt, *especially* if I tried to stretch.

On a walk one day, we came across a yoga studio just six blocks or so away from Marco's house. I put the name of the place and the website in my blackberry to check out their schedule later. I read up on the studio we'd come across as well as a dozen others in

Sacramento, because there are tons of different kinds of yoga. I liked the philosophy of the owner of the studio we had found nearby, and the studio practices Hatha Yoga in the Iyengar tradition, which seemed appropriate for me. This yoga is generally a slow-paced stretching also involving breath and mental awareness. It's supposed to be a good preparation for meditation.

Marco and I went for a free session together, and I signed up for an eight-week introductory yoga series for beginners. I also went to a Restorative Yoga series they had that used a lot of props (block and pads and such) so that you could be in the yoga position without straining your body (excellent for the chemo-abused body), and I tried Yin Yoga, which is particularly slow-paced and involved holding poses for five minutes at a time—holding the pose to allow the mind.

I've been doing yoga for, I don't know, just a few months, so I am not an expert, but certainly the meditative savasana my yoga instructor gives us at the end of each yoga practice is very calming, peaceful, and serene. While that doesn't relieve neuropathy pain, the entire yoga practice definitely has a mind-calming effect on me. In particular, I try to forget about pain or emotional strains and just think about the position, how to hold my muscles there, and breathing. I try to *not* think about anything at all, and just let my mind "be."

MEDITATION

I can't really claim to meditate per se. I don't really know how to meditate by myself, though I do have a couple of guided meditation CDs that I like. I think the only time I'm really in a meditative state is during that little time at the end of the yoga practice that I just mentioned, savasana. However, that meditative state can be mind-blowing in its stillness, so I'm still practicing it. It has helped me better maintain or find calm when I feel myself getting upset, so I use it as another method to keep my physical pain and the strain of controlling it from infecting others with negativity.

Besides yoga, I ended up with a couple pseudo-meditative practices during treatment though. One was watching my fish. My aquarium has an infinity edge so that the water flows over the glass walls of the aquarium, making a waterfall sound all the time. Even before I had fish, I liked to close my eyes and listen to the water. I love water. The sounds of a waterfall (common on hiking trails near my house), or water running over rocks in a river (also pretty much a constant out where I live), or ocean waves crashing or rolling gently onto a beach like at my first place in California, are all sounds I can feel peaceful listening to. So listening to the waterfall sound of my new infinity edge aquarium is rather meditative in and of itself, if you can get your mind out of the physical pain and focus on the sound and flow of the water.

When the neuropathy started getting bad and constant, I could not escape the pain. There is no escape, no drug stops it, yoga and meditation can't disconnect my mind from it, and even sleep is fitful because the burning wakes me up if I move and put my palm under the pillow or my toes are pressed too heavily by the covers. If there is a meditative state deep enough to escape neuropathy pain, I have not yet found it. But listening to the waterfall and watching my fish lazily wave their huge fluffy fins has become a kind of meditation for me. An hour of that and you can kind of forget the rest of the world exists.

The second meditative approach I practice is the one I learned from yoga, which is simply a deep cleansing breathing, focusing your attention on following the breath into, through, and out of your body. I use this a *LOT* when I'm around other people and the neuropathy pain spikes up for no reason (or for a reason—like standing up or touching something). A neuropathy breath (triggered by a jolt of burning pain) is more of a sudden intake though, a gasp, and usually my eyes bug out a little (open excessively wide) for a moment, until I can catch that gasp and swallow down the pain enough to take a slow, calming breath. Even taking just one deep slow breath like I learned in yoga can calm me away from panicky fear when there's bad news, or calm me away from what would be a regrettable reactionary response, like responding in kind if someone says something mean or derogatory. Though it's not an escape from pain, a world of bad feelings can be skirted with one deep calming breath.

Charka Balancing

I found a pair of CDs by Deepak Chopra that guide you through a visualization to balance your chakras (the seven energy centers of the body). Experts may or may not consider it meditation, but this is an interesting exercise or practice. Like everything else, it did not impact the neuropathy, but it did help me feel like I have more energy in my body, which is a great thing when you're feeling beaten down with fatigue. Most days I take a nap after I get back from radiation, but napping or resting quietly with my fish doesn't necessarily help me gain back energy that has been replaced with cancer treatment fatigue. I haven't tried the chakra balancing as a way to generate internal energy for yoga (I should), but I do use it when I know I'm going to need energy for something else, like the Wednesday night milonga at Cell Block, or hanging out with Babysitter Brian on a Tuesday night, or going to play dominoes or scrabble with friends some evening. A few hours before whatever it is I'm going out for, I spend an hour in the cat/music room doing the chakra balancing visualization (I've never do any of this stuff in my office because Marco is right there and it's just not peaceful).

I can't make any scientific claims on this, nor do I know if it may help other cancer patients in the same way, but for me chakra balancing usually helps me have more energy. I just have a little more energy in general on days I do chakra balancing, and I feel more like a body than a collection of parts in a faulty machine.

Neuropathy Massage

Another friend of mine used to date a guy (talk about a roundabout connection!) who is a physical therapist and does physical therapy massage. He works with diabetics, and went for specialized training in a particular foot and hand massage for diabetic neuropathy. Apparently diabetic neuropathy can be just as awful as chemo-induced neuropathy, but the diabetic has the advantage that changing diet and aggressively managing the diabetes can "cure" the neuropathy.

I haven't had the nerve to contact this guy yet. I can't even touch my feet, so the thought of someone squeezing or applying pressure to massage my foot sounds like agony, not relief.

I'll put this on the to-do list right below acupuncture.

Visceral Manipulation

Now I'm trying something even more out there, but very real. I had my second session with Don Curtz yesterday. I'm trading tango lessons with him in exchange for sessions of this kind of New Age physical therapy for your insides, called Visceral Manipulation. Don is all into this German New Medicine, which purports that cancer is the body's reaction to conflict and distress in your life.

The first session started with me lying on the massage table like for a regular massage except I was in my t-shirt and jeans instead of under a sheet like in most body massages. He started withholding the weight of my head in his hands and sensing out the tension in my neck, which is something of a wind vane pointing to areas of the body that are out of whack.

While stretching the muscles in my neck and gauging the connection into my body, Don was telling me how he got into this line of work, and his perspective that traditional Western medicine treats the human body (and the person) clinically, like a machine, unimportant as a human being. He feels that approach devalues the patient as a person.

Marco shot into my mind with deadly speed and precision as if from a sniper's rifle.

Don had just summed up exactly how I feel with Marco in five little words: "unimportant as a human being." I feel unloved, because he told me he doesn't love me, that he can't love me, at least not the current version of me. After the last workshop we taught together right before chemo, he terminated our professional dance partnership because he says I don't have the experience to match his (don't get me going on that unsubstantiated slap in the face). Our "romantic relationship" is on hold until cancer treatment is over to see if we are compatible without the strain of a potentially terminal illness overshadowing everything. I am just someone he "lets" live in his house. He likes being the "caregiver" because it makes him an authority over me. When I gave him $300 rent for having the cats in the house, he said "But now I have to give you your rights!" He was laughing, but he took the money. Marco is perfectly willing to let me pay for everything and accept money out of my savings that he can apply to his already dirt-cheap rent. All this instantly flashed like a lightning bolt in my mind, forcing me to recognize the base truth: he's never thought of me as an equal, not as a partner, not as a girlfriend, not even as a roommate, and certainly not as a person.

Don felt the immediate reaction as my muscles stiffened ever so slightly and I pulled in a quick breath with that flood of thoughts. Naturally, he asked what I was thinking about at that moment. I told Don that I agree with him and that "I definitely feel like I've been treated like a machine for the past six months." I left it at that, without comment on his real point of devaluing the patient as a human being.

The session went on. It was interesting, and odd, just like you would expect from a California New Ager. I read up on visceral manipulation and the New German Medicine earlier but I had no idea what the treatment would actually be like. The descriptions just didn't make sense without a way to visualize what actually happens.

After feeling out my neck and shoulders very similarly to a Swedish massage, Don then had me stand up to look at my posture and balance (haha, Cynthia balanced, that's funny). Then he stood behind me and told me to let myself fall back and he would catch me. You know, like in those goofy team-building exercises they do where you're supposed to trust the person that you won't hit the ground. Well, I trusted Don just fine because I've danced with him, so I let myself fall back. In the process, I also instinctively move my left foot back slightly, which told him that I am innately left-handed and right-brained. Neat way to confirm that, eh?

Then he had me lie down again. Now the visceral manipulation part starts. He said the indications were that my spleen and liver are not positioned properly. Here's where I didn't get it when

I was reading about visceral manipulation—that is literally what it is. Physically manipulating your viscera, (viscera being your internal organs, specifically the organs in the abdominal cavity). The visceral manipulation is like a massage in your abdominal cavity. Seriously!

He lifted my ribcage slightly on one side while apply a gentle firm pressure that kind of pulled down some organ, then he shifted that slightly toward the side where he was lifting my ribcage. Then, still holding up the ribcage to maneuver slightly underneath my ribcage, he applied pressure in from my side. This was all done with very gentle but firm and constant pressure. There was no "massage" kind of action like when they work out tensions in your back muscles or such. He was just, literally, manipulating my viscera to be in positions more conducive to reducing strain, stress, and pain.

It's kinda out there, but if it helps with the neuropathy I will be thrilled. It takes multiple sessions because you don't want to shift very far in one session. I guess that can make people really emotional. Crazy stuff.

It's been more than six months, and I'm losing my grip on who I am. As Don made me realize so vividly, my confidence and self-esteem have really taken a hit in the last six months—from living with Marco, from not feeling well—from all the side effects I guess, both physical and emotional.

Chapter 24.
Getting Emotional

CANCER—DAY 195 THURSDAY, NOVEMBER 5, 2009

I had a total meltdown last night about Cell Block. All day I couldn't decide if I were physically OK to go dance in San Francisco, and Marco kind of talked me in to thinking I was not doing well enough to dance (because of the neuropathy burning in my feet, and general radiation fatigue). He said that "we" should just stay home and watch a movie and play World of Warcraft (WoW). It turns out he was only being that way about it because he actually wanted to take my car to go by himself, leaving me cooped up at his house. When I finally agreed with him that I should stay home and, to be nice, offered for him to take my car and go without me, he *did*. Then he got mad because of the expression on my face (I was a bit ruffled that he would say "we" should stay home all day and then leap at the chance to take my car without me tonight) and he said something about how I'm so selfish and he can't wait for me to leave.

Needless to say, I thrust my car keys in his hand and begged him to just go. Why I thought it would be nice to have a quiet evening home with Marco, I can't tell you now. I think what bugged me is how he kept saying all day that "we" shouldn't go to the milonga, and then suddenly he changed that to telling me that *I* shouldn't go to the milonga but he *should* go, once I agreed I was too tired for it. I played WoW for a while, then went to bed in the cat bedroom so I wouldn't have to see him when he got back in the wee hours of the morning.

He had suggested I call Brian to come hang out with me while he went to Cell Block, and I never responded to him about that. It's hard to explain to Marco that Brian thinks so very highly of me that it can actually be a bit difficult. From Brian's perspective, I can apparently do no wrong, but I know with absolute certainty that I am not perfect, so there's no reason for Brian to act like I am. But Brian is just so good-hearted that he even seems to see my faults as admirable qualities. He's the polar opposite of Marco, who seems to think I can do no right, at least not now, in cancer treatment. And to go from Marco to Brian and back to Marco, well, that makes being here with Marco all the more pathetic and depressing.

I'm also afraid to tell Brian or my parents (or my brother or any of my close friends) how awful the emotional non-love situation has become. There would be a mob of people flying out here to tear Marco apart for emotionally abusing a cancer patient, especially their beloved Cynthia, if they knew what it's really like here. I tell everyone "I'm hanging in there," and that's literally what it is. I'm just getting through each day as it comes, and trying to control my emotions so I don't inadvertently set Marco off because he sees tears on my cheeks and thinks I'm trying to put a guilt trip on him.

When I'm alone, I don't bother trying not to cry anymore. I'm in pain all the time and, let's face it, I'm emotional. I try to hide it from him and just generally stay out of his way while I count down the days I have left, willing myself through it.

Every day takes its toll though. And I can't help getting more emotional with the constant neuropathy pain and the unending nature of it. I just have to remind myself to breathe and stay calm, to not let my emotions get the better of me so I can still interact with other people in a positive way rather than a negative one.

CANCER—DAY 196 FRIDAY, NOVEMBER 6, 2009

Oh boy. The last time Seoul was out here in my Volcanoville house, she was still more of a kitten and could fit behind the couch . . . but tonight she got stuck! I'm home in the forest for just one night, having a little break between radiation this morning and the milonga tomorrow night. I brought home some office stuff I don't really need to keep in Sac now, and the cats. Mizzou looked at me in disbelief (Seriously! Mizzou has great facial expressions) when he realized I was opening his cat caddy in my house instead of yet another foreign place. It took him about ninety seconds to make sure the house was still in order and settle back in to his usual position for that time of day, meaning, on a cat bed on top of my desk looking out the window to my backyard and the forest.

Seoul, on the other hand, has now spent half of her life traveling with me or living at the kennel or penned up in the cat room at Marco's house. Brian jokes that Seoul has become "institutionalized." Ha! He's right though. Seoul doesn't have the sense of "home" that Mizzou does. Mizzou owns this roost, that's clear. You know, Mizzou is as stubborn as the day is long. It's one of the reasons he's so good for me though, especially now, when I need to constantly muster up more inner strength and stubbornness to get through the next month of treatment.

Oh right, my story. Seoul and the couch. Wow, is it ever hard to keep my chemo brain focused long enough to get a complete thought out without taking myself on a tangent I can't find my way back from!

I have this huge heavy comfy corner couch with a slightly arched back so there's a little space at the floor behind the base of the couch. The space is just big enough for a kitten to have a little hidey-hole to run and hide in. But Seoul is teenage-cat size now, though she doesn't seem to know it yet. She just went behind the couch as usual and you wouldn't believe the racket coming from back there as she tried to turn around, which of course there wasn't space for. Her collar was jingling and scraping the wall, and then it went silent. Creepy. So I call her name a few times and it's still quiet but Mizzou has started moving along the top of the couch, following sounds too soft for me to hear, and next thing you know Seoul creeps out from behind the couch with a bum right foot, holding her front right paw up to her chest and moving gingerly and lying down really slowly . . . poor thing. I've checked her all over and she doesn't meow in pain, so she's OK, just sore in that paw from squishing herself up to turn around in her little trap. But she's learned not to go behind the couch anymore!

I'm only home for one night. I'll go back to Sacramento tomorrow and probably be there for at least the next couple weeks without coming home again because there's so much tango going on the next couple of weekends. But it was sooooo nice today to be able to drive home and NOT get carsick!

Most of the chemo side effects are gone completely. I can eat whatever I want now (tomatoes and milk in particular had suddenly become poisonous for me during chemo but now they're happily back in my diet). Now my food doesn't have to be bland and mushy, though I still can't have anything actually hot or cold, everything cooked has to be cooled quite a bit before I can eat it, and drinks like hot tea need to be near room temperature for me. Apparently that goes with the whole neuropathy thing. My hands are crazy-sensitive to hot and cold, I can't hold a hot mug, or wash dishes in hot water by hand (even with gloves), or pick up a glass of ice water if it's sat long enough to get the whole glass icy cold. Nor can I drink ice water. But room-temperature water is great! It tastes just fine to me now, no more nasty blood-water taste.

It's really nice to be home with the cats. They're settled in which makes me feel more settled, too. It'll be a quiet cozy night catching up on *Dancing with the Stars* for us!

CANCER—DAY 197 SATURDAY, NOVEMBER 7, 2009

I pondered this for almost two weeks . . . I am supposed to teach a graduate course in San Francisco starting the first week in January. It starts just a couple of weeks after radiation finishes, and I've been worrying that I won't really be up to making the drive into to The City every Wednesday night for four months, and that it will seriously impede recovering my energy after treatment. When I mentioned the class to my mom, I could hear in her voice that she was not pleased to hear I was planning on teaching one night a week in San Francisco starting in January besides going back to work consulting right away. Mom knows my over commitment tendencies so well . . . and worries too much.

Anyway, I finally decided yesterday to ask the university to let me teach just the cyber (online) section of the course and not have the S.F. section or else give the S.F. section to another professor. The nice thing about the cyber section is that, being online, I can do the work in little pieces and on the weekend to spread it out more and not wear myself out with it. The problem for the university (this is my opinion, not necessarily their opinion) is that I wrote this Business Intelligence graduate course for the university and have been the only person teaching it since 2005, so trying to get someone else up to speed in a short period of time could be fairly onerous.

So, after hanging the mouse pointer over the Send button for probably twenty minutes making sure this was really what I wanted to do (it could, after all, potentially end my tenure as an adjunct professor), I sent an e-mail to the department coordinator telling her I was concerned about all the drive time and my health following treatment. She replied with a nice note saying she completely agreed that my health was the first priority, and she forwarded my message to the department head to see what he wanted to do. Then I received a very nice note back from the department chair saying they'll cancel the S.F. section and that he's glad I can teach the cyber section, and, here's the teary part for an emotional cancer patient, he wrote "Cynthia, we care for you and we value your participation in our department. Take good care of yourself and keep in touch."

I never really expected a company or a professional organization or an educational institution to "care" about me so much. I mean, family, sure, everyone's going to be really concerned and asking frequently how I'm doing, but the response from people I know professionally has been seriously eye-opening. It probably shouldn't be . . . professionally I'm involved with many people I've known and respected for years, and many of them are good friends that I always make time to hang out with even though I only see them a few times a year at best. I know I would be very concerned about their health if they were ill. Still, I have a hard time getting my head around the idea that soooooo many people are sincerely concerned about me and reading my Web log and writing little pep-talk notes to me to "hang in there" and sending cards and text messages and on and on.

That has been seriously comforting and it's definitely made a difference for me; it's so easy to feel all alone in something like this, trying to take care of myself without disturbing my "caregiver," living it out day after day, and I can certainly feel alone. I can only feel alone until I turn on the computer or open the mail though, where there's always another note or card from another person wishing me well. It's amazing.

CANCER—DAY 198 SUNDAY, NOVEMBER 8, 2009

I came back to Sacramento for the Saturday night milonga, and I have a couple of brief mixed-together stories from the milonga last night . . .

There was a guy in town from San Francisco; he stopped in for some dancing on his way back from Tahoe. I remember seeing him in San Francisco at Cell Block and I think we've been introduced, but we've never danced together. But anyway, he's really *really* good, and last night he asked me to dance and we had two crazy tandas. It was so much fun! He led things I'm sure I've never done before in my life. That's the awesome thing about being a professional dancer and follower. Guys can lead pretty much anything with me, and the really good tangueros actually make up moves when they're dancing with me, to see what happens. We play.

Cute side story . . . there's a guy here that is pretty much the Godfather of Sacramento Tango (dubbed Tango Bear). He's my absolute favorite person to dance with for valse and milonga (the two fast and syncopated Argentine Tango dances) because he can actually lead the complicated little rhythms that are in milonga and valse. [I should explain that the word milonga can be used in two ways in tango. "A Milonga" is what a tango dance gathering is called, like how people refer to going "clubbing" for a certain style of dance. A milonga is a formalized event with all the social graces and traditions of Buenos Aires Argentine Tango. For example, you never, *ever* teach something during a milonga. If the guy tries something and it doesn't work with that partner, it is rude for him to try the same move over and over again. If he keeps trying to force it, he's being rude both to his partner and the dancers around him because he's interrupting the flow of the dance floor. After dancing tango a long time, taking several trips to Buenos Aires, and developing a serious respect for the history of the dance, I find it a bit insulting if a guy tries to lead something that doesn't work at a milonga and then keeps trying to force it instead of leading something that he can actually lead such that I can follow. It's takes two to tango, and it's incredibly rude to assume you are correct and your partner is wrong if something doesn't work. If I can't follow something, then don't try to lead me to do it again, at least not at a milonga. There is a more casual tango dance event called a practica, which, as it sounds, is an opportunity to practice tango and it is not considered rude to stop with your partner and try to figure out how to do something new together. OK, so, enough of etiquette. Argentine

Tango actually refers to three Argentine dances: tango, valse, and milonga. Each has very different music and rhythms, though it's hard to distinguish one from the other when you're new to Argentine Tango.] The rhythms in milonga and valse are hard to lead to, and often a guy will dance fixed patterns regardless of whether or not the action fits the music, and I have to guess what steps they're *trying* to lead. Though I keep my smile on and do my best to follow, it can be very, very difficult, and even frustrating, which I never, ever, let a guy see in my face or my movement because the more novice the dancer, the more encouragement he needs. What can I say? I'm a dance teacher. My goal in dance (besides challenging myself to always improve in my technique) is to encourage everyone to dance and to keep dancing, to not give up just because the dance is difficult at first. Dance is good for the soul as well as the body. Tango Bear and I share that philosophy as instructors. He being vastly more experienced than I.

In all of Sacramento, no one is as fun for me to dance with as Tango Bear for the difficult and complicated dances. My story about Tango Bear isn't actually about dancing with him, though. Once, a long time ago, I sat down next to Tango Bear after a tanda with someone who was still in the early stages of learning tango. Tango Bear was chuckling. I knew what he was laughing at, but I had to ask "What's so funny?" He said, "It's like watching someone who just learned how to drive a Volkswagen bug trying to handle a Porsche." I was in awe of receiving such an amazing compliment from the person I respect most in all of SacTango, but I couldn't resist the opportunity for a snappy comeback, so I raised one eyebrow and asked him "Am I the Volkswagen, or the Porsche?"

Back to the present . . . after dancing with the great dancer from San Francisco, I went to sit next to one of my tango friends, Dietrich, and commented that I had just had one of those dances where you don't care if you have another one all night, it was that fantastic. (I'd had a wonderful tanda with Dietrich earlier in the evening, we have great floor chemistry, so I don't think he took the comment about the San Francisco guy as a slight to his own dancing.) I chatted with Dietrich for a tanda, and she of course asked how I was doing and I remember telling him that going to the milongas really takes it out of me and I'd probably spend almost all of today resting, sleeping or napping, to recover. I remember it now because that's almost entirely what today has been. Recovery. From just a couple of hours at a milonga, not even dancing very much. Sheesh.

As for the San Francisco guy . . . I was talking with him again later in the night, as Marco and I were leaving, and he asked me what the free milonga on Friday is for (I'm throwing a party/milonga for my Sacramento tango friends next Friday to thank everyone for being so caring and supportive throughout my treatment, and to celebrate being done with chemo). When I told him it was the party I was throwing to thank everyone for their support during chemo, he said "I didn't realize that was you! Well, I've been reading about you, and I'm glad I got to meet you." I asked him to please come back for my party on Friday if he can. What got me emotionally is that he said he had "read" about me (my blog? the SacTango e-mails about the party? who knows), and here is this fabulous dancer from San Francisco saying how great it was to meet me, when I had felt the privilege was all mine, to have danced with him. Very cool, all around.

CANCER—DAY 199 MONDAY, NOVEMBER 9, 2009

Alone, I have these breakdowns. Emotionally, I mean. I'm trying to stay positive, and that wears me out and next thing I know I'm having a meltdown, feeling awful either about how I feel physically or about how I've let it affect me or what it's done to Marco's life, keeping him from doing things he'd rather be doing than babysitting a cancer patient (which he doesn't even have to be doing but he says he's doing it). The guilt is the worst.

Marco is thinking about learning the bandoneon, which is an accordion-like instrument that is the heart of tango music and fairly rare (and expensive) in the States. There's a guy that sells them though, and he offered to meet Marco at a place in San Francisco the day after my port removal surgery. We don't know what condition I'll be in, if I'll be fine or on painkillers or what, so we don't know whether or not I'll be up to the drive and dancing afterward to go with Marco or if I can be left alone at the house or what. Brian is going to be out of town, so that's not an option, and Marco needs my car to go see the bandoneons, so I can't go home to my house in Volcanoville and leave him without a car. I didn't realize at first that Marco was talking about going to San Francisco; I thought he was meeting the guy at a place here in Sac and I thought, well that's no big deal, he'll be gone maybe an hour the day after surgery and I'll be fine to be left alone for an hour since it's incredibly unlikely there will be any health emergency. While explaining that the meet-up is in San Francisco at Cell Block, Marco said "If I have cancel and reschedule, oh well, but I want to do more dancing too, even if you can't."

That put me on this massive guilt trip about how I've interrupted Marco's life with all my mess. The worst meltdowns are over things that I really, REALLY want to be doing that I can't or shouldn't do, that Marco either goes to alone (which can leave me jealous that I can't go) or he stays home with me and piles on the guilt, telling me that I am selfish and I don't appreciate the sacrifices he's making for me. Sometimes I think it was a big mistake to be here and torturing myself with the things (mostly dancing) that I can't do. But how could anyone have known how damaging chemo was going to be to my body? When I was deciding whether to stay in Sac or go to Nebraska to stay with my parents for treatment, I never considered this potential situation where I'd be so physically incapacitated for so long, unable to dance, unable to walk, unable to even stand up for any duration, without pain. It's been much worse than I would have ever anticipated mentally, physically, and emotionally.

I apparently cover it up pretty well with everyone except my parents. My parents know me well and they can hear how I'm truly feeling in my voice even when I'm saying things that are upbeat and chipper. They hear tension in my voice, but that doesn't tell them what's going on, and I just blame it on the pain if Mom asks what's wrong.

With Marco, well, because he's around all the time, there's no real escape or hiding, so he sees the struggle of my recovery from the emotional strain of trying to be "doing well" for everyone else at the milongas or parties. With everyone else I see, it's pretty much a temporary act of pretending to be doing well for just a couple of hours at a time, but that completely wears me out and takes me a day or more to recover from.

Kind of like now. I have to leave for yoga within the next five minutes or so, and I really don't want to go because I don't feel up to the emotional cover-up, swallowing down the neuropathy pain, but I know I have to do it, it's the right thing to do even if it's difficult (it's the right thing to do in part because it gives Marco a little break from me, and in part because it forces me to keep trying to be normal and I really do achieve some calm there). So I keep struggling and I keep trying. Off to yoga I go.

CANCER—DAY 200 TUESDAY, NOVEMBER 10, 2009

I had dinner with Brian while Marco was teaching tonight. I finally broke down and told him everything about what's going on with Marco and his temper and his frustration with me being around. Brian did exactly what I knew he would do, which is exactly why I had avoided telling him all this time.

Brian insisted that I move out immediately and go to his house. The primary problem there, and the reason I didn't just go live with Brian this whole time is that he doesn't have anywhere to put me (no spare room) and I'd be on the futon couch the whole time, occupying the only piece of living room furniture and feeling always in the way because he also has a housemate, a doctor who works nights and is home during the day. Now I don't really want to move my stuff to Brian's with just four weeks left and then move it home. I'd rather just move back home to my house, but that is also a fairly major endeavor for someone with chemo/radiation fatigue. The drive in for radiation every day looms fairly daunting when I long to be at my own house. All that driving, every day, tired enough to fall asleep at the wheel. I would also feel really bad leaving Marco without a car since his was stolen and he's been using mine for everything for the past however many weeks. Finally, because Marco and I have been keeping up this public "act" of the mutually supportive couple in love, moving out now would shock everyone and make Marco look bad even if I didn't tell anyone why I left his house with only a few weeks of radiation left. And it would be mean to suddenly leave him without a car, which I don't really want to do.

But Brian's house is completely open to me and his housemate is aware that I may suddenly appear and be their houseguest for the rest of radiation, even though Brian may be in and out of the country for work. So at least I have an escape route for when Marco finally says something so mean I just have to leave regardless of the trouble that causes for him in not having a car or how it may create gossip in the tango community. I'm trying to be nice and stay out of his way and let him do whatever he wants like I'm not even there, right down to telling him to just take my car anytime he wants without asking me, so hopefully he'll be able to keep his anger and frustration under control just a couple more weeks. He is completely, totally burned out on the whole cancer patient thing. I'd say I'm burned out too, but I don't have the luxury of allowing myself to burn out mentally check out. I have to finish treatment, so I'll just keep going along as best I can for this short while longer.

It's reassuring to know I can go to Brian's at the drop of a hat though. That was actually true all along, but I feel better knowing that if it happens it will only be for a few weeks and not crowding them for months. It was an enormous relief to finally admit to Brian how Marco is treating me. I think I've been keeping up a good front with everyone, keeping everything in, so having dinner with Brian and letting some of it out really helped. The more I told Brian, the more emotional we both became. Best friends are like that.

CANCER—DAY 201 WEDNESDAY, NOVEMBER 11, 2009

It's been a long morning. With fatigue really kicking in, it's getting harder and harder to get out of bed to get wigged and over to radiation every morning. I'm still managing to make it in time, but every day I'm a little closer to being late.

A little while after my radiation this morning, I had my weekly appointment with the radiation oncologist. No new news, I'm getting more burned of course, and she told me another skin gel to buy that's supposed to help with the sores I'm developing in addition to the sun burning thing. I have a sore in my radiation area that itches like crazy, so I'm supposed to use cortisone on that.

Today after seeing the radiation oncologist I came to the infusion center for the blood draw they need every three weeks. (You have no *idea* how much blackberry journaling I do!) They draw the blood through my chemo infusion port. But the port keeps getting clotted up so they can't get blood from it. When that happens (which is the case every single time I go for a blood draw now), they inject this de-clotting agent called TPA into my port and I sit and wait. Last time it took two hours and two TPA injections to clear, but after all that, it worked. I don't know how long it will take today, but it didn't work right away today so they TPA'd it and now I'm just in the infusion center blackberrying away and waiting for the TPA to work. I've been here about an hour already.

This is a really nice infusion center. It's new, and each patient is in a little three-sided room with a curtain, a big cushy reclining chair, and a cable flat screen TV. I'm not in one of those rooms today though, because they're all full. Instead they put me in an unoccupied office next to the chemo rooms. No big cushy reclining chair for me! I would definitely be napping right now instead of journaling on my blackberry if I were in a cushy chemo reclining chair.

I get my port taken out in a minor surgery next week, instead of waiting until after radiation. There may be one more blood draw in December that will have to be done through my arm (yuck!), but I wanted to get the surgery done earlier so that if there's any difficulty using my arm it will have a chance to heal before I fly home for Christmas and have to haul luggage around. I originally thought I would have the port removed the week after radiation is done in December, but this way it will have more time to heal and I can leave earlier to go visit my parents. I also wanted to have the port removed during this calendar year so more of the cost will be covered by my health insurance. Good ol' Cynthia Swan, ever the practical analytical planner.

Someone was telling me about a woman they know who has been diagnosed with breast cancer but she doesn't have health insurance. I can't imagine how horrible that would feel, to be told you have cancer when you don't have health insurance. The costs are ridiculous. Like there's not enough to worry about when you have cancer.

They just checked my port, and the TPA hasn't worked yet. They'll check again in half an hour, and TPA it again, probably. More waiting. Uff da. I am sooo ready for a nap.

CANCER—DAY 203 THURSDAY, NOVEMBER 12, 2009

I just got home from yoga. The neuropathy pain was just awful today because I did too much last night.

I went to the Cell Block milonga in San Francisco for just a couple of hours last night. I think I only danced with four guys the whole night, and I sat out a LOT more than I danced. Even so, it still takes *such* a physical toll on me that I find it hard to believe myself. Just walking from my office to the bathroom hurts with the burning in my feet, and a couple of hours in three-inch heels and doing a little tango, well, it quickly becomes unbearable and I'm done for the night. Then I get to sit there and watch my friends dance and be jealous that other people can dance without being in gut-wrenching pain. All the while I'm smiling my fake smile and making small talk, trying to be normal and keep a good face on for everyone. Last night my hands got worse too, and the radiation burn was really getting to me, and by the time we got back to Sacramento it was so bad I couldn't sleep most of the night. It's getting to the point where I associate dancing with pain instead of the serene and playful unity you can have in tango.

I don't care what the doctors say about how neuropathy can be permanent. I cannot imagine this burning stabbing gut-wrenching blinding neuropathy pain lasting forever. It just *has* to get better, or else I'm going to go crazy, because the pain is making me hate doing the thing I love doing most.

I spent most of today day on the LoveSac, hurting too much to do anything, resting and napping. Into the afternoon the burning was a little less, and the stabbing prickly thing had stopped in my hands, so I was determined to go to yoga and to ride my bike there. It was a beautiful day and since Marco's car got stolen we've had just my car and last week he skipped his yoga so I could drive my car to mine in the cold rain. Tonight I wanted to ride my bike so he would take the car and go to his yoga. When Marco skips yoga he gets more crabby, so it's easier all around to do what I can to get him to go, right down to pushing my car keys into his hand and saying I *want* to ride my bike to my yoga (even though it's a cold and rainy night in late November).

I switched to an earlier yoga class tonight. The later class is an introductory one, and last week was the last intro class, so this week I graduated to a real regular practice. The time passed quickly. At the end, during savasana ("corpse pose" for final rest), Kym (my yoga instructor) read a few sentences from a book or a poem, I'm not sure which. But it really got to me emotionally and brought out the tears. It was about the bud and how even things that don't bloom in flower have a bud and do blossom, and it ended with something inspirational about how we as beings rebloom with self-assurance, or something like that. My eyes welled up with tears as she read it, but I didn't really lose it until I got back to the house (Marco wouldn't be back for another hour). I locked myself up with the cats and let it out. I just bawled, releasing more pent up emotion than I thought I had locked up.

Kym's poem really got to me because that's what I feel like it's going to take when cancer treatment is over. I'll go back to my "regular" life, consulting, teaching (grad school, probably not dance), resting peacefully in my forest . . . I will go back to my old life, but it will never be quite the same again. I will never be quite the same again.

When treatment is over, I'll be starting a new life, reblooming, I hope.

Chapter 25.
Tenacious C

CANCER—DAY 204 **FRIDAY, NOVEMBER 13, 2009**

A Special "Gracias" Milonga
Friday, November 13, 2009

Cynthia Swan would like to thank the Sacramento Tango Community for its heartfelt support during her battle with breast cancer by hosting a very special "gracias" milonga!

Location: River Tango

Old Sacramento

Date: Friday, November 13

Free Milonga: 9 p.m. to midnight

DJ: Marco Sasielli

Food & beverages also provided

Come dance the night away and help Cynthia celebrate completing her chemotherapy treatments!

CANCER—DAY 205 SATURDAY, NOVEMBER 14, 2009

Last night was amazing. I can't believe how many people showed up for my Gracias Milonga. Actually, I don't even know how many people there were. I tried to count heads in the group photo we took and it's something over 55. So cool.

And people brought me stuff! I got three bouquets of flowers, and Shaina brought me this beautiful calendar of Renaissance paintings called Beauty & Grace because she said it reminded her of me. How nice is that?

And uff da, Debra (the owner of the tango salon and a dear friend) made this little speech after the group photo to thank me for the milonga and to say what an inspiration I am to have kept attending milongas and supporting the tango community with my involvement even during cancer treatment, and now, even bringing together elements of the tango community that had not shared the dance floor in over a year (people came from all over, from all the studios, regardless of any competitiveness between studios, because I go to all the milongas rather than patronizing just one studio). Debra's speech was a tear-jerker and it really choked me up. Then everyone kept clapping and clapping and clapping and *clapping* until all of us were in tears, including the men, I swear.

This seems strange to me to say, but having cancer actually restored some of my faith in people in general. I didn't even realize how jaded I had become from seeing how poorly so many of us treat other human beings, until I had this experience of having so many people be so wonderfully supportive to me throughout my ordeal.

I stood chatting (and danced) too much, way beyond what the neuropathy in my feet would allow, and I'm really paying for that today. But man, it's so hard to NOT dance! Even when it hurts, I just have to tango.

The radiation burn hurts all the time now, and I'm sore all through my radiation area, on the inside too. Now if I put my right arm straight up over my head, like in yoga, it pulls on the skin and muscles of my radiation site, and boy oh boy is that uncomfortable. I had one excruciating hug when someone lifted me up off the ground last night, and I kind of yelped like a hurt puppy and it took me a few seconds to recover my composure. At first I thought I was going to faint from the sudden sharp pain, but that passed, thank goodness, and I was able to swallow down the pain that wanted to scream out of my body. I told everyone I was all right, it's OK, I'm all right, I'll just sit for a bit, I'm fine, I'll be fine, don't worry.

I had some really, really fun dances and a beautiful romantic tanda with one of my favorite tangueros (like me, he's been to Buenos

Aires many times and he can sing the tango songs in Spanish under his breath, somehow adding to the moment without disturbing it, which is part of his charm). Everyone had a great time. There were even some friends from San Francisco who made the drive out to come to my milonga, how cool is that? Oh, and from Reno, too! People came from all over to show their support. It was unbelievable.

CANCER—DAY 206 SUNDAY, NOVEMBER 15, 2009

There was another milonga last night, a special one-year anniversary at Firehouse 9, and I was determined to go no matter how bad the neuropathy was. Apparently the Tenacious C side of me still has a fair amount of tenacity so I can stubbornly persist in spite of myself. After dancing too much Friday night, I pretty much couldn't even walk Saturday morning, and I was in tears most of the night when I should have been sleeping. So I spent Saturday resting

Last night I danced several tandas in a row with my friend Dietrich (I forget how many songs we danced, I kind of lost track because we were having such a good time). Dietrich hadn't been able to come to my milonga on Friday, so he made it up to me at the Firehouse 9 anniversary milonga. I did dance just one other song with one of my former students, and that was it for me. I don't think Marco danced at all, now that I'm trying to remember it. He just took photos and video and visited with people. Luckily for my feet, they had several special little things going on for the anniversary party: they had a live violinist perform with electronic backup. The live music was good and looked enjoyable to dance to too (I stayed seated, watching the violinist), and there was a harp/violin performance that was amazing. They did a champagne toast which took some time, so I didn't have to just sit out avoiding cabaceos the entire time (because of my feet and hands and radiation burn) longingly watching other people dance. Other than dancing with Dietrich, I was in hard-core non-cabaceo mode all night.

When I'm sitting out, I watch the floor pretty closely most of the time, usually focused on the footwork. I can't help it. Even when I'm chatting with someone, I'm usually watching the dance floor, studying technique and embellishments, taking mental notes of things I want to try to play with or improve in my technique. Watching the floor is also my tactic when I need to rest and not dance (a year ago you would never see me do this, because I danced all night). I keep my eyes focused on the dance floor, watching people's footwork, so that I don't make eye contact with any guys, since looking up would suggest I am open to receiving a cabaceo. Some of the guys are crazy quick with the cabaceo, assuming that the slightest glance in their direction *is* a cabaceo, so when I need to sit out I tilt my chin down and don't make eye contact with anyone, not at all, not even close.

CANCER—DAY 207 MONDAY, NOVEMBER 16, 2009

The police found Marco's car! We just got back from seeing it at the towing impound yard. His car is seriously totaled.

Marco wants a minivan now, to be able to haul workshop stuff around and to get more people in the van for tango trips to San Francisco and such. But of course a minivan costs more than his car was worth, so there's the whole financial thing to work out, the question of getting the bandoneon, and knowing this house is still going into foreclosure at some point. Marco doesn't know if there will be a garage for his workshop at the next place or how much it will cost and so on and so on. Lots of life stresses for Marco on top of dealing with a fatigued, neuropathized, radiation-burned cancer patient living in the house. I don't quite know how he deals with it all, mostly by bottling it up, from what I can tell. As much as he can, anyway. Even when he's ignoring me, the negativity seems to emanate from him in waves of frustration and discontent.

CANCER—DAY 208 TUESDAY, NOVEMBER 17, 2009

The port-removal surgery went fine today, except that I had some internal bleeding afterward so it got more swollen and painful than they would have hoped. Boy, am I ever tired of hearing medical people use the word "hope."

The bigger problem is that I have spent my entire evening heaving my insides out from the anesthesia (again!). I'm trying to drink lots of water, but man, I can't even keep that down. Ugh.

CANCER—DAY 209 WEDNESDAY, NOVEMBER 18, 2009

I called in sick to radiation this morning. I was so miserably nauseous all night that I didn't sleep well, and I ended up staying in bed until nearly two this afternoon. I can't actually skip a day of radiation though, even if I'm sick. So I'm going to be here (in the radiation waiting room) a while. They didn't actually have any appointment openings this afternoon, so when I called early this morning to cancel and they told me to just come in whenever I could and they'd work me in. How nice is that?

Yes, I have often felt like a piece of faulty equipment getting repaired by the medical mechanics, but then there are times like this when the medicos do something very kind and you don't feel like a machine for a moment.

I'm still shaky and haven't tried to eat since all the throwing up last night, but it's been 24 hours since the surgery now, and I haven't thrown up yet today. Early this morning I had some water that turned my stomach, but I kept it down and I managed to have a cup of tea after sleeping practically all day. No Cell Block for me tonight. Good night for Marco to take my car and get out of town for an evening, methinks. If I can stay awake and touch the keyboard, I'll be gaming tonight. Anyone up for World of Warcraft?

CANCER—DAY 210 THURSDAY, NOVEMBER 19, 2009

All right, Mizzou has finally had it with being locked up in a bedroom. Last night he decided it was time for a prison break. Unfortunately it backfired on him . . .

I couldn't stomach real food yesterday after the anesthesia on Tuesday, so I cooked a mushy, bland tuna hot dish for dinner. This is actually a treat for the cats because I always squeeze the tuna juice into little dishes for them to drink and they love it.

Well, I couldn't hold both bowls and open the door at the same time, so I set one bowl down in front of the door and opened the door just enough to slip my hand in to turn on the light. The width of my wrist, apparently, is shockingly also a width that Mizzou can slam his 14 pounds through with amazing stealth and speed. (Just ask Angelina's little dog, Bay Bear, about the time Mizzou bolted through a practically closed door to pounce on Bay Bear and scare the little Pomeranian to death!) But, this was hilarious . . . as soon as Mizzou bolted through the door he slammed on the brakes, slipped on the rug, and whipped a U-turn to come back for the tuna juice, which of course I set down inside the door so he went right back in. Ha!

Mizzou made another break for it when I opened the door this morning, but I was ready for him and caught him on his way out. Time to get us all home to Volcanoville for a night, methinks.

CANCER—DAY 210 FRIDAY, NOVEMBER 20, 2009

There was a guy in the radiation center elevator this morning whose hair looked just like mine. Chemo-pattern baldness, as I've come to think of it.

My hair is a fine fuzz, and I think it's coming in pretty dark, from what I can tell. But the sides and back are of a more normal "density" than the top. On top I have this oval where there just isn't much hair growing yet. It's the same patch that fell out first, so maybe there's a correlation there. I hope the top starts filling in a little before Christmas. Right now I'm still in wigs and hats all the time. The radiation techs get a kick out of me wearing a completely different wig every single day, though. They say they like my attitude . . . "Wigs are the only good thing about chemo!"

Cancer—Day 212 Sunday, November 22, 2009

We played World of Warcraft all day with a couple of Marco's friends (like, seven hours straight), so there wasn't much to fight about. This morning when Marco was waking up, I made him breakfast, so he was a little affectionate for a few minutes after that, but now I think we're back to him just tolerating me. I think.

I haven't talked to him about moving out early. I don't know how to bring it up. When he's not being a selfish jerk complaining that he has no freedom and needs more space, we can get along all right and the situation is tolerable. Mostly he just ignores me and I just stay out of his way.

Do I really want to go to the City tonight? With radiation first thing in the morning? Not really. Maybe I should move over to Brian's tonight while Marco goes to the City? I am ready to leave, I want to leave, to hell with the gossip.

Darn. Marco can't go to the City without my car. And I can't move my stuff to Brian's house without my car, and Brian is out of town. But man oh man is it getting difficult to be here with Marco and the heavy loathing of Cancer Girl just seething from his pores. OK, maybe not *loathing*, but there is definitely a massive negativity apparently caused by my mere presence. He hasn't quite gone past the point of no return with the malcontent that seems to be always coming my direction, though I am now ready to leave at any moment if he gets too mean. It's hard to say what "too mean" is though. But with three weeks of radiation left, I don't want to make a hullaballoo of moving out and having everyone all worried about why I did. The false front has been out there so long now, and I don't want to embarrass Marco or make him look bad. I just want out, and I'm almost counting down the minutes now. Just get through the next sixty seconds, Cynthia, it'll be fine. OK, just another sixty seconds, see, you can do it. Now, another sixty seconds . . .

Cancer—Day 213 Monday, November 23, 2009

Ugh, this is just so *miserable*! I stopped and bought cat litter at the pet store on the way back from radiation, and by the time I got here I was so exhausted I couldn't even stand up and I just managed to get my shoes off before I collapsed in a ball on the LoveSac in my office, right by the door. I couldn't even walk to the bedroom to take my shoes and wig off first (I don't usually nap in the wigs, they get itchy and that often wakes me up). I can't believe how tired I am. And everything hurts, my feet and hands burn with neuropathy, the radiation burn and its little scabby sores is tender, and the port surgery site and all around it is bruised and sore. The surgery site looks pretty nasty too. The entire scar line bled through the steri-strips and you can see where the bruising goes all the way down and then deeper into my chest toward my heart, everywhere the port tube was inside my vein down into my heart.

I ended up having this major meltdown today, crying because I just can't stand it anymore and I'm weary from trying to be the strong person everyone always knew me as before. But I just don't seem to have any strength left. I don't even feel strong enough to call my parents back from yesterday, because I know that hearing in their voices how much they care about me and believe in me will just start me crying again. The idea of another three weeks of all this (or longer, since it's not like I'll miraculously be completely healthy the day radiation is over) is just unimaginable.

After a meltdown, I get upset with myself for having given in to it. So many countless people have cancer and go through this every day, and here I am crying about pain and fatigue like I'm the only person who's ever suffered through it.

I completely lost it on Marco a while ago and was sitting on his office floor just bawling and telling him all stuff about the pain that I've been covering up even around him. He was actually in a supportive mood and he patted my back and reminded me in a positive tone that it's only three more weeks, not so much longer really, and eventually I calmed down. You can only cry so hard for so long before that exhausts you too and your body just doesn't have anything left in it at all. It's a weird kind of emptiness.

At the beginning of all this I was thinking I'd be strong through treatment, that I'd keep working at least part time, and I'd be, well, doing something with the time. Now I think back over the last 213 days and I don't know where the time has gone. Looking back, I realized that I don't really even remember chemo (not that I particularly *want* to remember chemo, I know it was awful and I have been careful not to re-read that section of my journal). When I'm frustrated by the incapacitation like this, I get all down on myself and I think I haven't learned anything, I didn't get stronger as a person, I didn't accomplish anything in my career or my life or with who I am as a person, and after all this time of doing nothing during treatment, here I am now, so fatigued and worn out that I'm having a really hard time even seeing the light at the end of the tunnel. I know it's there and I can tell myself it's close and getting closer, but wow, does it ever seem far away, and I wonder just how I'll get there.

Just do it, Cynthia. Break it down, get through each thing as it comes. Minute by minute the clock is ticking ever closer to the moment treatment will be finished and you are going home. It's coming—the end is there even if you can't quite see it. You can do this, Cynthia. You have to.

CANCER—DAY 214 TUESDAY, NOVEMBER 24, 2009

Here's some news . . . Marco is going to Phoenix for work and his company's Christmas party during my last week of radiation. So it will be very quiet around here while I'm packing up the last of my stuff from Sac to move it home to Volcanoville. He'll be in town on my birthday (Monday the 7th), though I don't know that he wants to do anything different than our usual I-go-to-yoga-early-you-go-to-yoga-late-so-we-don't-really-have-to-be-around-each-other Monday night routine. That Monday may very well be my last yoga class before moving back home, and it definitely won't be a bad thing to go to yoga on my birthday instead of spending it with Marco.

CANCER—DAY 215 WEDNESDAY, NOVEMBER 25, 2009

I saw the radiation oncologist yesterday and she said I'm taking very good care of my skin (in terms of the radiation burn). The skin is burned, has sores, and is peeling, but apparently it could be a whole lot worse! I'm hoping that it won't get much worse. Only two weeks left, after all. I can hang on another two weeks. I can.

I made a comment to the radiation oncologist about the fatigue and told her about how tired I was Monday after running an errand on the way home from radiation and she was all like, yeah, that's totally normal, you pretty much just have to deal with it, take naps as often as you need to, and don't expect it to start improving until about three weeks after radiation. On the positive side, that does work out perfectly (if it's true) since I am determined to go back to work on January 4th no matter what.

CANCER—DAY 217 FRIDAY, NOVEMBER 27, 2009

Yesterday was a quiet Thanksgiving Day . . . we slept in *really* late, and I didn't do a thing except rest and mess around on the computer a little until it was time to get ready to go to Thanksgiving dinner in the evening. We went to a little tango get-together that was very enjoyable. I almost didn't make it there, I was in tears on the drive over because I was having a really hard time getting in control of the pain, which was especially bad in my feet at the time. But I got it together and had a good time, ate too much turkey, and I lasted over three hours in the company of others before I really couldn't hold on anymore and just had to leave. Marco is starting to understand -- when I stop smiling, go completely silent, and stop making eye contact with anyone, the pain is in control over me and I'm done for. But I held out for three hours, which is quite the extended duration these days.

It's a game face thing, I've always had it. I sometimes think I learned it from my mom, but it's probably from having been a performer all my life, in music growing up, public speaking as an adult, teaching grad classes, dancing competitively and for shows while teaching dance classes . . . in some way or another I've been in front of people most of my life. It's ironic, because I was painfully shy growing up. But in terms of any kind of performance or presentation, I think the underlying notion is that just because you feel awful doesn't mean you have to make anyone else feel awful, and so, as much as possible, you grin and bear it rather than take out whatever's wrong on the people around you. I've always done that for work and speaking engagements—it's not like clients need to know you don't feel good or are having a bad day. Same thing with the grad classes. Teaching dance it's the same concept but a more visible impact because you can't let illness slump down your posture or reveal a reduction in your energy level. I've learned how to put on that I-love-what-I'm-doing-and-who-I'm-doing-it-with smile and keep it on through hours upon hours of lessons when I don't feel well or am really stressed or tired. It doesn't matter if your feet hurt, if you are sick, or if you're just plain worn out. The last student of the night deserves the same attention and pleasurable dance lesson that the first student of the day had with you. So, I have a game face, especially for dance. But these days I can only keep it up for so long before I can't do it anymore, and then it's time to disappear to recover for the next thing.

I didn't think ahead to this, but our hostess at Thanksgiving dinner last night asked to go around the table and each of us say what we're thankful for. I was to her right, so after she spoke, I was first. Oh boy, that was an emotional moment for me, and of course all I could choke out was that I was thankful for this community and just being able to be here and to be able to spend time with friends, then, teary, I turned to Marco, who had comfortingly taken my hand. It was Marco's turn. He said something about being thankful for me and that I was doing so well . . . I have to admit I was dumbfounded by his sincerity and it really got to me. Of all the things he could tell this whole group that he's thankful for . . . well, it was definitely an unexpected moment of tenderness to hear him say something about being thankful about me. Later I realized that Marco has a pretty clear delineation of my Jekyll & Hyde. He's fed up with Cancer Girl, but he's thankful for, and cares quite deeply about, Cynthia Swan. Interesting, that the bipolar existence of normal identity and cancer identity seems to reside in both cancer patient and caregiver.

One more Thanksgiving story, sort of. On Monday at yoga my instructor, Kym, was already in a Thanksgiving mood, and at the end of the practice while we were in savasana she suggested that we perhaps take a moment to think about something we were thankful for. I immediately thought of my parents and how much they love me. It was such a strong emotional pull that it instantly brought me to tears. Even when they don't know it, they are the underlying emotional support when I have to reach deep inside myself for more. I am truly lucky to be so loved and so blessed.

CANCER—DAY 218 SATURDAY, NOVEMBER 28, 2009

I don't always feel weak exactly, but I often feel like I don't have any strength left these days. It's a strange kind of completely-worn-out feeling. It's like I can't quite believe myself when I tell people all the things you're supposed to assure people of when you're in cancer treatment: "I'm doing ok." "It's almost over." "I'm hanging in there." "I'm going to be fine."

I've been wondering for quite a while now what "fine" really means, and when I'll actually be there. (Like, what if the neuropathy really is permanent and I am in pain the rest of my life, never to dance pain-free again? That is my most scary thought now.) If I could just get my head around it I'd probably decide that being "fine" is a state of mind and is whatever you make of it. But then I wonder about specifics. Here I sit in my own back yard, in this place of peace and beauty, but I'm feeling lost rather than at peace in the beauty of the moment.

I used to think I was good at living in or appreciating the moment, but now I have so many days like this where I feel kind of lost in life. I forget to breathe.

Right now the lake is calm while the trees whisper with the wind and scent the air with purity. Life is everywhere. That's something I need to remind myself of. This is what I need to remember when I have to tenaciously conjure up more inner strength to get through another day of treatment.

CANCER—DAY 220 MONDAY, NOVEMBER 30, 2009

Radiation is constant and monotonous. The only change is the progression of the burn. My radiation oncologist said that monotony is part of the reason people get fatigued by radiation, because it's draining to keep going through this treatment regimen day after day week after week.

I think being in pain all the time is what's been so fatiguing for me. So, nap time it is.

CANCER—DAY 221 TUESDAY, DECEMBER 1, 2009

They changed my radiation today. For the first 28 treatments, they were doing a proton radiation, and today they changed to an electron radiation that they're going to do for the next two weeks . . . they call it a radiation "boost." There was some confusion as to the technical details for my radiation boost, so one of the techs was running back and forth to my radiation oncologist confirming the setup while they had me on the table this morning (oy vey, is that thing COLD!). The notes in my chart were conflicting. There was a note for them to use the same bolus as before, which is circular and about two inches in diameter, not too bad in terms of the size of skin patch getting the extra burn. But the doctor told the tech to radiate the entire electron field, which is essentially the entire area that's been burned already and that didn't make sense with the small bolus. Bummer is that it turns out that they had to use a new bolus that is absolutely huge, and they used three long strips of tape to secure it, so all three of my worst burn spots had to have tape *peeled off* after the radiation treatment, taking some skin with it. Awful! I hope tomorrow the tape won't be as sticky . . .

I actually had the *best* evening last night. Yoga was cool because Kym was focusing on the hyoid bone in the top of the neck, and thinking about moving that bone really helped stretch my spine and I feel better somehow. Then I had dinner at Brian's house. He grilled steaks and opened a great bottle of wine and we spent the evening remembering all these great stories of fun adventures we've had together. All the way back to the first day we met, which was so much fun we laugh ourselves silly in the retelling of the tale. It felt soooooooo good to laugh. It's amazing what one evening with your best friend can do for morale.

CANCER—DAY 222 WEDNESDAY, DECEMBER 2, 2009

Uff da, the neuropathy has been worse with the cold weather (it's been in the low 50s), especially in my feet. I hope it won't get much worse when I go to Nebraska where it's truly *cold* this time of year.

Last week sometime (I think) I uploaded a few family photos to my Facebook. Which got me looking at some of my other Facebook photos, like from dancing West Coast Swing (WCS) for the filming of *Love 'N Dancing*. The second weekend of the filming, I was partnered with Edward Lee, one of the WCS champions (oooh, now there's a smooth lead for you). We had a blast hanging out that weekend, besides all the fun (amidst some dreary repetitiveness) of the movie filming. So anyway, to finally get around to the story that all this Facebook photo stuff made me remember today . . .

I was on a long road trip when I went to Albuquerque for the filming. During my road trip, I would work from whatever hotel I was at during the day and then drive to a new town in the evening. I took the cats with me, the traveling twosome, Mizzou and his minion kitten, Seoul. For the movie filming in Albuquerque, they put us up at a nice desert resort, 5-star. I had a ground level room with a huge patio to work from and it was just beautiful. However, the first day there, when I walked in from the patio for a break the cats were being all freaky. Suddenly Mizzou *bursts* after something that had been hiding under the footstool and was startled by my entrance. It was crazy. Mizzou followed every zigzag and circle and kept right up with this insanely quick Speedy Gonzalez. When the mouse disappeared behind the headboard (a 2-inch gap), Mizzou could only take up his vigilant watch again. (Seoul studied Mizzou's technique and took notes from the safety of the ottoman. She a curious cat, but not brave like Mizzou, at least, not yet.)

When they brought room service later, I asked the girl if mice were common out there because of being in the desert, to which she said they do catch one once in a while. She sent two maintenance guys over, and they moved the bed and all the furniture away from the walls but didn't find the mouse. I honestly wasn't too concerned. Mice can flatten themselves to slip under doors, but I knew Mizzou would get the mouse if it idiotically decided to venture back into Mizzou's territory.

Which it did sometime the next day. When I got back from the first day of filming that weekend, there was the mouse, dead on the floor by the ottoman. Mizzou looked very satisfied with himself, lounging on the bed like the king of the realm he is. Seoul, still a small kitten then, adoring and in awe, was lying nearby but respecting the space Mizzou commanded. Seoul was star-struck by Mizzou the Mouse Killer.

I put the mouse in a Ziploc bag and put it in the garbage can, then met up with Edward and Benji (yes, Benji Schwimmer, the guy who won *So You Think You Can Dance*) and the two stars of the *Love N' Dancing* movie we were dancing for. A maintenance guy walked by, and I told him about the dead mouse and asked if they wanted me to do anything in particular with it. He said he'd send someone to my room to get the mouse. Then, of course, I had to tell the whole story to everyone in the hot tub. The funniest part is that Tom, the lead actor, was all freaked out that there had been a mouse in my room. It was ridiculously funny, how nervous he looked at the prospect of a mouse running around in a hotel room. Now *that* was some fun storytelling, to get such a reaction from a grown man about a mouse!

Ahh, memories of a different life.

CANCER—DAY 223 THURSDAY, DECEMBER 3, 2009

Last night we went to Cell Block and looked at a couple bandoneons (the bandoneon is the elemental accordion-like instrument in tango orchestras). Marco got to play them, and the guy who's going to teach him to play was also there and played them for us as well (it was amazing to sit two feet from an astounding professional bandoneon player working the instrument in his hands) and he told us his opinion regarding which would be the best instrument for Marco. The first one was newer and a little cheaper because it was made after World War II (post-WWII bandoneons just don't sound as good as the ones made in the 20s & 30s, seriously). It was black and in very good condition inside and out, and mechanically sound. The second one, a dark cherry wood, was made in the 30s and had a more resonate, richer sound compared to the black one, which had a brighter sound. Based on the sound and character of the instruments, I would have gone for the older, richer-sounding, more expensive bandoneon if I were buying it. But that one was also appreciably older, and while it had tons of character, it also had its signs of aging, and would be more difficult for Marco to learn on because the key tension varied fairly significantly. The newer one had very even key tension, and that was what ultimately convinced both of us that Marco should go with the newer one, which will be easier for him to learn on.

The guy who was selling them wasn't pushy at all. He loves these instruments and he seemed to genuinely enjoy just having someone be so interested in seeing them and taking them apart and comparing them. When Marco told the guy he was interested in the black one, the guy told him he'd hold it for Marco for a month to give Marco time to think about it. I liked that, because I know Marco needed a week to move cash around to make the purchase (the higher priority and more pricey need right now being for Marco to get a car to replace the one that was stolen).

The polar opposite of my opinion—that the guy was pleasantly non-pushy—Marco was turned off by that very fact. He thought the guy should push for the sell, and since the guy didn't push Marco to buy the instrument then and there, now Marco's being a bit waffley about the purchase. Interesting. That is definitely not my approach, but then again, I wouldn't go looking at fine instruments and opening them up to expose the insides to contaminating air particles and such unless I was already completely committed to buying one to begin with. I don't know if Marco is also questioning his decision to get a bandoneon as well as a car, or if he is really only concerned that the guy wasn't pushing him to buy the instrument.

It was an interesting reminder of how different we are, and also an important realization for me to remember what kind of person I am—decisive, dedicated, motivated, and committed. Once I have analyzed every aspect, determined my feelings, and made a decision to do something, I do it. I don't waffle and I don't give up. That's how I got the nickname Tenacious C. That's the inner me that's going to survive it all, because Tenacious C is determined to do so.

Chapter 26.
That's a Wrap

CANCER—DAY 224 FRIDAY, DECEMBER 4, 2009

Marco bought a new car today! Well, not brand new, but a good replacement to his stolen and totaled Acura. It's been six weeks since Marco's car was stolen. I think Yoda (as I affectionately refer to my Toyota Camry) is relieved to be getting a break from being the only vehicle for both of us. It's too late to keep me out of the cold and fog riding my bike to yoga all this time, but at least Marco won't need my car anymore, and I don't have to worry about whether or not to offer to loan it to him while I'm away visiting my parent at Christmas like I had almost decided to do. I've never had a "shared" vehicle before, I've always had my own car, so this has been an interesting six weeks of compromise, or something like compromise. It's do-able, but I would be lying if I said we could easily have only one car between the two of us indefinitely. That is definitely *not* the case. The ever-independent Cynthia Swan most definitely prefers having the freedom to come and go as she pleases with her own car!

I had an unexpectedly candid talk with Lisa at the wine club party tonight. Marco was avoiding me, and I went into the bedroom where the coats were to get in control of the neuropathy pain and to compose myself from feeling rejected by the guy who, to this point, has been pretending to be my boyfriend for months. I was sitting there in the coat room blackberry journaling and feeling pretty bad about how terrible the relationship with Marco had become, and who walks in but Lisa, the woman who had breast cancer two years ago and is a strong survivor. She was incredibly encouraging at the beginning when she heard about my diagnosis, and we've had many good talks as I went through treatment. She came into the coat room while I was sitting in there last night and, seeing my facial expression and guessing the situation, sat down and asked me what was wrong. I couldn't speak. All I could do was burst into the tears I had been so vigorously trying to control. I felt awful. But she's been through the same thing, the same way, except that she suffered through it alone while living with her now ex-husband. Same kind of person as Marco, her ex-husband, so Lisa seriously gets how I'm feeling. And knowing all that about her, I couldn't hide how I was feeling from her.

I said simply "Marco is mean to me." I didn't know what else to say. But Lisa said she understood completely. She told me how when she diagnosed, Marco was pretty unsupportive, breezing through the standard lines of "You'll be fine, this is just a bump in the road and life goes on" and then immediately changing the subject to something he wanted to talk about.

She also said—very positively—how it's only a week more and I'll have time with my family to think and decide what I want, and what I want my life to be like. Lisa also pointed out that we had no real relationship when the cancer started, so the relationship had no foundation on which to survive together, and it will be no loss in my life if he is not a part of it in the future. Ironically (or not), that was just what I needed to hear at that moment so I could pull myself together to put on The Act for a couple more hours and get through the evening.

CANCER—DAY 225 SATURDAY, DECEMBER 5, 2009

I thought I was going to stay through in Sacramento this weekend for tango, but instead I drove home to Volcanoville today, and when I got here it was just gorgeous out! The weather in Sac has been cloudy, cold and wet, but at home it's fifteen degrees warmer with that perfect California blue sky the state is known for. Just beautiful. And the cats love being out here, having an entire house to roam around in and even getting to go outside when I lie in my hammock. Seoul's gotten a little clingy . . . when I first got home with them, the first few hours, she followed me around from room to room as I put things away and such. She didn't settle in until I sat down and stayed put for a while. She and I had a nice nap on my big comfy sofa.

I'm skipping the Saturday night milonga and the Sunday night milonga. This weekend I seriously needed the peace and solitude of my home in the mountains much more than I needed to push myself to put on The Act to be with other people and telling them I'm OK while my feet are in burning agony inside my tango shoes. I attempt to tango, a few songs in a night, but mostly these days I'm just sitting out and chatting with people. But right now I'm relaxing on the couch and just enjoying being in my own home for a couple of nights before the last week of radiation.

CANCER—DAY 226 SUNDAY, DECEMBER 6, 2009

Now that it's almost over, I've been pondering . . . how did I survive all this? There were actually a ton of different little things I did to get through it day after day after day. My head kept swirling around with this all day yesterday, wondering how it all fits together, just *how* I survived to this point, days away from being done with radiation, done with the worst of cancer treatment (I hope).

So many cancer survivors say the emotional support from their caregiver was an important factor for them. In my case, my "caregiver" was an additional challenge. A big challenge. So, no emotional support there. I did have a lot of emotional support from countless other sources, though.

I had a lot of emotional support and love from my family and friends, as you would expect, but also more than I would ever expect.

My mom was constantly calling, telling me about how her friends were always asking how I was doing and how supportive everyone was being. There were only a few people I would talk on the phone with, and even fewer now because it's gotten harder and harder to hide pain and emotion in my voice. I think I only talked to my brother voice-to-voice once or twice during treatment, but I talked with my mom and dad, and Artie's mom, frequently. I'm not really a phone person though.

Rather than talking on the phone though, I have been using every other communications technology to the max. I have friends all over the country and overseas because I've moved and traveled a lot, and it made me smile when, while I was instant messaging with a friend in India, Brian texted me "Oktoberfest! Just had to send a quick hug and a smile to my Cynthia!" from Germany. I have no idea what time it was for either of them, but it was like I was getting 24-hour online support from my friends.

People that I only know professionally have shown themselves to be wonderful friends that I didn't even realize I had, sending e-mails and cards and flowers and such. I mean, I've always liked and enjoyed my colleagues (I figure, we only have so much time in this world, better to spend it with people you respect and appreciate), but I never expected the kind of constant and personal support I have received from people I've only known in a professional setting.

I was on Facebook at some point practically every day trading messages with people and posting photos of each new wig after I'd been out to a milonga or to a wine club party. I think I have more than a dozen wigs now, all different lengths and styles and colors. People ask why I have so many wigs, and I tell them that "Being bald is the best part about having about chemo, and changing wigs is the only fun thing about having cancer!"

I tweeted frequently (short posts on Twitter), trying to keep upbeat by tweeting amusing little things that happened or that occurred to me as I was going through something. Like after the first MRI, I tweeted something like "Did you know there are 2,639 buzzes and clunks during an MRI? Seriously, I counted!" I also tweeted to give everyone quick status updates, like on chemo day, "At least they make you woozy before infusing you with chemo poison," or "Just had first radiation. You should see this machine, it's like the back end of a rocket!!" I played online Scrabble with a group of friends, and I traded Facebook flair and Facebook "pokes" with others. People I hadn't talked to in years were constantly sending me Facebook messages, like my high school boyfriend's sister. Talk about a fun person I hadn't had contact with in years! Which reminds me of one other person I *did* talk to on the phone . . . *uff* da . . . the first post-diagnosis conversation with my high school boyfriend was seriously emotional because we were both kind of upset by the whole thing. We hadn't talked in about two years, though, so it was also a ton of fun to catch up on each others' experiences and stories, to remember good old times, and to laugh.

Especially after college, I've made a concerted effort to listen more than I speak in a conversation. People will tell you amazing things if you just shut up and stop thinking about yourself and what you want to say next. That little practice turned out to be extremely helpful during treatment. I tried to get into other people's stories as much as possible to distract myself from dwelling on my own current situation. That saved me from a lot of self-pity, though it got harder to pay attention as the neuropathy worsened. The pain also kept me from talking though, so I guess that one's a wash—at least I was *trying* to listen rather than talk to hear my own voice. Whether or not I heard and understood what was being said was probably debatable.

I ended up having these long e-mail conversations with other women with breast cancer who read my blog. Ironically, I now have numerous friends that I've never "met" who are now a part of my emotional support network. The women that contacted me would tell me about their own treatment experiences and ask me questions. That did a lot for me too, actually, because it made me think about what I was doing to get through it, in order to encourage them that they can get through it too. Same thing with women who called me on a referral from the cancer center for, well, peer counseling I guess. I'm not a licensed counselor or anything, but if someone contacted me, I would just talk (or instant message or e-mail or whatever) with the woman and try to be encouraging and supportive, and be an open ear for the things she couldn't say to her spouse or family or friends, like her worries and fear.

One thing I did not do much was go to breast cancer support group meetings. Marshall had separate support group meetings for patients and caregivers, and I often wished Marco would go to the caregiver ones because he could have vented his frustrations to a supportive audience, but I can't judge him harshly on something I only did for a month myself. I liked the women in the breast cancer support group and the conversations were mutually supportive in a way, but the more difficult treatment became, the less I wanted to talk about what I was going through. I would have been fine just listening, but they go around the room one by one and each person says something about where they are in treatment or how many years they've been a survivor and whatever they're dealing with at the moment. I could listen to other people talk, I could engage in conversation, but I did not want to talk about my treatment or side effects or pain any more. I was doing everything possible to not even *think* about any of that, so after a month or so I stopped going to cancer support group meetings. Maybe after treatment I'll give it another try, when I'm a post-treatment survivor.

My yoga class was a kind of group therapy, because everyone has problems, not just cancer patients. So I often stayed late after yoga talking with the other people that had been in my yoga practice, asking them about their lives and just, well, talking. Yoga in and of itself has been great for helping me stay calm when I otherwise would not be able to, but the people in my yoga sessions were like a special little support group, just because of what we were experiencing together in yoga.

I was online much of the day, and people would instant message me though a widget I put on the blog page of my website. My cousins did that a lot, and that was another way I met other women with breast cancer. One woman instant messaged me to say she was diagnosed that very morning, she had just spent four hours reading the entire *Cielem'el Cancer Journal*. She read *every word* that I had written and put in the Web log, and she simply wanted to thank me and tell me that reading about my experiences was inspirational to her for facing the upcoming months of her own treatment. My response was "Holy cow, you read my ENTIRE blog in one sitting? That's amazing!" She told me what little she knew about her diagnosis (the doctors don't really know much about squat until your surgery when they can test lymph nodes and such). She then told me she's afraid of what's coming but she was inspired by my story, and I reassured her that she will get through it and not to be frightened of the process and just keep going and she'll make it. The conversation ended with an upbeat dialog about wigs, I think.

Shifting away from emotional support a little bit . . . I did a ton of research online, all the way through. The very first night after my gynecologist had found the lump and ordered tests for the next morning, I spent most of the night online reading everything I could with the tidbits she had given me so far and learning how the tests were done and how to read the films and just, well, everything. I have been like that all the way through, every day. Every time there was a new side effect, every time something unexpected happened in treatment, and before whatever was coming up next in treatment, I was online digging and learning about breast cancer. I don't really like the saying "Knowledge is power," because it seems to imply that by knowing more than someone else you are better than the other person, which I find a bit disturbing. I believe, as human beings, we should always treat everyone with the same level of consideration and respect. So I don't like saying knowledge is power, but I do appreciate knowledge. I research and collect facts to no end. I am a data pack rat and I enjoy learning and figuring things out, analyzing or trying to look at a situation from a different perspective. I tried to learn about cancer from any and all sources, be it from cancer websites, survivor stories, medical journals, the Chicken Soup books—you name it, I was reading it. Academic, personal, emotional, supportive, critical . . . there are so many ways to look at this thing called cancer and this experience called treatment and how we become survivors. "Knowledge is power" doesn't begin to address it. My approach became more of a Sun Tzu thing: "Know thy enemy." It's easy to think of cancer as the enemy, and the more I learned about cancer, the less afraid I was. I probably should have become *more* afraid, but, it is what it is. The more I know about what I'm getting myself into, the less afraid I am to do it.

Journaling did a lot for getting the hard realizations and most depressing emotions out of my head so I could at least function. My cancer blog has been about 200 pages or so, but my private journal since diagnosis has more than 450 pages to it. I write in my private multi-level security-protected saved-to-thumb-drive always-on-my-person digital journal to get the bad feelings out, get the pain out of my head by shoving all that into my journal, putting it in my pocket, and mentally locking it away from my active thoughts as much as possible. My journal is also full of little gems and stories about anything good that happened, all the wonderful notes I received from people, and, well, a lot of pep talk to myself. I go in there and I write in third person telling myself to get off my damn bum and go to yoga, or stir up my gumption, put on a wig, and go to the milonga. I used my public blog to keep telling the story with honesty but without the ugliness, censored. Writing the blog kept my family and friends informed, but for me, it was both a release and a continual reminder—I was trying to survive with grace, looking for a positive perspective on each thing that happened so I wasn't all depressing in the online journal—or I would tell funny stories along the way to distract myself and everyone else from the worst aspects of cancer treatment or the experience.

I did everything I could to keep a positive outlook and demeanor. The first thing was keeping a smile on my face no matter what. At first I managed to keep the spark in my eye too, but that light went out pretty quickly once chemo started. No one else seemed to notice that but me, though. I bet my mom will be able to tell when I explain to her what to look for in my expression, comparing photos from last spring to now. But when I was down one day and told my mom on the phone that my spark was gone, I think she took it more metaphorically than literally, as I meant it.

Once I was in chemo, instead of just always smiling, it became "a wig and a smile." People would say things like "I just don't know how you get through it!" Smiling (of course), I would say something like "A wig and a smile can go a long way to making yourself feel normal."

Another, potentially less positive "positive" perspective that I use on myself comes out in two sayings I use a *lot*. "It is what it is," and "It could be worse." I have said "It is what it is" so many times now that I really do have myself convinced of the truly positive perspective of the saying. If you can accept that it is what it is right at this moment, then you can see this moment as a starting point for moving forward. That one does a lot for me. If I keep moving forward, I'm not going backwards, right?

The "It could be worse" motto is, admittedly, not as positive an approach. Telling myself that other people have it worse than I do is a pretty negative way to look at it, like other people suffering is a good thing in some psycho Nazi way. When I use "It could always be worse" on myself, I'm trying to remind myself to be grateful for all the good things that I *do* have—wonderful parents, lots of people who care about me, a beautiful peaceful national forest to go home to some days, a roof over my head so I don't have to drive for hours for radiation, good memories, whatever. I've read that gratitude is the strongest emotion, even stronger than love, and I believe it. When you go through your day looking for things to be grateful for, the opportunities are endless, and the effect is utterly inspiring. I have countless blessings to be thankful for every single day, and if I can make myself pay attention to that and be grateful and express gratitude to others, it makes me feel better as a person even if it doesn't change my situation or make me feel better physically or feel less neuropathy pain. Spend a whole day finding reasons to say thank you to people and see how you feel that evening. Pretty freaking amazing, floating on air, buoyed by gratitude.

Lovely as that sounds, there are plenty of times when that just seems impossible to do and I turn to other means of surviving. As things became more and more difficult, I spent more time trying to find the calm I vaguely remembered having at my home in the mountains before all this happened. During treatment I would sit and listen to the waterfall sound of my aquarium and watch my fish for hours on end, just breathing. Thinking about breathing, even, to distract my mind from the pain as much as possible.

In the last three weeks or so, I started counting my breaths. "Getting through it" became so compartmentalized that I was taking it one breath at a time, literally. Early on there were these big chunks of time to get through. First surgery, then chemo, then radiation, and —whoohoo!—there's the finish line! In chemo I first broke the time down into months, then number of infusions, then number of weeks. During infusion week I would take it one day at a time.

The most difficult countdown has been getting to this point, right now, today. Last week, as the living situation with Marco became pretty much unbearable and the neuropathy was just burning away and that pain was completely boggling my mind so I couldn't even think, I *really* got into the countdown. I told myself to just get through this day, and deal with tomorrow, tomorrow. But that was too long a time, too daunting to demand of myself. I started telling myself, OK, Cynthia, breathe, just get through this morning of radiation, then worry about getting through the afternoon, then deal with getting through the night. It became hour by hour, my little breakdown for counting the passage of time. There have been times in the last three weeks when I've counted the seconds to try to not think about anything else. When the neuropathy pain is absolutely awful, I start thinking in seconds. One second at a time, count to sixty, when the pain is unbearable. Now take a calm breath and let the seconds tick by. It takes me about five seconds to take one calming breath. That means twelve breaths to get through the next minute. I can take just twelve breaths without going to pieces, right? OK, now take another breath, Cynthia. Good girl, now do it again, good. Breathe in, breathe out. Breathe in, breathe out. Twelve times and you are another minute closer to surviving through the bitter end. Survive, that's all you have to do. Just survive. Don't worry about cancer recurrence or the next dreadful treatment. Just survive this day, this hour, this minute. Just take a breath, Cynthia. Breathe, and the seconds will pass.

But now we're just down to tricks I use on myself for "just surviving" as I think of it, just getting through it. Strokes of a paintbrush. So where's the big picture?

I have two answers here, but I cannot separate them—they are completely entwined in me. First, I made this promise to myself right at the beginning that I was *not* going to make other people miserable, that no matter what happened I would not become this "poor me" soliciting pity from others or making other people feel bad for not being sick like me or not being sympathetic or whatever. I made a commitment to myself at the outset that I would do this thing while being as kind and thoughtful of others as I possibly could. Whenever I saw any other people, *any* other people be it friends or a grocery store clerk, I put on the smile and tried to be normal and make pleasant conversation. That was the bare minimum of the promise I made to myself. And, let's face it, Tenacious C didn't get her nickname by giving up just because there's been a setback, like severe side effects. Just because something has gotten harder to do does not mean I should quit. I don't give up just because something is hard or difficult. Catching a snag or bumping into a wall doesn't mean stop trying, it means try harder.

This is where it ties together. I refused to give up tango. When I refuse to give up, that's when Marco calls me Tenacious C, which is making me smile as I write this.

I gave myself what I felt was an ambitious growth goal of going through cancer treatment with grace and kindness, and tango became the where and how for gauging my progress (if any, or at least making sure I wasn't moving backward). The goal became more and more difficult as things went wrong or the pain became unbearable, but that didn't mean I could just give up on myself. I made a promise to myself. *Myself!* If I can't keep a promise I make to myself, what good can I possibly do for anyone else? OK, OK, slow down here. Truth—I know I haven't always been good for Marco. I've tried, and I've made a lot of mistakes, sometimes just by being me and having *that* be wrong for him. But he's also told me many times that the situation itself is stressful and therefore frustrating for him and he didn't blame me for that. He always refused me leaving when I said I could go stay somewhere else so he wouldn't have to deal with it anymore. If he was so stressed and frustrated by the situation, and I was offering him an easy way out, why didn't he take it? Maybe he wanted find a little Tenacious C in himself, or have some of my tenacity rub off onto him. He was at an interesting crossroad in life when we met. Through some setbacks and twists of life, he seemed to feel that he had failed himself in the past, not achieved his goals as it were, and here was his crossroad: it was time for him to take a stand and believe in himself, or give up and well, not believe in himself and just accept, I don't know, mediocrity. I think that's how he described it—his fear was mediocrity and because he hadn't met certain financial or family life goals that he set for himself wayyyyy back when, he was questioning himself as a person, losing faith in himself. So here he is at this cloudy amorphous place in his life, and then he meets me, quite likely the most tenacious person he's ever known (I'm not boasting, that's what he says made him want to do the whole caregiver thing, giving himself a chance to be tenacious and committed to a purpose, to a good and noble purpose). That could be an interesting conversation after Christmas, asking Marco how he looks upon the experience with hindsight, going all the way back to what his life was like before he ever met me at all.

Whoa, OK, that was a tangent. Interesting thoughts and perspectives to ponder later, but off the subject. Besides, it's getting late and I've been writing practically all day (with lots of little breaks so my fingers endure the neuropathy). But I'm close to something, I'm really close to the most important thing, the real "how" of this whole thing, the challenge and the growth experience and everything that my life has been since that phone call long ago telling me it *looked* like cancer.

Simply put—I believe in myself. I believe in myself because my parents believed in me whenever I wanted to try something new growing up. And they somehow knew how to challenge me so that I would try, *really* try, without getting so discouraged that I gave up. That's how music became such a big part of my life, starting, gosh, in kindergarten. Playing the piano was difficult, I had to practice a lot, and my mom would make me sit at that darn piano every day while she made dinner and if I made a mistake she said "That's OK honey, do it again, you'll get it," and when I played something right she'd call out "That was beautiful!" Oh yeah, and when I sat there glaring at the keys because I was frustrated, there was her voice from the kitchen teasingly calling out "I don't *hear* anything . . . " essentially guilting me into plunking on the keys again even if it was just one stupid frustrating note at a time. It was hard, but I loved it. And when I started playing the flute and later got a music scholarship for college, it was *hard.* My college flute instructor was a drill sergeant and the pieces she expected me to master required hours of practice every day, every single day. But I could see where it was going, and I loved it. I also became more practical and got a degree in economics so I could get a "real" job after college instead of being a starving artist. But the point is, the goals were hard to achieve but I believed in myself, I kept trying, and I didn't give up on myself, which evolved into the tenacity Marco has so often admired since we met.

Like music was for me in school, tango became my sincere avocation (as opposed to my vocation in consulting, as my dad would say). It's complex, it's hard, and when it's right it is absolutely unlike anything else in this world, two people moving like one person. One heart, four legs.

As treatment knocked me down with side effect upon side effect, as the fatigue piled on and then the neuropathy threw me upside down and sideways, I gave up more and more of the activities that had been my reason for staying in California for treatment in the first place. But not tango.

In a way I've given in to the physical challenges of the chemo side effects because I don't dance every song of the entire night like I used to. In another way (at least this is what I tell myself), I haven't given in to the disease or the treatment, because I keep going.

I put on the wig and the smile. I go to the milongas where I tango a tanda or two if I can stay in control of the neuropathy pain. I get (and keep) myself in "kind" Cynthia mode talking with other people, encouraging them in whatever they're doing, asking them questions about their lives and smiling and laughing as much as possible—all at the milongas. I've been going to milongas every week, usually twice and sometimes three times a week since chemo (once a week at best during most of chemo). I've been staying very active in the tango community, putting on the wig and the smile and spending time with people in the tango community. And somehow, by trying to convince them that I was all right, I was convincing myself of that as well. As the neuropathy became unbearable, I danced less and less, but I still went to the milongas. The bottom line is that I refused to give up tango. I would not let cancer or pain take that away from me.

In a way, that's been a bigger part of how I've gotten through this than I expected. I love being home, but with radiation every weekday and most of the milongas being on the weekend, I had to choose between going home or staying in Sacramento to go to milongas even though going home would have been the easier choice (and probably better for my relationship with Marco). But I can't drive four hours from home for tango like I did before treatment. And I could not give up tango, so I gave up coming home instead. This is one of the few weekends since finishing chemo that I finally chose home over tango. I'm glad I did because I wanted the space and quiet to think, to muster up that last little gulp of strength to get through the last week of radiation, and breathe in the beauty of this place. I get lots of good clean energy from being at my little place in the national forest.

Staying at home, or (more likely) going to stay with my parents during treatment would have been easy. At least, it would have been easier than this. But without the challenge and a way to get there, what was the point of having a goal? The goal was kindness and grace, cancer was the challenge, and tango became the means to get there.

CANCER—DAY 227 MONDAY, DECEMBER 7, 2009

It's my birthday. I had forgotten it's my birthday, until I got part-way to town where there's cell signal and my cell phone started dinging and donging with all the text messages people had been sending me all morning to wish me a happy birthday. It was going off again and again all afternoon with each new happy birthday note. Technology can be so fun!

My parents called this morning but since there's no signal way out at my house, they got my voicemail. Instead of just leaving a message, they *sang* "Happy Birthday" to my voicemail. Too cute!

After my last yoga class, Marco took me out for dinner and a movie. We haven't done that in a long, long time. In the restaurant after dinner, the restaurant staff all came out clapping with a dish of ice cream for me and they shouted to the entire restaurant that it was my "21st" birthday, and they made the whole restaurant shout "Yee Haw!" to me. Marco was so sneaky. I had no idea he was slipping off to talk to the staff when he got up to use the restroom early in our dinner. The surprise made it fun though!

CANCER—DAY 228 TUESDAY, DECEMBER 8, 2009

What an insane day. I spent the entire day packing up my office and disassembling my office furniture. (Well, the entire day after noon, that is, since I can't seem to get out of bed until the last possible minute before having to go to radiation, and then I nap when I get back because I'm so tired, but anyway, it was Radiation Girl's version of the entire day.) Brian came over with his truck to take the last of my stuff (all the big stuff, including my aquarium) to my home in Volcanoville while Marco is out teaching tonight. Marco only wanted my stuff moved out by the end of the year, but since I'm leaving Thursday right after radiation to fly to my parents' to surprise them by coming home early for Christmas, and I'm not coming back to California until after New Year's, I wanted to get everything out now, before I fly out. I've been gradually moving stuff back home for ages, a carload at a time every time I went home. Marco probably would probably be OK with my stuff being at his house until sometime in January when I should have more energy for packing and moving (and hopefully less neuropathy killing my hands), but you know, once someone bluntly asks you when you're going to move your stuff out after your treatment is over, well, it just doesn't feel good to stick around or leave anything behind after that kind of conversation. So I finished packing everything today—books, clothes, office furniture, aquarium—and by the time Brian showed up I was done *in.* My hands were toast, just little claws that couldn't grip anything, and I was exhausted. Brian had to load everything in the truck by himself (Marco was busy working at his computer). Then up at my house Brian unloaded everything and got all the heavy stuff (the office furniture) put away in the garage for me, and he moved a bookcase to the guest room to make room in my living room for the aquarium, which he also put into place for me . . . he even nailed up the artwork I had framed while I was at Marco's house. (Now *there's* a benefit of being six and a half feet tall, you don't need a ladder to hang artwork!) I tell ya, Brian is one of a kind, one of the best friends a person could have. Bummer he's moving to Denver next month to live with his fiancé, but YAY for him that he's getting married next year. It's always neat to see a happy person made even happier by the one they love. That's Brian.

My last radiation session is on Thursday. Then I'm flying to Denver, and on to Sidney. Originally I wasn't supposed to fly home for another week or two, but then, sometime in November, I think, I decided there wasn't much point to staying any longer than absolutely necessary at Marco's, so I changed my flight up to the 15th so I could be home longer. As Marco got more and more burned out in my cancer treatment, I started missing my family more and more, and when this thing came up that Marco had to go to Phoenix the last few days of my radiation, it just didn't make sense to stay around Sac even one more weekend to dance when I could already be with my family, where I am so longing to be right now. So last week I changed my flight AGAIN, and bumped it up to this Thursday, a few hours after my last radiation session. But I didn't tell my parents, I didn't tell anyone who was connected to my parents in any way and it's not on my website, only my local Sac friends know I'm flying home right after my last radiation.

My parents don't know. They still think I'm not flying home next Monday because I need one last weekend to go to the milongas and see my friends one more time before I leave for the holidays. My parents should be pretty darned surprised when I ring their doorbell Thursday night! I do that sometimes, surprise them by showing up early for a visit, and they always love the surprise. Their friends ask them when I'm going to be back in Sidney next, and my mom tells them "You never know, she could appear on our doorstep tomorrow!"

I am so relieved to be going home, *soon*. Lately, whenever things seem really difficult, I keep telling myself it's OK, I'll get through it, I just need to keep up appearances for one more week, now just a few more days, now the countdown is in hours and next thing you know I'll be in Nebraska watching a movie with my dad or visiting with my parents at wine time or whatever, something pleasant and non-cancer. Somehow that's made the last week or two sufferable. I am soooo ready for this to be over . . .

CANCER—DAY 229 WEDNESDAY, DECEMBER 9, 2009

The days have counted down and it's time for some goodbyes. After treatment I'll be working again, from my home in the mountains, and I don't expect to be driving down to Sac for things like afternoon yoga. It was sad to say goodbye to my yoga class friends on Monday, but I put off saying goodbye to my yoga instructor, Kym, until my last full day in town.

I had the most wonderful lunch with Kym today. I haven't gotten to spend a lot of time with her, but over the weeks there have been a lot of really vulnerable moments when she asked how I was doing and we talked about where I was in treatment or how I was doing emotionally or whatever. She's perceptive, and she had correctly assessed the reason Marco changed to a different yoga studio and she thought it was better for me to be at yoga by myself anyway. We'd talk for just a moment before or after a yoga session sometimes, but most days it was just a smiling heartfelt hug of support as I left. Kym felt like a good friend even though I didn't know her well, and we wanted to get together and have lunch before I left for Christmas. We had a fabulous conversation about really interesting life stuff. Kym actually had scoliosis of the spine and the doctors were going to put her through numerous painful surgeries but with her yoga practice she has not had to have a single back surgery. Kym also went through some really trying times with the Christian church after she realized her internal gender identity in her late teens. In a way, music and meditation saved her. She would sit on her front porch with her guitar for hours, sometimes playing, sometimes not, just letting her mind be quiet. It was fascinating to hear about. Today she's very spiritual and has a great energy about her and it was really, really nice to spend time with her on my last full day in town.

She gave me a little card that was so beautiful, about how my life is moving from winter into spring. And she made a point of telling me again at lunch that she just finds me so inspirational. It's really something, that so many people have used that particular word to describe me in the past six months. I never would have thought it of myself. With the cancer, all I've thought I've been doing is surviving, just getting through it, and not always gracefully at that. But lots of people have said how inspiring I am, even though I don't have a clue how it happens. What a wonderful thing to be to people. I don't think of myself as inspiring because it's just too huge to comprehend, inspiration. It definitely feels wonderful to help someone though, especially when they're facing something as challenging as a cancer diagnosis. But you know, it also feels wonderful to do something as simple as donate stuff to charity. There's just something joyous about potentially making someone else's life easier or happier simply by giving away stuffed animals or toys or nice clothes. My mom volunteers in a charity store kind of place called Helping Hands or something like that, and she told me a wonderful story about a man that came in wearing rags with six dollars in change that he had scrounged together so he could go to the charity store and get a suit because he had a job interview. They managed to get him everything he needed with those six dollars, right down to his socks. And, here's the best part, the guy came back a week later to thank them because he had gotten the job and it was going to change his life. How's that for an amazing impact from people making simple donations to charity?

Marco left for Phoenix this morning. He's been nice to me since I came back to his house on my birthday, night before last. At dinner on my birthday we talked about the tango workshop we are teaching together in January, and he said he's hopeful about our relationship once there isn't this cancer thing hanging over it. Overshadowing it, I think that's how he feels about the cancer and our personal relationship.

I can't resist being hopeful, but I'm not holding my breath on the possibility that our relationship suddenly reblooms when I'm done with treatment. Technically, I won't be out of treatment for at least another five years anyway, if you want to be nitpicky about it. In all honesty though, I think living together during my treatment revealed enough about each of us and our relationship that even though we're still a couple today and say we will still be so when I return in January, well, it's just impossible to say what the future holds. It's weird though, I just can't help being hopeful about Marco. I remember what he was like before I was diagnosed. I was different then too, and I know how the ongoing strain affected us both. Who knows, maybe Marco is right and the only thing wrong with our relationship was cancer. I'm not really thinking about that now, though. I'll cross that bridge when I come to it. As life-battered Scarlet O'Hara would say, "Tomorrow is another day!"

Saying goodbye today, Marco was hugging me, and he gave me lots of little kisses and hugged me some more, and I said "I'll miss you," which is true, I *will* miss him. I moved my head back to give him a kiss goodbye and I realized that he was crying. I definitely wasn't expecting that. How strange, that I, the now freakishly emotional cancer character, would be calm, while the strong silent type is in tears. I asked him what was wrong but he said he didn't know. So I held him a little bit and told him everything is fine, it's OK, and after a little bit he quieted down and we said goodbye and he left.

I had no tears to shed. I went straight back inside, and the first thing I did, before Marco was even out of the driveway (not smart, but he didn't come back in so, no harm no foul), I went straight to the cat room and opened the door to let the cats out to roam. Then, tired and drained, I went to sleep (in the cat bedroom). When I woke up later, Seoul was sleeping under the bed and Mizzou was sleeping in the window of the room just like he's been doing for the last two or three months. Here they had the entire house to roam around in all morning, but there's no furniture and nothing to play with and no other windows with sunshine, so they actually both went BACK into the cat room to sleep. Sheesh. They could have been roaming freely this whole time and it wouldn't have bothered Marco because they aren't interested in hanging out in a cold empty house, they prefer their warm little bedroom!

Chapter 27.
Fade to Black

CANCER—DAY 230 THURSDAY, DECEMBER 10, 2009

It's dark outside. There's no one here. Everything is packed and gone, and the house is empty. On my last walk-through, making sure I haven't left a single thing behind, I was surprised when I felt the tears brimming. Then I realized what this moment is.

The end.

The end of surviving what at times I didn't think I could, the end of a brief life I wouldn't wish upon my worst enemy, the end of an emotional experience I never imagined I could endure. But here I am, and onward I go. And I finally remembered my favorite saying of all.

Every ending is also a new beginning.

Postlude. The Tanda Continues

My journey did not end on that day in December, of course. The last day of radiation and the three weeks visiting my family in Nebraska was simply the brief cortina played while one tanda ends and another begins. I can't help thinking of this whole experience as a tango with cancer, flowing like a tanda like at an Argentine milonga.

In the first song of a tanda, you get a sense of the person you are dancing with, unsure at first, but gradually feeling out how to dance with this partner. Finding out you have cancer is like being thrust into that first song without a shred of preparation, and you have to find your feet and quickly figure out how to tango with the cancer beast.

Going through cancer treatment was much like the second song of a tanda to me. You now have some idea how this tango partner moves, but finding the balance of partner, music, and movement requires careful attention and constant readjustment.

After chemo and radiation, my life settled into a different rhythm. The neuropathy pain is still severe, so my life has adapted to accommodate that. It's the third song of my tanda, when I've figured out how to adjust to my partner and am actually dancing with my partner and allowing him to lead without losing my own sense and feeling of the music, my sense of who I am.

Being a cancer survivor is a new kind of life, a new beginning. The song may change but the music still plays and there is more dancing to be done. The tanda is a journey of exploration, adaptation and connection. Surviving is like that. You learn that life is a journey, not a destination.

ABOUT THE AUTHOR

Cynthia Swan grew up in the Midwestern United States and moved to California after graduate school. She has been a national and international public speaker since 1995, and founded her own consulting company, Cielem'el, in 2003. An Argentine Tango enthusiast, Cynthia also became a professional Ballroom, Latin, and Argentine Tango dancer, competitor, and instructor.

Diagnosed with breast cancer at the age of 32, Cynthia underwent multiple biopsies and surgeries as well as chemotherapy and radiation treatment. Still dealing with chemo-induced neuropathy today, Cynthia's unwavering spirit continues to encourage and inspire others as she travels the continent meeting a wide variety of audiences to share experiences of survival, inspiration, and hope.

Cynthia's first Argentine Tango was in Buenos Aires in 1997, when she was taken onstage from the audience at a tango show and was amazed to find herself dancing ochos, molineras, ganchos, and boleos without a clue how the tanguero made it happen. A management consultant traveling throughout South America on business at the time, Cynthia never forgot the experience, but temporarily set aside the thought of dancing to complete her education and pursue her business career. Over the years she has returned to Buenos Aires multiple times to develop as a tanguera and appreciate Argentine Tango.

While consulting in supply chain management and teaching graduate courses in business intelligence and information systems, Cynthia began her dancing career in early 2003 as an amateur with Arthur Murray Dance Studios. Dancing in three competitions in four months as an amateur competitor, Cynthia won the top student award for her division at all three competitions, over 100 first place awards, top solo routine awards for Argentine Tango and Cha Cha/Hustle, and placed twice in the top three in the American Open All-Around (a competition across all nine American-style Ballroom and Latin dances) before going pro in June 2003.

As a dance professional, Cynthia has performed in numerous professional shows and pro-am competitions/shows. Her students have won dozens of first place awards, as well as the Silver Pro-Am American Open All-Around. Cynthia also won the top teacher award at the 2005 World Pro-Am Championships in Buenos Aires, Argentina. Though not always a dancer, Cynthia has been a performer her entire life, performing her first piano recital in kindergarten and eventually becoming a professional pianist, flutist, and singer, with the pinnacle of her singing career occurring on the main stage at Carnegie Hall followed by a six-week European tour and the CD release "U Singers - Live in Europe."

A DVIDA certified NDCA professional in the Ballroom and Latin dances since 2003, Cynthia also completed her Argentine Tango certification with the University of the Tango in Buenos Aires in 2007. Cynthia's love of dance is contagious, and her ability to break down technical elements for any dance level, combined with her teaching ethic for students of all levels to have fun while learning, gives her students self-confidence that is evident both on and off the dance floor.

Though no longer a dance instructor due to severe chemo-induced neuropathy, Cynthia is still a tanguera, dancing Argentine Tango as much as possible in venues across the county and occasionally in her favorite city, Buenos Aires.

Additional information regarding Cynthia Swan's book tour, speaking engagements, Cielem'el, and preview content of *My Tango with Cancer* is available at www.cielemel.com. Requests for book signings or speaking engagement in specific cities or venues should be directed to info@cielemel.com.

ORDER INFORMATION

Copies of *My Tango with Cancer* may be purchased online at:
www.cielemel.com or www.mytangowithcancer.com

Inquiries regarding other formats such as eBook, large print, or bulk order discounts for *My Tango with Cancer* should be sent directly to GoBeyond Publishing at info@gobeyondpublishing.com.

GOBEYOND PUBLISHING
401 E. 8TH ST., STE. 214-547
SIOUX FALLS, SOUTH DAKOTA 57103
WWW.GOBEYONDPUBLISHING.COM
INFO@GOBEYONDPUBLISHING.COM

BOOK DESIGN BY C.L. MILLER

Made in the USA
Monee, IL
04 November 2026

67384092R00223